Praise for *Fibroids*

"Skilling, who suffers with fibroids herself, has written a comprehensive guide that defines the condition, its symptoms, and the myriad possible treatments. She includes chapters on diet, sex, pregnancy, and emotional issues . . . Skilling liberally sprinkles her text with stories from women and their doctors, including their successes and failures with different types of traditional and alternative treatments. . . . [T]his book is recommended for public libraries and consumer health collections."

—*Library Journal*

"Skilling has suffered from fibroids herself, and she produces a practical and understandable book on this complaint that affects so many women and, hence, their partners and family members."

—*Booklist*

D0965150

About the Author

JOHANNA SKILLING wrote *Fibroids* for women who, like her, have been frustrated by inconsistent treatment recommendations and information about fibroids. Johanna is also the author of *The First Year: Fibroids*. For more information, visit her Web site at www .fibroidguide.com.

Johanna's work has also appeared on beliefnet.com, and "New Morning," a daily program on the Hallmark Channel. She lives and works in New York City.

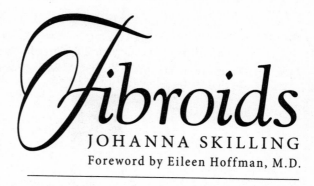

Fibroids

JOHANNA SKILLING

Foreword by Eileen Hoffman, M.D.

THE COMPLETE
GUIDE TO
TAKING CHARGE OF
YOUR PHYSICAL,
EMOTIONAL AND
SEXUAL WELL-BEING

MARLOWE & COMPANY

NEW YORK

FIBROIDS:
*The Complete Guide to Taking Charge of
Your Physical, Emotional and Sexual Well-Being*

Copyright © 2000, 2006 by Johanna Skilling
Foreword copyright © 2000, 2006 by Eileen Hoffman, M.D.
Illustrations by Scott Fowler

Published by
Marlowe & Company
An Imprint of Avalon Publishing Group Incorporated
245 West 17th Street • 11th floor
New York, NY 10011

AVALON
publishing group incorporated

The Library of Congress has cataloged the previous edition as follows:
Skilling, Johanna
Fibroids: the complete guide to taking charge of your physical, emotional, and
sexual well-being / by Johanna Skilling; with a foreword by Eileen Hoffman.
p. cm.
Includes index.
ISBN 1–56924–620–3
I. Uterine fibroids—Popular works. II. Title.
RC280.U8 S566 2000
616.99'366—dc21   99–056897

This edition
ISBN 1-56924-322-0
ISBN-13: 978-56924-322-0

9 8 7 6 5 4 3 2 1

Designed by India Amos, Neuwirth and Associates, Inc.
Printed in the United States of America

Fibroids are the commonest tumours in humans.
—RESEARCHERS AT THE UNIVERSITY
OF NEWCASTLE, AUSTRALIA

[T]hose conditions that are most prevalent . . . represent
the most significant health issues for American women.
—NATIONAL INSTITUTES OF HEALTH

ᓚ Contents ᓭ

～ *Foreword* ～

IN THE LONG history of medicine, issues that specifically affect the female body, with the exception of pregnancy, have not been studied extensively. It's only in very recent days that the medical establishment has begun to view women's bodies as more than male analogues with child-bearing capacity: that is, to see us rightfully as unique, holistic human beings whose uteri, breasts, ovaries, and hormones are part of a delicately balanced, whole-body system.

Still, our fragmented medical system often classifies women, and handles our health care, on the basis of the single defining issue of our ability or desire to have children. Many doctors view the uterus and ovaries as dispensable if we don't plan on having children or if we're past our child-bearing years. Many women also subscribe to this notion, accustomed as we've become to centuries of male-dominated medical and cultural values.

These cultural attitudes about women, our child-bearing potential and ability, and the uterus itself are encapsulated in the issue of fibroids. Long defined by the accurate but emotionally charged word "tumor," fibroids are a common occurrence that affect some women greatly and others not at all. Fibroids have been used as a justification for removing the uterus, and often the ovaries, of at least 200,000 women every year in the United States alone, adding up to one million fibroid-related hysterectomies every five years. In some cases, this drastic approach is medically necessary; too often, it is not. Other therapies are becoming available on a more widespread basis for women with fibroids; however, given the misconceptions and, until now, the lack of a truly comprehensive resource for women with fibroids, we have to be vigilant to make sure that we are not getting swept up in the excitement of new but unproven possibilities.

Fibroids are probably the least studied and most common growth that human beings can have. They're a quintessentially female problem in that they affect the organ that biologically makes us uniquely female. When you are dealing with fibroids, you may be dealing with issues as diverse as infertility, heavy bleeding, and emotional distress. Having fibroids can lead us to question the deepest feelings we all hold about our own femaleness, our identities as women, partners, mothers, and lovers.

How we treat fibroids is also a feminist issue, as it calls into question the research and medical care women receive from the general medical establishment. In a holistic, woman-centered approach to medicine, fibroids are just one part of our physical makeup. The question of treating your fibroids raises the question of treating *you* and determining what is best for your body, mind, and spirit, both now and in the long run. Thus, treating a woman with fibroids means treating the whole woman, not just her uterus. Our current life choices and medical decisions can and often do have a decisive impact on the rest of our lives. As doctors begin to define the new discipline of woman-centered medicine, we are expanding our focus from the reproductive organs to include hearts, bones, lungs, colons, and bladders—as well as the psychological, behavioral, social, and cultural arenas in which each of us exist.

One of the fundamental questions I try to answer in my own practice is, How would medicine be different if it functioned as an advocate for women? And how can we as patients and practitioners make this happen in our own lives?

One of the best things you can do is to be a full partner in your health care; becoming educated about your body, your fibroids, and the treatment options available is your first step toward being your own best advocate.

As I contemplate the impact of this book, I imagine you—and your female friends, relatives, and colleagues—showing up in doctors' offices, clinics, and hospitals, asking educated questions, making demands, and requesting information. If every woman with fibroids took this approach, just think of the changes that could ensue, not just for the care and treatment of women with fibroids, but for woman-centered medicine in general.

And that would be good for all of us.

EILEEN HOFFMAN, M.D.
New York, New York

⌒ *Introduction* ⌒

"WE KNOW SO LITTLE"

THE UNIVERSITY OF Texas in Smithville.

The National Institute of Environmental Health Sciences in Research Triangle Park, North Carolina.

Brigham and Women's Hospital in Boston.

These are the nerve centers of fibroid research in the United States. Yet when I asked a lead investigator if she could tell me what she knew about fibroids, she said simply, "We know so little."

I was disappointed and dismayed. If a scientist on the front lines of fibroid research felt that she had no information to share, what hope was there for a book like this?

That was in 1999, when I was researching the first edition of this book. Even though that same investigator wrote those very same words about fibroids in 2005, the reality is, there's been an explosion in research, political action, not-for-profit associations, books and articles, all dealing with fibroids. There's so much new information, in fact, that it was time to update this book, with information from the worlds of research, medicine, surgery, alternative therapies, and more.

I started writing this book because I found so few answers to my own questions when I was first diagnosed with fibroids. I talked with doctors, nurses, physicists, geneticists, clergy, healers from nonmedical disciplines, authors, activists, and psychologists, all of whom added to and burnished our understanding of fibroids, their effects and treatments. I read dozens of books, and scanned hundreds of articles and Web sites. But the fact is, my original and best resource for information about fibroids and treatments was other women—women who've been where you are now and who were willing to share what they've been through and what they've learned.

The women whose stories are told throughout the book make up a pretty diverse group: Some are single, some have partners, some still want children, some don't. The youngest woman I spoke with had problems with fibroids in her early twenties; the oldest was in her sixties. They come from a variety of ethnic and religious backgrounds; some have a strong belief in Western medicine, others have a preference for "natural" remedies. But they're all women with busy, everyday lives—and they're all women with fibroids. I enjoyed meeting, speaking with, or corresponding with each one. These are women you'd want to sit with over coffee and trade recipes with—not recipes for low-fat cheesecake or pasta primavera, but rather, recipes for holding your own against a tide of medical opinion, trusting your instincts, and handling the hard times. Some of the stories are fun, some are difficult, some have happy endings, some don't. But all are real. And together they paint a textured landscape of life with fibroids: the good, the bad, the ugly, and sometimes, even the beautiful.

When the women I approached for interviews asked me what I was doing, I said my goals were twofold: First, to create a "support group in a book," so that at two in the morning, instead of lying awake and anxious, someone could pick up this book and feel a sense of comfort and support, and second, to build a resource of current information about fibroids and their treatment.

Since the first edition appeared, the conversations have only continued. At times, I've felt like I was part of an old-fashioned quilting bee, where each person comes with her bits and pieces of material, contributing to a rich and unique new work. I like the image of quilting: The end result is both beautiful and comforting, an emblem of the work of many hands, traditionally women's hands, and a reminder of how women work and contribute and talk together, sharing information, compassion, and stories.

This book is the product of our collective wisdom. But each of us may feel ignorant and, sometimes, alone. We need each other, sharing our questions as well as our answers. That's what this book is all about—helping to collect and share information about what it's like to be a woman with fibroids and, in the process, helping each of us feel more in control of our own bodies, our own destinies.

C'mon . . . Are Fibroids Really That Big a Problem?

At a minimum, fibroids are thought to affect one woman in every four. But fibroid researchers believe the number may as high as—are you sitting down?—more than three in four. According to the most recent U.S. Census, there are 108 million women over the age of 18 in this country; that means that anywhere from 27 to 81 million women in the United States alone may have fibroids.

According to Dr. Nelson Stringer, author of *Uterine Fibroids: What Every Woman Needs to Know,* "fibroids are the most common tumors" of women around the world. Fibroids are also the single biggest reason for hysterectomies in the United States, accounting for about 30 percent of these operations. Based on that estimate, over 200,000 hysterectomies are done for women with fibroids every year; the annual cost for inpatient care alone is well over $2 billion.

In addition, as most of us know all too well, fibroids are the reason for any number of other inpatient and outpatient procedures, as well as tests, visits to the doctor, and over-the-counter and prescription medications. As many as one in five visits to gynecologists may be for fibroids. The economic impact of fibroids is even greater when you consider that women affected by symptoms lose time from work or feel less effective on the job.

There are also costs that don't involve money. The emotional and physical symptoms of fibroids can affect our well-being and the quality of our relationships. They can call into question how well we take care of our children, if we have them, and how well we take care of ourselves, how we ask for help, how our partners, friends, and family react to the dilemmas that fibroids create.

Don't Doctors Have the Answers?

Doctors and scientists have discovered some remarkable things about fibroids in recent years. We know that certain chromosomes seem to play a role in how our bodies develop fibroids; there is an increasing body of information about how estrogen and other hormones work in our reproductive systems and the role of these hormones in the development and growth of fibroids. Techniques that preserve the uterus are being practiced by an ever-expanding number of doctors, and researchers continue to explore the possibilities of less invasive, more effective therapies. We'll spend time on all these things later in the book.

But do doctors always understand and explore what may be important to us? I think not. For instance, I asked several doctors how fibroids affected women's sexual response. None of them had ever asked their patients any questions about sex. Similarly, I asked these doctors—all warm, intelligent, highly trained—whether they could explain to me the functions of the uterus beyond childbearing. Most could not. In one conversation, I asked a doctor whether a new technique he was exploring would change the way a woman's body feels to her. He stopped and thought for a moment. "I never considered that," he said. "I'll have to ask."

How Will We Learn More?

A very interesting thing emerged over the course of my conversations with doctors. Many of them started exploring new therapies, new techniques, and even new attitudes after their patients pushed them in that direction. Over and over, I heard some variation on this sentence:

"I never thought of it, until one woman made me realize that I needed to pay attention."

Change doesn't always come easily. One well-known doctor told me that he initially refused to do the procedure for which he is now best known. The patient who wanted the procedure went elsewhere and came back to tell him about her successful result. That made him think about how he could better serve his patients, and it opened up a new field of expertise for him.

On other fronts, individual women have created wonderful resources for collecting and sharing information, particularly on the pluses and minuses of surgical techniques. The National Institutes of Health, and the Office of Research on Women's Health in particular, consider research on fibroids "among the top priorities for women's health research." There's even a bill in Congress to fund research and education about fibroids and fibroid management.

As we continue to learn about the whys and hows of fibroids, we can become ever more confident, clear, and outspoken about the information and outcomes that we want for ourselves. We can make the wheels of change turn even faster—but it will take determination, commitment, and—as always—a lot more questions.

~∂1c~

Fibroids Defined

WHAT ARE FIBROIDS EXACTLY?

The most common pelvic tumor in women.
—*JOURNAL OF OBSTETRICS & GYNECOLOGY*

The most common neoplasms of the female pelvis.
—AMERICAN COLLEGE OF OBSTETRICIANS
AND GYNECOLOGISTS

They're just one more damned thing.
—VALERIE

THEY DON'T ENGAGE your physical senses: You can't see them, smell them, or touch them. They're something "other"—of you, but not you. They appear and grow and sometimes die inside you, following their own mysterious life cycles, mirroring your own age and stage of life.

The clinical reality is simple. Fibroids, also known as *leiomyomas*, are solid lumps of muscle and connective tissue, almost always benign, that grow in and around the uterus. But the emotional reality of fibroids is incredibly complex.

Fibroids are a fact of life for women of all races and ages, all over the globe. According to the Center for Uterine Fibroids, a division of Brigham and Women's Hospital in Boston, over 70 percent of all women are affected by fibroids; the National Institutes of Health says the figure is as high as 77 percent for women of childbearing age. Fibroids are the reason that a quarter of a million women in the United States have surgery every year and countless more take drugs that fundamentally affect their hormones. Fibroids may never cause a problem, or they may be responsible for some of the most difficult chapters in a woman's life: hemorrhaging, miscarriage, life-altering surgery.

Fibroids hit us at a basic, primitive point, both physiologically and psychologically. The uterus is the keeper of the species, of our immortality; it gives us our capacity to bear children and thus to be mothers, grandmothers, ancestors. To many women, the uterus fundamentally defines their femininity, desirability, and identity.

Fibroids can threaten all these things, especially if you only know enough about them to make you scared. Fear can make your fibroid problem bigger than you are, allowing it to take over your life and thoughts in predictable and unpredictable ways.

But as with any potential threat to our health, safety, or happiness, the more we know, the less we fear. The more we know about our fibroids, the more we can understand our choices and the more control we can have over our situations.

There's a lot to learn about fibroids: who gets them, where they come from, how they grow, how they die. There's a lot to learn about how they make us feel physically and emotionally; how we treat them, if we treat them; how our diets might affect them; and how they affect our relationships and connections with ourselves.

Here are some of the things fibroids are *not:*

o Malignant (99 percent of the time, anyway)
o A punishment for bad sex, too much sex, or no sex
o Aliens from another planet (though they can feel that way, especially if you've seen too many aliens-from-another-planet movies)
o Dermoid cysts (the kind with hair and teeth)
o A death sentence
o An end to your fertility
o A reason for immediate surgery
o Something you should automatically ignore and forget about

Who Gets Them?

Maybe the question should be, who *doesn't* get them?

The American College of Obstetricians and Gynecologists points out, in its booklet *Getting the Facts on Fibroids,* that "as the 'Baby Boomer' generation reaches middle age, more and more women are experiencing the condition of uterine fibroids." Over 70 percent of all women develop fibroids before age 50; for African-American women, that number rises to 80 percent. As an article on a leading hospital's Web site almost comically states, "There are no known risk factors for developing uterine fibroids, other than being a woman of reproductive age."

Although most sources say that 25 to 30 percent of women develop fibroids, small fibroids may be present in virtually every woman by the time she reaches menopause. (Contrary to popular belief, fibroids don't go away at menopause, though they often shrink.) Fibroids create problems for up to half of the women who have them; the rest may never even know they're there.

Doctors have long pointed toward family history as the reason some women are affected by fibroids. The National Institute of Child Health and Human Development (NICHD) tell us that women who have fibroids are more likely to have mothers, sisters, or daughters who have fibroids as well. This is supported by a Russian study, which indicated that women who have a family history of fibroids are twice as likely to develop them than women with no family history.

African-American women are three to five times more likely to get troublesome fibroids than are white, Asian, or Hispanic women. African-American women also tend to develop fibroids at an earlier age than white women and are more likely to have anemia and pelvic pain. I've been told anecdotally that Jewish women get fibroids at a higher rate than the "average," and while that is not supported by research, scientists acknowledge that there may be various groups of women who are more affected by fibroids than others.

IRIS: *I remember having a conversation with my mother about all of this and she informed me that her mother had a hysterectomy in her late thirties because of excessive bleeding. Mom said the doctor who performed Grandma's hyst said that he had never seen such a deformed mess as her uterus. Keep in mind this was in the early 1940s, and she lived in a rural area. My mother and I assumed that my grandmother had fibroids.*

KACI: *My mother had fibroids, I was her only child, and I'm willing to bet her sister had them too—she never had kids, and getting the sort of medical care available today was not an option 50 years ago for young black women.*

Other risk factors for fibroids, apart from accidents of birth, may include being overweight or childless (okay, so it sounds a little like being punished twice), or being between 30 and 50 years old.

Believe it or not, smokers may have less risk, as do athletic women, women who have used oral contraceptives, and women who have had children.

But apart from the literature, I've spoken to women who are thin or have had children (or both), those who are in their twenties or in their fifties, and they've all had fibroids. If almost 80 percent of us get them, that's a whole lot of women.

What Causes Fibroids?

BONNIE: *I was told that holding grudges caused these fibroids to occur.*

MARY: *My first ob-gyn examined me and shook his head. He told me that despite the "numerous abortions I'd had," yes, I was pregnant, but I had tumors. I was FLOORED. I had NEVER had any abortions . . . I'd never been pregnant before . . . and WHAT TUMORS? He was very chauvinistic and insisted that this was the price I had to pay for my promiscuous early years!*

BETH: *I discovered that I'd been sexually abused. I think that the fibroids were partly caused by my blocked memories.*

The fact is, fibroids originate from a single cell gone wild. Although any two of your fibroids may be different, each fibroid is a clone of a single cell that has somehow has gotten the wrong signals about how it's supposed to grow. The technical term for this is a *monoclonal tumor.*

But how do you get fibroids in the first place? The answer may lie deep within our genes.

> Genes keep us alive, but sometimes they go wrong and
> cause disease, or make us more susceptible to ill-health.
> —THE HUMAN GENOME PROJECT

A few years ago, a group of 42 women agreed to have their DNA sampled: each of them had fibroids, as well as an inherited skin condition that causes benign skin tumors. It turned out that almost 60 percent of the women had something else in common: a mutation in a gene called FH (short for *fumarate hydratase*)—a mutation not seen at all in a control group of 150 women without either condition. In 2002, researchers announced that mutations in FH could cause fibroids.

Dr. Cynthia Morton, Director of Cytogenetics at Boston's Brigham and Women's Hospital, and one of the country's foremost researchers on the genetic causes of fibroids, including FH, says it's only the first example we'll see of "inherited predisposition genes" for fibroids.

Dr. Morton and her colleagues successfully demonstrated that the FH mutation on a gene could be inherited—but just having the mutation isn't enough to cause fibroids. According to Dr. Morton, "If you inherit this liability, you'd tend to develop the condition earlier in life than someone who doesn't have a predisposing gene."

So what's a genetic mutation? Sharon Begley, a science reporter, likens them to "typos" in our DNA, which can alter a gene's intended purpose, much like typographical errors can change the meaning of a sentence. (To put this in some perspective, according to the Human Genome Project, "there are 3 billion letters in the DNA code in every cell in your body." Just think of the possibilities for things to go wrong: like me, you may be amazed that we stay as healthy as we do.)

To help visualize how we acquire genetic mutations, think about your skin. As we age, we go from baby-smooth perfection to a catalogue of bumps, bruises, cuts, scars, freckles, wrinkles, which is how our genes react to a combination of heritage, environmental "insults," like too much sun exposure, and the not-so-simple process of aging.

As Dr. Morton explains, "As we live, we accumulate genetic mutations. A predisposition to fibroids is the result of both inherited mutations in genes and mutations along the way."

As of this writing, FH is the only gene proven to be related to fibroids, but it won't be the last. In 2003, scientists at the National Institute of Child Health and Human Development, and the University of South Florida, Tampa, announced that they'd identified an additional 145 genes that contribute to the development and growth of fibroids. (By the way, don't blame your mom: your dad passes down some fibroid-related genes, too.)

Beyond mutations, scientists are investigating how our genes may be switched on or off, making us more, or less, susceptible to disease, including the development and growth of tumors like fibroids. In July 2003, researchers launched The Human Epigenome Project (HEP) to study what some scientists have called "the missing link between genetics, disease and the environment."

What does all this mean for us? According to Dr. Morton, understanding our genetic heritage will "change the paradigm for managing treatment." In the future, you'd have a conversation with your gynecologist about your family history, followed by a simple blood

What Do Fibroids Look Like, Anyway?

DR. BRIAN WALSH of Brigham and Women's Hospital in Boston says that fibroids "are like a Superball." Unlike other growths, fibroids tend to be firm and well defined; under the microscope, the borders are clear and sharp. Compared to malignant tumors, even the color tends to be different: fibroids are white, tan, or light pink, while cancerous tumors tend to be more gray or yellow. If fibroids are like hard rubber balls, cancerous tumors have been described as "fish flesh."

test. Then, Dr. Morton says, "The genetics might help us deliver the appropriate choices for medical therapy."

Over time, one of those choices might include "smart" drugs, targeted to treat specific genetic issues. We'll look at one such drug, currently in FDA trials, in Chapter 5, "The Best of the West."

What Makes Fibroids Grow?

If anything, this is even more complex than what causes fibroids in the first place. In the future, we're likely to find out that, like the genetic causes of fibroids themselves, the factors that make fibroids grow are as individual as we are.

One thing you've probably heard about quite often is the influence of estrogen on fibroids. It's not that if you have fibroids, you simply have more estrogen in your blood; studies have shown that women with fibroids have absolutely normal amounts of estrogen. But somehow, even though fibroids start from a cell in the uterus, they act like a sort of evil twin; fibroid cells behave very differently than normal uterine cells. They may use estrogen at a faster rate or attract estrogen more than normal tissue does. According to the Center for Uterine Fibroids, fibroids actually "have higher estrogen concentrations, bind more estrogen, have more estrogen receptors, and convert estradiol (a more active form of estrogen) to estrone (a less active form of estrogen) more slowly than normal myometrium [uterine tissue]."

Estrogen stimulates a hormone called *basic fibroblast growth factor.* If this hormone becomes damaged, possibly as the result of a problem at the genetic level, it can make smooth-muscle cells—the kind that make up fibroids—grow out of control. So fibroids may actually act like their own power plant, using the extra estrogen that they accumulate to make more basic fibroblast growth factor, which in turn helps produce more smooth-muscle cells.

Progesterone has also been identified as a factor in the growth of fibroids: Synthetic antiprogesterone therapy has been shown to shrink fibroids and relieve symptoms. A newer area being studied is how the amount of progesterone relative to the estrogen and other hormones in your system may affect your fibroids.

There's evidence that the blood vessels surrounding fibroids also go through a series of changes. Not only do your fibroids need blood to grow, but the same hormones that affect fibroid cells may also make the blood vessels around the fibroids larger. This brings to mind a classic chicken-and-egg question: Which comes first, the larger blood vessels or the fibroids?

A number of other natural chemicals have been tied to the growth of fibroids. Researchers are studying the influence of such things as prostaglandins, insulin-like growth factors, peptide growth factors, follicle-stimulating hormone, growth hormone, prolactin, epidermal growth factor, platelet-derived growth factor, and fibroblast growth factor.

Now, in addition to what fibroids have, what they're missing may also provide some important clues: new research shows that fibroids may lack a protein that keeps normal uterine cells from growing out of control. In a small but highly influential study, researchers found that fibroids have lower levels of *dermatopontin,* a protein that literally helps keep muscle cells in place, and may also help keep them from changing. (Low levels of dermatopontin may also play a role in the formation of *keloids,* overgrown scars that—as it happens—also affect African-American women up to three times more than other ethnic groups.)

The researchers who found low levels of dermatopontin in fibroids also noticed something else: seen under a microscope, the connective tissue inside the fibroids was, to put it bluntly, a mess. Normally that connective tissue—known as collagen—looks like a pattern of threads laid parallel to one another: very neat, very orderly. But the collagen in the fibroids looked like a big tangle of those threads. What's more, the fibroids seemed to secrete a substance that allowed more of the abnormal collagen to form.

Collagen, according to one source, "has a greater tensile strength than steel," and is "invulnerable" to many of the body's natural defenses. The same team of scientists plan to study the ability of anticollagen drugs to keep fibroids from growing, or to help shrink them.

Who Are You Calling a Degenerate?

Fibroids not only develop and grow, they can also deteriorate and die. When this happens, the fibroids are said to *degenerate*. Degeneration is sometimes referred to as *necrosis,* a term that indicates the death of clusters of cells inside your body. This process is normal: Two-thirds of all fibroids show some form of degeneration.

Reduced estrogen levels during menopause can cause fibroids to degenerate; a fibroid can also outgrow its blood supply. Degeneration can be a sign of infection, and some doctors think it can signal malignancy. There's disagreement, however, as to whether the fibroid "turns into" cancer or a new, malignant tumor forms. Doctors who believe that degenerating fibroids can become cancerous think that it happens about 1 percent of the time.

There's no specific timing for degeneration, and you may notice no symptoms when it happens. When fibroids degenerate, they can

A Fibroid By Any Other Name

WHERE I GREW up in Massachusetts, the road-naming system was a source of constant amusement. Every few blocks or so, the name of any good-sized street would change. Sometimes it would have two names at the same time. Sometimes you couldn't pronounce at least one of them. Sometimes a road sign would tell you that you were currently going both north and south at the same time.

So maybe someone from my home state was in the room when they came up with all the names for fibroids, which are also called tumors, fibroid tumors, monoclonal tumors, fibromyomas, fibromas, myofibromas, myomas, leiomyomas, and leiomyomatas.

None of these names signify anything more dangerous, unusual, painful, or frightening than "fibroids." Except maybe that your doctor has a preference for the polysyllabic. Or has friends in the Massachusetts Highway Department.

either calcify, meaning they get harder, or liquefy. You might bleed more during your period, pass clots, get a low-grade fever, or feel a tenderness in your lower abdomen.

In some cases, you may get a pain so severe that it feels like a knife going through you. Physically, it's similar to a heart attack (both attacks are called infarctions): The fibroid is not getting enough blood to survive, and a part of it dies. Unlike a heart attack, degenerating fibroids are not life threatening.

Even so, you may be in enough pain to go to the emergency room. If this happens, doctors may ask you for permission to perform an emergency hysterectomy. Keep in mind that, as bad as it can be, the pain of degenerating fibroids generally only lasts 24 hours. When it passes, you can make your decisions about further treatment calmly.

Where Do Your Fibroids Live? Meet Your Uterus

Considering that at least half the human race is female, it's a mystery to me that we seem to know so little about the uterus. The doctors I've spoken to agree that we just don't have a lot of information: There is more imagined about the uterus in art and religion than in the realm of science.

Even in the United States, a country that invented the term "multitasking," many doctors will tell you that the uterus has one function and one function only: providing the all-important home for developing babies. And we honor and respect that function. But wait, as they say on the late-night commercials, there's more.

DR. VICTOR REYNIAK: *The uterus is not just the place for the baby to grow. It's a very complex organ and very poorly understood—we don't know many things yet, but that will eventually be unmasked.*

LEONIE: *My belief is that if nature intended us to lose our uteri at menopause, they would shrink up and fall out. Since that doesn't happen,*

I have to assume that there are reasons for having a uterus beyond childbearing.

As Natalie Angier writes in her book *Woman: An Intimate Geography,* "the uterus has emerged as a maker as well as a taker. Yes, it responds to steroid hormones from the ovaries and other organs, but it also expresses hormones and releases them into the global marketplace of the body." The uterus produces proteins, sugars, and fats, as well as prostaglandins, which stimulate contractions of the uterus, and may well help keep your blood vessels from hardening.

Dr. Herbert Goldfarb, author of *The No-Hysterectomy Option,* suggests that uterine prostaglandins may also protect against heart disease. Dr. Brian Walsh of Brigham and Women's Hospital adds that "the story hasn't completely unfolded. For instance, there's a lot of work in terms of the uterus producing prostacyclins, which cause blood vessels to relax. Some people think it may cause the coronary muscles to relax, which would be a good thing."

> The womb . . . fabricates drugs that would
> be considered illegal in other contexts.
> —NATALIE ANGIER,
> *WOMAN: AN INTIMATE GEOGRAPHY*

In April 1998, researchers at UCLA reported finding a unique, natural antibiotic which, in laboratory experiments, killed even the infamous *E. coli* bacterium. The head of the research team called this possibly the most important of all the antibiotics our bodies produce, and pointed out that the largest concentrations were found in women's reproductive systems and urinary tracts, specifically, in the vagina, cervix, uterus, fallopian tubes, and ureters.

And that's not all. The uterus makes some of our natural opiates, and a substance called *anandamine,* a molecule almost identical to the active ingredient in marijuana—and chocolate. Now you know.

The uterus also plays a little-understood—and certainly little-discussed—role in sex and orgasm, which we'll talk about more in Chapter 9, "Sex and the Single Fibroid."

PICTURE THIS

In a sweet and unusual description, Dr. William H. Parker, in *A Gynecologist's Second Opinion,* says that "the uterus is a reddish-pink color, much like the color of the inside of your lips . . . Most women are surprised to see how attractive [their] organs actually are. The colors are quite beautiful."

The shape of the uterus is often compared to a small pear turned upside down. The wide part on top is called the *fundus;* the narrower part is called the *isthmus.* Together, these two parts are called the *body,* or *corpus,* of the uterus; this is the part that grows during pregnancy, and it's the place you're most likely to find your fibroids. The body of the uterus is nestled between the bladder and bowel, below the ovaries, and helps keep all those organs firmly in their proper place.

At the rounded part of the pear (the fundus), two thin tubes come out from either side; these widen and finish in a fringe, like the arms of an old-fashioned, romantic blouse. Those are the *fallopian tubes* (or *oviducts),* which provide the pathway an egg travels from the ovaries to the uterus.

At the opposite end—the "stem" of the pear—is the *cervix,* a donut of muscle that forms the opening to the uterus and connects it with

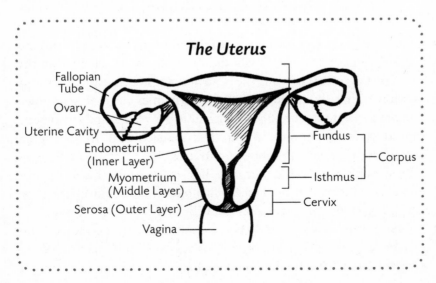

The Uterus

Fallopian Tube
Ovary
Uterine Cavity
Endometrium (Inner Layer)
Myometrium (Middle Layer)
Serosa (Outer Layer)
Vagina

Fundus
Isthmus
Corpus
Cervix

Why Can't They Just Name Them Like Hurricanes?

Where They Are	What They're Called	What Form They Take
On the outer wall (the serosa)	Serosal *or* Subserosal *or* Subserous *or* Subperitoneal	Pedunculated (a ball on a stalk) *or* Sessile (a ball)
In the muscle (the myometrium)	Intramural *or* Interstitial	Sessile
In the lining (the endometrium)	Submucous *or* Intracavity	Pedunculated *or* Sessile

the vagina. The cervix is connected to the pelvic bones and ligaments and helps keep our pelvic organs in place.

Of course, the uterus is hollow: If you're not pregnant and don't have fibroids, the cavity is just a narrow opening, but obviously both the cavity and the surrounding uterus can expand to accommodate one or more babies—or fibroids.

If you want to get a really rough idea of the size of your uterus, hold out your hand, and fold down your thumb and pinky. Your uterus is about the height and width of your middle three fingers.

If you want to be more exact, get a ruler (go ahead, I'll wait); the average uterus is 2 to 4 inches long, 1.5 to 2.5 inches wide, and 1 inch thick; it weighs about one-sixth of a pound, or 50 grams, if you're metrically inclined. If you've ever been pregnant, your uterus may be on the larger end of those dimensions.

Now remember, that's the size without fibroids, adenomyosis, polyps, or pregnancy, which rules out most of us right there.

WALLS WITHIN WALLS

Depending on what you read, you may get the impression that your uterus is nothing more than a simple bag of muscle. In German, you may be amused to learn, the uterus is sometimes called a "fruitsack" which reminds me, at least, of a brown paper bag. But the reality is much more delicate and interesting than that.

The uterus is composed of three distinct layers: the *endometrium,* the *myometrium,* and the *serosa.* These terms will become very familiar, as they intimately relate to the names of your fibroids.

If you go back to thinking about that upside-down pear for a minute, the "skin" is the *serosa.* This is the thin, tough outer layer; it protects the uterus and connects to the ligaments that support the uterus inside your pelvic cavity.

Under the serosa is the *myometrium.* This is the thick, middle layer of the uterus, most often called the *uterine wall.* It's composed of the same kind of smooth muscle as your heart, and like your heart, it is able to contract and expand according to signals sent by your body. You feel these contractions most often during your period, during childbirth, and during sex.

Under the myometrium, surrounding the cavity, is the *endometrium* (also called the *uterine mucosa* or *uterine lining).* The endometrium is the setting for the monthly cycle that culminates in our periods; it's also one of the areas most likely to be noticeably disrupted by fibroids. The endometrium itself is composed of two layers: the thin *basal layer,* which grows new blood vessels every month, and the *endometrial lining,* the layer of tissue that grows every month in preparation for pregnancy.

FIBROIDS AND UTERINE REAL ESTATE

Where in the uterus can fibroids grow? Anywhere they want to.

When it comes to fibroids, just remember what you've always heard about opening a business: location, location, location. Where they are—and often how big they are—will generally make a difference in how they may affect you. Of course, as fibroids grow, they may encroach on more than one part of the uterus.

While it's possible to have just one fibroid, it's more likely that you'll have several. Because they can grow at different rates, it's possible you could have one large fibroid along with several smaller ones, or even microscopic ones. On average, you can expect to have six or seven fibroids, growing either in clusters or singly, but doctors have found as many as 50 separate fibroids in one woman.

Most of the names you'll read or hear about for fibroids refer to the layer of the uterus in which they're rooted. But just to make life interesting, not everyone uses the same names for the different locations.

What really matters is that you know what your doctor means when he or she refers to one of these. Let's look at them one at a time, starting from the outside of the uterus and working our way in to the lining.

ON THE OUTER WALL: SUBSEROSAL, SEROSAL, SUBSEROUS, OR SUBPERITONEAL

These terms are used interchangeably to refer to fibroids located on the outer layer of the uterus (the serosa, or *peritoneum*). These fibroids come in two shapes: either a ball on a stalk *(pedunculated)* or just a ball *(sessile),* embedded in the wall.

Subserosal fibroids can easily push out the outer wall of the uterus, potentially pressing on other organs, such as the ureters or bladder. Sometimes these fibroids can get large enough to push against the wall of your abdomen, causing the kind of swelling that can make you feel "pregnant."

Pedunculated fibroids, growing on a stalk from the outer wall, can sometimes attach themselves to other organs or even the muscles in your pelvis. If these fibroids outgrow their original blood supply in the uterus, they may begin to draw blood from other organs, deserving their new name of *parasitic leiomyomata.*

Since subserosal fibroids aren't near the cavity, they generally don't affect your menstrual flow. As a rule, they don't even interfere with pregnancy. The main symptoms you can expect from these fibroids are pain or pressure.

IN THE MUSCLE: INTRAMURAL OR INTERSTITIAL

Intramural or interstitial fibroids are the most common types, growing in a ball-like shape inside the muscular wall of the uterus *(intra*

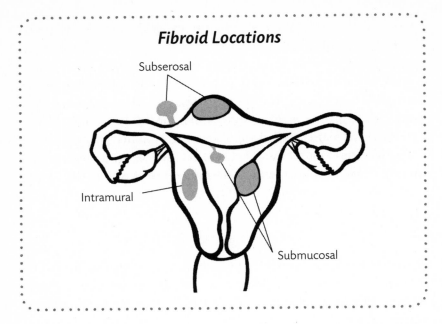

Fibroid Locations

Subserosal

Intramural

Submucosal

means "within;" *mural* refers to the wall). As intramural fibroids expand, they make the uterus feel larger; depending on how deep they are, they can distort the cavity of the uterus or press out against the outer walls toward the pelvis.

Small intramural fibroids may cause no symptoms at all. But as they grow, or as more fibroids form, they can make the cavity of the uterus larger, resulting in heavier bleeding during your period.

If intramural fibroids grow quite large, they can start pressing on the other organs in your pelvis or cause heavier cramps during your period.

IN THE LINING: SUBMUCOUS

Sub means "under," and *mucous* refers to the mucosa, the uterine lining, so you can tell that submucous fibroids grow just under the lining of the uterus. Although they're the least common type of fibroid (occurring about 5 percent of the time), they produce some of the most obvious symptoms: Since they interfere with the blood vessels in the lining, even a tiny submucous fibroid can cause heavy bleeding and prolonged periods.

Submucous fibroids also come in two varieties: sessile or pedunculated. While the stalk of a pedunculated fibroid is rooted in the lining, the fibroid itself hangs into the cavity like a light fixture dangling from the ceiling. Since pedunculated fibroids take up space inside your uterus, they are also called *intracavity fibroids.*

Intracavity fibroids can extend right through the cervical canal, which can cause infection and discomfort during intercourse. Since they're hanging freely, they may twist; this condition, called *torsion,* can cause severe pain. These fibroids are the ones that can interfere with pregnancy the most (for more information on this, see Chapter 10, "And Baby Makes Three"). Occasionally there will be fibroids in the cervix itself, but this happens less than 1 percent of the time.

So how can fibroids make you feel? There are a whole range of physical symptoms that you might experience—and a fair number of emotional issues that may come up as well. Let's start by looking at what, if anything, fibroids may be doing to your most tangible asset: your body.

~ 2 ~

Why You Feel the Way You Do

FIBROID SYMPTOMS

WHAT ARE THE symptoms of fibroids? For quite a few years, I had no physical symptoms at all. That's the case of many women who have fibroids: Research indicates that only 20 to 50 percent of those of us with fibroids have symptoms.

But while many women never experience a moment of discomfort from their fibroids, there is a real range of physical symptoms that you may have, all of which are basically a result of fibroids taking up space where they don't belong and causing one heck of a disruption.

The two most common symptoms of fibroids are uterine bleeding and pelvic pressure. But the symptoms can also include bad cramps during your period, loss of your period, anemia, pain in your lower abdomen, pain during sexual intercourse, pain in your lower back, difficulty urinating or increased need to urinate, constipation, fatigue, miscarriage, preterm labor, and infertility.

It's important to know that these symptoms could also signal other problems, such as endometriosis, polyps, or adenomyosis—and equally important to know that doctors could mistake one of these common conditions for fibroids.

JENNIFER: *I started having heavier periods in December, and told my gynecologist at my annual exam in April. She said it was nothing. I started to feel my abdomen bloating and couldn't button my pants for a few months afterward. In November I was having pain when urinating and sitting in certain positions, so I thought I had a bladder infection. My primary care doctor made me come in and felt an enlarged abdomen but didn't know what it was. He sent me for an X-ray and they found an enlarged uterus, so then they sent me for an ultrasound and found that I had fibroids and an ovarian cyst.*

No Symptoms, No Problem

ACCORDING TO NORA COFFEY of the HERS Foundation, many women discover they have fibroids during a routine checkup, or, as in my case, a medical appointment for something else. This is important: You may hear that you have fibroids, or "tumors," and panic. You don't have to: Many women experience no symptoms or problems with their fibroids and often need to do nothing other than get regular checkups.

GAIL: *My gynecologist had told me that I had a small fibroid, but nobody told me fibroids grow to big sizes, or that sometimes fibroids become bleeders, so a year and a half later, when I had my first bleeding episode, I was shocked.*

Some of the emotional issues are just as real as your physical symptoms: the anxiety of finding out that there's this unknown "thing" in your body; the fear of having something wrong with you, in particular, with your reproductive organs (or simply a part of your body that, for you, defines your femininity); the concern that what your doctor tells you might not be the whole story, and having to find out more from other sources; the embarrassment that you might feel telling your partner, family, or friends what's wrong with you; and the frustration of trying to explain it to them—and yourself—without adequate information.

For women who find out they have "tumors" during a routine examination and have no associated problems, the resulting anxiety itself can be a devastating "symptom." We'll talk more about the emotional effects of having fibroids in Chapter 3, "My Fibroids, Myself." For now, let's explore the physical symptoms.

Uterine Bleeding

Bleeding is by far the most immediate, the most visible, and the most frightening physical symptom women with fibroids can have. About 30 percent of the women who have fibroids have heavy bleeding. Typically, this means having extra-heavy periods, but any type of unusual bleeding is possible. Fibroid-related bleeding, according to an article in *Human Reproduction Update,* "is a significant medical and social problem for many women." So far, the article continues, "effective treatment strategies are limited by a narrow understanding . . . of this disease."

Like fibroids themselves, it's hard to talk about heavy bleeding; in a word, it's embarrassing. But heavy bleeding affects the whole body: in a study of almost 3,000 women, 70 percent of women with normal flows described their overall health as good or excellent, versus 55 percent of "heavy bleeders."

If you have prolonged periods, you may start feeling tired or worn down. If you have sudden gushes of blood, you may feel faint or light-headed; you may feel your heart palpitating, your skin may feel clammy. If this happens to you, try not to panic: find a place to sit quietly, drink lots of water, along with fruit juice or a sports drink, and wait until you feel you can safely stand up again.

If you feel very weak, or you've lost a truly excessive amount of blood, go to your doctor or a local emergency room to check your vital signs, including blood pressure and hematocrit (red blood cell) levels. If you suffer from regular bouts of heavy bleeding, you may want to stash supplies—tampons, pads, juice boxes or water, cookies, even a change of clothes—in the trunk of your car, or in your desk at work.

Heavy bleeding not only takes a physical and emotional toll: it also has an economic cost. Women who bleed heavily lose, on average, 18 days of work each year as a result, representing a possible loss in salary and a definite loss in productivity. And of course, there are the costs of frequent visits to the doctor, not to mention pads, pads, and more pads. And tampons: lots and lots of tampons.

BARBARA: *I went to England in March. On the plane I changed my "superplus" tampon every hour and used overnight pads. In London, I was at Harrod's, where you have to pay to use the bathroom. I was bleeding so heavily, I couldn't figure out how to go back to my hotel. I was in there for five hours.*

IRIS: *The fibroids didn't scare or worry me. What did worry me was all the bleeding. I was afraid of becoming severely anemic and having complications, or bleeding to death.*

The Monthly Machinery

To understand how fibroids can interrupt the normal mechanisms of your body, let's take a look at how your body sets up and controls the flow of blood to and from your uterus every month before menopause begins.

At the end of your cycle each month, when your period is over, your levels of estrogen and progesterone are at their lowest. Your hypothalamus, a command center in your brain, senses that it's time to start a new cycle and starts raising your estrogen level again.

As your estrogen starts increasing, arteries in the uterine lining actually start to grow. These new blood vessels build up a layer of fresh blood in the uterus, making the lining up to three times thicker.

Just before mid-cycle, a new egg is released and your body begins making progesterone. When the egg completes its journey through the fallopian tube and reaches the uterus, you're at mid-cycle.

What happens next depends on whether conception occurs. If the egg is fertilized, you continue making progesterone, and your estrogen levels stay high. If the egg isn't fertilized, your body stops making progesterone and your estrogen level goes down. Without the high level of hormones, the lining of the uterus falls away and blood flows freely into the cavity. This is what we see as our monthly period.

At this point, you produce yet another hormone, called a *prosta-glandin,* which makes the uterus contract. The contractions help push out the lining and squeeze shut the blood vessels in the uterus. And just like anywhere else in your body, your blood forms clots to help stop the bleeding.

And just think: If NASA had come up with this, it would have cost billions of tax dollars.

How Do Fibroids Cause Excess Bleeding?

There are four primary ways in which fibroids can interrupt your system to cause heavy or irregular bleeding:

○ Fibroids in the wall of your uterus can interrupt its normal, rhythmic contractions, meaning it can't squeeze shut the blood vessels in the lining as well as it usually does.
○ Fibroids in the lining can keep the uterus from closing the blood vessels around it.
○ The blood vessels that feed fibroids may become so large that the normal clotting action of the blood is no longer as effective.
○ A protein that reduces muscle tone in smooth-muscle cells may also contribute to uterine bleeding. Relaxed fibroid muscle may allow blood vessels to bleed more freely.

The latest information suggests that women with fibroids are not only more likely to experience heavy bleeding than other women, but the risk of heavy bleeding increases with the size of fibroids.

The worst culprits for bleeding are generally thought to be the submucous fibroids, those located in the uterine lining.While many sources say that bleeding is caused almost exclusively by submucous fibroids, the math doesn't add up: Only about 5 percent of fibroids are submucous, while 30 percent of women report having heavy bleeding.

WENDY: *I was having very bad periods. About a year ago, I was at work and I completely bled through my pants; I went to the bathroom and*

I passed this huge clot, but I didn't know what a clot was! I mean, I'd never seen that. I found this huge blood clot in the toilet and I was very freaked out. And I went back to my office and I just felt another rush, so I basically just bled through my pants again. I didn't really know what was going on because my symptoms up until then had been pretty mild.

Bleeding may also have a number of causes other than fibroids. Polyps and endometriosis, like fibroids, can cause what doctors call *functional bleeding*—that is, bleeding related to an obvious physical cause. Heavy bleeding could also be a sign of endometrial or cervical cancer, especially after menopause. Doctors stress that any postmenopausal bleeding must be considered a sign of cancer of the uterus until proven otherwise. Since most uterine cancers bleed early, you can get an early diagnosis if you pay attention to your symptoms.

A Little List of Bleeding Terms

Ovulatory bleeding: Your normal period, occurring every 21 to 40 days

Intermenstrual bleeding: Bleeding between your periods (breakthrough bleeding)

Menorrhagia: Prolonged, heavy flow during your period

Hypomenorrhea: Light periods at normal intervals

Hypermenorrhea: Heavy periods at normal intervals

Polymenorrhea: Periods at shorter than usual intervals, every 21 days or less

Oligomenorrhea: Long gaps between your periods, from 41 days to 6 months

Amenorrhea: No periods for at least 6 months

Metromenorrhagia (or metrorrhagia): Heavy bleeding at unpredictable intervals

Spotting: Light, irregular flow, including light pink or brown staining

Dysfunctional bleeding is bleeding without an immediately obvious physical cause. It may be due to hormonal fluctuations, thyroid problems, or something else happening in your body that's not directly related to your reproductive system.

Before you or your doctor automatically assume that your fibroids are causing your bleeding problem—or that they're the only reason for it—be sure that you can rule out any other possibilities.

CAROLYN: *Some time ago, I began to have longer and longer periods, where they were noticeably longer to me, and heavier flows. When my period was running nine or ten days and flooding most days, I finally went to an ob/gyn. He told me, and I quote, "All women think they bleed too much."*

Anemia

If you're bleeding too much, you may be a candidate for anemia, a condition that develops if your body doesn't have enough iron.

Without enough iron, your body doesn't use oxygen as efficiently. The Centers for Disease Control says that only 25 percent of us get enough iron in our diets: Iron deficiency anemia, while present in only 3 to 5 percent of women, can become more likely if in addition to too little dietary iron you're also losing an unusual amount of blood.

It's not just heavy periods that can make you anemic. Fibroids seem to need more blood than normal tissue, and studies show that arteries actually grow to feed the fibroids more—taking vital nutrients away from the rest of your body.

It's important to note, however, that having fibroids—or even heavy bleeding—does not automatically mean you have, or will get, anemia. Ask your doctor to check your iron levels at your regular checkups to be sure.

LAURA: *On the scale they measure your iron, you should be a 13 or something like that, and I was a 7. I was freelancing, so it really slowed me down—I spent days in bed with towels between my legs. One night,*

How Heavy Is Heavy?

DOCTORS DEFINE ABNORMALLY heavy bleeding as menstrual blood loss greater than 80 milliliters: This is two to three ounces, or about a quarter of a cup, which is also the amount of blood loss that starts resulting in anemia.

Sometimes it's hard to tell if your blood loss over the course of several days equals a couple of ounces or not. Studies suggest that half of the women who report excessive blood loss have actual measured losses that are normal.

In practical terms, saturating a pad at least once an hour means that you're probably losing too much blood. Some doctors suggest keeping a kind of visual diary of pad saturation—that is, drawing an outline of each pad you use, and filling in the amount of blood. For an accurate record, note the date and time of day you change each pad.

Some brands of tampons list their absorbency: a little math can help you figure out if you're bleeding more than you should. The following chart is based on absorbency rates published by o.b. tampons.

Tampon type	Absorbs Approximately		Number of tampons saturated equals
	In grams	In ounces	
Light flow	6–9 grams	0.2–0.3 ounces	3–5 per ounce, 6–10 per ¼ cup
Super	9–12 grams	0.3–0.4 ounces	about 3 per ounce, 6 per ¼ cup
Super Plus	12–15 grams	0.4–0.5 ounces	about 2 per ounce, 4 per ¼ cup
Ultra Plus	15–18 grams	0.5–0.6 ounces	about 2 per ounce, 4 per ¼ cup

I went to a party and I had a little accident, and I remember thinking, I'm wearing black jeans, I just have to say good-bye to people and hope no one noticed I was a mess from the waist down. I went out to my car, found a plastic bag to put down on the seat because I had blood halfway down to my knees, and I got home and got in the bathtub with my jeans on. I turned the water on and I just sat in the bathtub and cried.

IRIS: *I had iron deficiency anemia. At times the bleeding and clotting were so heavy that I would fill an adult diaper within half an hour. I found that sanitary pads were worthless and had switched to adult diapers to contain the "mess." I had very little pain, just normal cramping, but I had a feeling of constant pressure, and the clots were sometimes so large I could feel them ease out of me. It was very discomforting. I worked a full-time job as an office manager at the time, dealt with the public a lot, and hosted community social events. I missed very little work during all of this but was very tired most of the time, due to the anemia, insomnia, etc.*

ROBIN: *I went to a dermatologist for my hair loss—it turned out to be connected to severe anemia.*

Cramps

Cramps are so common that, ironically, they're not even listed in the indexes of many popular women's health books. But cramps are more than just an inconvenience: As many as one in ten women are temporarily disabled during their periods. And while we may think of menstrual pain as being routine, there is evidence that pain may weaken the immune system, lowering your resistance to all kinds of disease.

Just as with bleeding, there are two kinds of cramps, or, if you feel like talking technically, *dysmenorrhea*. Again, knowing the reason for your cramps can help you and your doctor pinpoint accurate treatment methods.

Primary dysmenorrhea is caused by prostaglandins, the hormones that make your uterus contract during menstruation. If the contractions are very strong, they can temporarily cut off the blood supply to your uterus. This deprives your uterus of oxygen, which in turn creates the pain you feel. "Sometimes," write Dr. Niels Lauersen and Eileen Stukane in their book, *Listen to Your Body,* "the uterine contractions [during menstruation] can be more pronounced than they are during childbirth." It's possible that women who have very painful cramps produce higher than normal amounts of prostaglandins. Most women who have primary dysmenorrhea have had it most of their lives.

If your cramps started later in life and have gotten worse over time, you may have *secondary dysmenorrhea,* that is, cramps with an obvious cause, such as fibroids, pelvic inflammatory disease, or endometriosis. These conditions can also cause cramps during intercourse, or even during times of the month when you're not menstruating.

Fibroids can cause or make cramps worse if they prevent your uterus from contracting normally. This is especially true of intramural fibroids, those that grow inside the wall. As Dr. Stanley West, author of *The Hysterectomy Hoax,* explains, "When the uterus contracts, it contracts uniformly, so if you've got fibroids in there, the contractions are going to be disjointed, which can cause pain and severe cramps."

FELICE: *Over the years, I took various over-the-counter painkillers. All along, the various doctors I saw said it was no big deal to have such bad cramps. I know now that this is not "normal." One doctor told me to take double doses of Advil, which seemed to help for a while, but eventually the pain got worse. I was then given a prescription for naproxen sodium (Anaprox). It worked for a while, but I eventually needed to raise it to a double dose. The double dose usually works so that I can somewhat function, but a couple of months ago the cramps were so bad that it was ineffective, and after I called my primary-care provider, she sent a prescription for something called Ultram, which finally did the job.*

CAROLYN: *I used to lose 10 to 15 days a month to pain, and massive amounts of ibuprofen were all that made me functional. And by that I mean meals on the table and the clothes washed. NOTHING else much got done on my pain days. It really affected my quality of life—not to mention my family's.*

Pain or Pressure

About four months before I started writing this chapter, I started noticing that I was always slightly in pain in an area low down on my abdomen. It was faint, like a slight tension headache, but it dawned on me that it just wasn't going away.

Simply put, Mother Nature did not provide for fibroids. The uterus is supported by a network of ligaments and muscles. As the fibroid grows and the uterus stretches, there's more strain on the muscular support structure you have in your abdomen. Think about the way your arms feel when you carry a heavy bag of groceries—that's what can happen to your pelvic muscles when they have to support a heavy fibroid.

Women with fibroids are almost three times more likely to report pelvic pain, as well as pain during sexual intercourse, than women without fibroids. Keep in mind, of course, that there are many sources of pelvic pain: even if you have fibroids, make sure that your doctor doesn't overlook other possibilities.

Fibroids can also cause a feeling of bloating, and being, well, bigger.

JENEANE: *My abdomen was hard. No matter how many sit-ups I did or how much dieting, this hard bulge just wouldn't go down.*

SHARON: *I knew I was gaining weight despite my dieting, plus I had to go to the bathroom every two minutes, but I didn't really have any other symptoms. A few things got me worried: I was doing some exercises lying on the floor and I felt something like a lump in the carpet, but the lump was in me! Then, not long after, I saw an article on the Internet about the warning signs of ovarian cancer, which included a bloated abdomen and increased frequency of urination. So, after the holidays, I made an appointment for a checkup.*

As soon as he examined me, the doctor said I had a huge mass, and that it was probably a fibroid. Fortunately, he sent me right then to have a sonogram to confirm the diagnosis.

KIM: *It affects the shape of my body, but most of the time I'm not thinking about it. Once in a while I will: One of my many jobs is acting, and I go for costume fittings and have a 2-inch waist and 45-inch hips!*

Pressure on Your Bladder or Bowel

As any woman who's been pregnant knows, the uterus and the bladder are kissing cousins inside your abdomen. A larger uterus makes your bladder smaller, forcing more frequent trips to the bathroom, often for minute amounts of urine.

Pressure from a large uterus can also squeeze the ureters, the tubes that transport urine from the kidneys. This can reduce flow, and in serious cases, if urine backs up into the kidneys, can lead to kidney infection and damage. In extreme cases, large fibroids can result in kidney failure.

The symptoms you might feel include an increased need to urinate, sometimes really badly, sometimes without being able to go at all or just a little. Or you might experience *urinary incontinence—*leaking— when you sneeze, laugh, or exercise hard.

WENDY: *I never used to have to get up to go to the bathroom, ever. I'd sleep through the night, I'd wake up when I woke up. And now I wake up almost every day, whenever, 5 o'clock, 6 o'clock, and I'm sure that it's because of my fibroids.*

DARBY: *I seem to get constipated every month about a week before men-struating. It seems that my uterus becomes enlarged, or at least it feels that way, and I pee all the time and my bowels feel compacted. When I do defecate, it is with great effort and the results are very thin. Sorry to be so graphic, but this is clearly a fibroid-related problem for which I am hoping to get relief.*

ELLEN: *I was periodically very constipated, which would end in massive bouts of diarrhea. It turned out I had a fibroid the size of a fist pressing against my bowel.*

You're probably getting the picture by now. The bowel is also in that remarkably small space inside us. A larger uterus can put pressure on your bowel, which may mean that your body can't eliminate waste properly. And what's the result of that? Tiredness, irritability, uncomfortable feelings of fullness in your abdomen, constipation, and possible intestinal obstruction.

Pressure inside the abdomen is a big reason many women seek medical relief. While the symptoms may be "no worse" than if you were pregnant with a fetus the size of your fibroid, the difference, of course, is that the fibroids won't be delivered after nine months—or give your parents something to brag about.

Fatigue

Fatigue is one symptom of fibroids that took me by surprise; in fact, as many as 70 percent of women with fibroids experience it. But I don't know any adult, male or female, who doesn't suffer from fatigue. We live super-stressful lives, often to the point where many of us don't have time to sit down and simply relax. So if you have fibroids, why would you think that's why you're tired all the time?

Well, there are a few reasons. First, as we discussed, fibroids demand a constant supply of blood to stay alive; they're like little muggers, stealing parts of your blood supply that your body had other plans for. If your fibroids are causing you to bleed heavily, you may be losing too much blood and iron, which can also create fatigue.

The second reason fibroids can be fatiguing is that they're an extra weight. Not when they're small, but if they get to the size of a four-month pregnancy, for instance, you're carrying around a couple of extra pounds just in fibroid weight. Some women claim that fibroids caused them to gain weight, and while that's not documented scientifically, it's an article of faith for the women who go through it. Even if it's not much, even if the fibroid adds only an extra five pounds, your body has to work harder.

Third, if you're spending time worrying about having fibroids or treating them, that too can be tiring. Anxiety uses energy.

ANGELA: *For a couple of years before my hysterectomy, I was just so tired by the time I got to work in the morning. I would think, I really want a*

month off from work! But after I had the surgery and was back at work,
I had much more energy.

I used to go to a coffee bar every morning on the way in to my office
because I wanted that jolt, because I was dragging. And I rarely go in
there anymore.

DARBY: *I keep feeling, gee I'm getting old, but that's not me, 42 is not old.*
You don't get this old this quickly, feel this tired all the time.

Infertility and Miscarriage

Most of the doctors I've spoken with told me that fibroids are not a
major cause of infertility, affecting perhaps 5 percent of the women who
can't conceive. On the other hand, if fibroids are making it impossible
for you to get pregnant, it's a pretty big problem indeed.

If you do become pregnant, fibroids can present a new set of issues.
Fibroids in the cavity are known culprits in miscarriages, as well as
in premature labor and other complications. We'll discuss the issue
of fibroids and infertility at length in Chapter 10, "And Baby Makes
Three."

Can Fibroids Kill You?

A sad case made the front-page headlines in New York City several
years ago, when a young woman walked into a New York hospital
for a "routine" removal of a fibroid. This woman was married to her
high school sweetheart, had a good job, and every reason to expect
a fulfilling future. The doctor was not familiar with the equipment
being used in the operating room. The equipment was not properly
used; the young woman died.

The situation was tragic, but most of the people I spoke with agreed
it was not specifically about fibroids: It was about a doctor who was not
experienced in a surgical technique, and who, it turned out, was on

What Else?

YOU'D THINK ALL this would be enough, but fibroids have some other surprises in their bag of tricks.

- ○ Large fibroids can compress the blood vessels, which can lead to varicose veins, swelling in your legs, hemorrhoids, and pain during sexual intercourse.
- ○ Fibroids can put pressure on nerves, causing pain in the lower back, pain in one or both legs (sciatica), or numbness in the legs.
- ○ Pedunculated fibroids, the kind that grow on a stalk, can twist and cause extreme pain; this is called *torsion*.

probation for other patient-related problems. Perhaps, though, it also underscored the arrogance of a doctor treating a common problem among women.

The death rate for hysterectomies is about 1 in 1,000. Casualties among women of color or of lower economic status are two to three times higher, suggesting a range of issues that need to be addressed by doctors and hospitals.

The lesson is this: There are some tragedies that none of us can avoid. But we can do our best to protect ourselves and our sisters, mothers, partners, and friends by finding out as much as we can about the risks of each procedure, as well as the experience and reputation of our doctors, before we consent to any kind of surgery. We'll talk more about choosing a doctor in Chapter 5, "Best of the West."

Because when it's your body, no procedure is "routine."

When It Just Isn't a Fibroid

As we've discussed, other conditions may cause the same types of symptoms as fibroids. It's important for you and your doctor to be able to rule out these other causes before proceeding with treatment, especially if that treatment includes surgery. On the other hand, if the fibroids don't seem to be the culprit behind your symptoms, you shouldn't assume that your problems have no physical cause.

Typical conditions that can mimic—or coexist with—fibroids are polyps, endometriosis, adenomyosis, and a blood disorder known as von Willebrand's disease.

POLYPS

Uterine polyps are fleshy, generally benign growths that grow from the lining of the uterus into the uterine cavity. Malignancy has only been reported in 6 out of every 1,000 cases.

Polyps are almost as common as fibroids: They're responsible for fully 25 percent of all cases of abnormal bleeding. Polyps can cause prolonged, heavy bleeding before menopause, bleeding after menopause, and breakthrough bleeding in women on hormone therapy. So even if you have fibroids, if you're bleeding, you should find out if you have polyps as well.

As a bonus, since polyps are almost always in the uterine lining, they're relatively easy for a doctor to remove with a hysteroscope (see Chapter 5, "Best of the West").

ENDOMETRIOSIS

Endometriosis is another common disorder, affecting over five million women in the United States and Canada alone. According to Kate Weinstein in her book, *Living with Endometriosis,* it's second only to uterine fibroids as the most frequent cause of hysterectomy in premenopausal women: Endometriosis accounts for 18 percent of hysterectomies every year.

If you have endometriosis, pieces of your uterine lining have somehow migrated to other parts of your pelvis. The symptoms of endometriosis mimic those of other conditions: pain, difficulty during sex, irregular bleeding, and infertility. Unfortunately, the only definitive test for endometriosis is *laparoscopy,* a surgical procedure that allows the doctor both to see whether there's a problem and to take a biopsy sample in order to examine the tissue for evidence of disease. For more on laparoscopy and biopsy, see Chapter 4, "Testing . . . Testing . . ."

ADENOMYOSIS

With *adenomyosis*, another benign disease of the uterus, parts of the endometrium migrate deeper into the uterine wall. Dr. Robert Worthington-Kirsch, an interventional radiologist in Philadelphia, Pennsylvania, says adenomyosis is "sort of like endometriosis within the uterine muscle. It is not—to my knowledge—precancerous. However, it does cause lots of pain and abnormal bleeding."

Diagnosing and treating adenomyosis becomes more complicated when you consider that it's rarely the only problem: 50 percent of women with adenomyosis also have fibroids. Many have endometriosis or polyps as well. All of these conditions, as we've seen, can cause bleeding or pelvic pain. As with endometriosis, the only certain way to get a diagnosis of adenomyosis is through a surgical biopsy.

Nobody knows how you get adenomyosis. Like fibroids, like polyps, it's an amazingly common condition: Although perhaps 20 percent of women have symptoms, microscopic analysis of uterine specimens reveal that as many as 65 percent of all women have it. As a rule, adenomyosis tends to show up in women between 40 and 50 years old; about 80 percent of women with adenomyosis have at least one child.

LAURA: *This gynecologist examined me and said, "Oh my God, you really have something going on in there." She said, "Your uterus is huge, but it's soft: It can only be adenomyosis. You'll just have to get a hysterectomy." Adenomyosis usually happens with perimenopausal women who've had multiple children, and I was 25 and had no kids. It turned out I had a fibroid the size of an orange buried inside the wall of my uterus. The doctor who finally found it said it had been there a long time.*

FELICE: *In May I went back for another exam, and the gynecologist felt that the uterus seemed larger. So I had another ultrasound that showed that the uterus had increased to about a 16-week-sized pregnant uterus, and in the posterior of the uterus was an "ill-defined solid-appearing mass measuring up to 9 centimeters." The ill-defined mass meant that there were no defined borders, which is what "classic" fibroids normally have. This is why adenomyosis is considered a likely possibility—it's "woven" into the uterine wall, unlike fibroids that have a distinct edge and are encapsulated. So we had an MRI done in order to try to get a better picture. The MRI didn't shed any new light on the matter—just that there was a mass on the posterior and off to the right somewhat and it looked like adenomyosis.*

VON WILLEBRAND'S DISEASE

According to the Centers for Disease Control (CDC), about 3 percent of women have an inherited disorder called *von Willebrand's disease,* which, like hemophilia, makes your blood clot more slowly than normal. If you have von Willebrand's disease, it's likely that you've always had heavy bleeding during your periods. Other possible symptoms include frequent, heavy nosebleeds, a tendency to bruise easily, and bleeding when you brush your teeth.

A study reported in *The Lancet* found that 13 percent of women with excessive menstrual bleeding had an undiagnosed case of von Willebrand's disease. Another 4 percent had other clotting problems, including factor XI deficiency, platelet dysfunction, or the presence of the gene for hemophilia.

The doctors conducting this study recommended strongly that women with heavy bleeding be tested for these problems before agreeing to invasive procedures. A simple blood test can measure whether your blood clots normally.

~ 3 ~

My Fibroids, Myself

FIBROIDS AND YOUR FEELINGS OF IDENTITY

I was diagnosed with a fibroid tumor that made my
uterus about thirteen weeks' size. . . . At first I was
saddened and didn't want anyone to know about
it. I grieved for the loss of my "normal" uterus.
—DR. CHRISTIANE NORTHRUP,
WOMEN'S BODIES, WOMEN'S WISDOM

The fibroids were part of my life that I had to cope with.
They physically controlled me. I think part of the problem
was that I couldn't trust my body, how it felt. It was very
unpredictable—I couldn't trust my body to be consistent.
—ANGELA

FIBROIDS ARE AN interruption—not just of your uterus, your blood
flow, your physical well-being, and your schedule, though they are
often all of that. Fibroids can interrupt and change how we feel about
ourselves. While any kind of illness can be an interruption, fibroids
can challenge us in unique ways.

In a very real sense, fibroids mark a transition from being a woman
with a healthy, functioning uterus to being a woman whose fertility

and, perhaps, femininity are on the line. When I was first diagnosed with fibroids, I was told that I might need a hysterectomy. I immediately felt a threat not just to my ability to have kids but to my identity as a woman. I was ambivalent about having children, but the idea that I would have no choice was almost unbearable.

Beyond the biological aspect, the idea that I might be judged, categorized, and possibly rejected by potential mates, relatives looking for the next little leaves on the family tree, or even friends focused on the joys of family life, challenged my identity in ways that made me question everything that makes me worthwhile over and above my ability to reproduce.

All of us handle transition and change differently, but because having fibroids can touch on some of our deepest feelings about womanhood, motherhood, sexuality, and mortality, the sense of loss can be profound.

In *Necessary Losses,* Judith Viorst writes, "The changes in our body redefine us. The events of our personal history redefine us. The ways that others perceive us redefine us. And at several points in our life we will have to relinquish a former self-image and move on."

Learning that we have fibroids, experiencing the symptoms, and making treatment decisions are some of those defining points.

LAURA: *My fibroids were threatening my organs and my fertility. You have no idea what your organs mean to you until they're in danger . . . what they mean to your identity, what they mean to your identity as a woman.*

I just couldn't separate what makes me a woman from what makes me a person—it was completely integral, more than I had ever guessed—and so it was more threatening than I could even fathom.

LEONIE: *The first time I was told about the fibroids and to expect a hysterectomy in the near future, I remember a sense of loss and sadness. My femininity and identity felt very threatened by the loss of my uterus. I think that even if I wound up having a hysterectomy because*

The Power of the Uterus

YOU MAY FIND that having fibroids gives you a strange new
sense of connection to your uterus, that mysterious, hidden part
of ourselves. Psychologists believe that even if we're not aware
of it, most of us connect very strongly to ancient myths, traditions, and symbols. Although most definitions of the uterus today
are fairly clinical, the uterus was once a powerful symbol of life,
rebirth, death, and sex—a connection with the greater forces of
nature.

The Sanskrit word for temple was "womb." In ancient Greece, the
words for "fish" and "uterus" were the same: Fish is still thought by
some to be an aphrodisiac. Native Americans saw the earth as the
womb from which all life emerged and all life returns; Christianity,
of course, tells us that the human womb nurtured and held the
Son of God.

So does it come as any surprise that the uterus in our own
bodies should be important to us? Or that fibroids cause a
threat that can feel inexplicably emotional? Or even that science—still—may have a stake in rooting out the ancient power of our
bodies?

---

*of something that really required it, such as cancer, I'd still have a very
difficult time coping with it emotionally. It's a major loss, and I think I
would grieve for it in the same way as any other major loss.*

HILLARY: *There's just no way I want to lose my uterus, just no way. It
just seems so quintessentially a female part to me, on every level. It's
about sex, it's about being female, it's about who you are.*

LINDA: *Everyone has their own psychology of what's important and
what isn't. I think the loss of my uterus might be more traumatic than
the loss of a breast.*

Only the Lonely

Part of who we are and how we define ourselves is how we interact with the people around us. Having fibroids can change who we are in relationships, whether with a partner, friends, or family members; it can even affect the relationship itself. Some women who've had difficult pregnancies because of their fibroids report that their marriages are closer than ever; other women, whose fibroids affected their sex lives, energy, or lifestyle, say that their partnerships suffered.

Women who are single while they're dealing with their fibroids may feel closer to friends who offer support. Unfortunately, it may not be surprising that a number of single women feel alone and isolated as they struggle to make decisions affecting their future.

Making decisions about treatment can be stressful, lonely, and complex. Whether or not you have a current partner, you may have to face a number of life issues. You may find yourself thinking about a changing body image. You may come up against challenges to your feelings of self-esteem, self-confidence, and independence. You may need to explore your feelings about having more children—or any children. You may find yourself thinking about what you've achieved, what's left undone, and how the quality of your relationships affects your overall quality of life. You may, in short, find yourself smack in the middle of a midlife crisis well before you feel like you've hit midlife.

ROBIN: *My partner tried to be supportive, but if you're in a partnership, it's not one person going through it—both people have their issues. That's a hidden aspect of having fibroids that nobody seems to talk about much.*

KATE: *The year before my surgery, I would lie awake in bed at night and feel the big bump in my stomach. I had a lot of uncertainty about what to do and felt very alone with the decision process.*

SHARON: *I find myself thinking that since I went to all this trouble to save my uterus, maybe I should see if still works. It's very irrational, I don't* *even know if I could get pregnant. Right now, I'm sort of coasting, trying to heal, and hoping I'll get back to my old self at some point.*

It has been a real watershed, though, and has brought into sharp focus the fact that I don't have a lot of time before menopause, and how do I want to use that time? I don't know how many of these issues come up with any major surgery or if they're connected to this particular problem. Right now, I just have a lot of questions, and no answers.

LEONIE: *One of the first things I felt was that younger women were more valued than older women; after all, if I had been younger, the MDs could have understood my wanting to keep my uterus! This made me really angry, and I also felt it was humiliating. It was like being told, "Well, you're not worth enough to spend the effort to keep you intact."*

If I Wanted to Fight Aliens, I'd Be Sigourney Weaver

Ever felt like fibroids were little aliens living in your body? That's probably one of the most common comparisons I've heard, and not just from women who have them—even some doctors refer to fibroids that way. It's weird to find out that there is something living in your body that isn't supposed to be there, like one of those gleeful little monsters from *Ghostbusters*.

A growth in the uterus is especially confusing for those of us who spent the first half of our adult lives trying to avoid pregnancy and the second half trying to have children. This intruder is something we could neither prevent nor plan—and if it could suddenly appear on its own, what else could it be capable of? How much can it really change us, age us, hurt us?

Nora Coffey of the HERS Foundation makes the point that if 80 percent of women have fibroids, it's not "abnormal;" in fact, quite the opposite. "We need to understand," she says, "that fibroids are not a disease, they're just part of our genetic blueprint." But so far, that's not our collective training.

KATE: *I was afraid that my body was out of control—and it felt like aliens were growing inside me.*

JENEANE: *When the fertility doctor showed me, using her hands, how big my uterus was, I started crying. I thought, I can't believe I have this monstrosity inside me. I had visions of cutting myself open and cutting the fibroids out. I felt like I had foreign objects inside. I looked at them as being very separate from me.*

BARBARA: *About seven years ago, my doctor decided it was time for my fibroids to come out. I could no longer sleep on my stomach, I could feel them, I was gaining weight, I had this giant ball in my stomach, 21-week sized. I could feel this thing distorting my body.*

FELICE: *When I told my mother I had fibroids, her first response was "Get this thing out of you!" So the first thing I needed to do was educate my mom.*

Who's in Charge Here?

So fibroids are one of the things in life—like losing a job, a relationship, or the waistline of our youth—that can make us feel like we've lost control. And aren't we supposed to be in control of everything? Isn't that the mark of our success? But these hidden intruders can make us question our competence. More than one woman told me she wanted to be rescued and—given the confusing array of medical choices—that she just wanted someone else to make the decision for her.

Fibroids may be one of the first big changes in our bodies, except for any pregnancies, that we've experienced since our early teenage years. And just as those changes confused and surprised us then, having fibroids can shake up our grown-up confidence and self-esteem. Dr. Leon Hoffman of the New York Psychoanalytic Society says, "Any time the genital part of a person's body is damaged, which is so important, a sense of self-esteem is involved. There are all kinds of psychological consequences not appreciated by gynecologists."

So there may be some moments when we wonder whether our fibroids are our fault—whether we could have done something better, smarter, differently. Unfortunately, a lot of self-healing "experts" out there reinforce the idea that we're responsible for creating our fibroids. Personally, I don't buy it: This tactic only seems to add unfounded accusations of inadequacy, blame, and guilt to a situation that's distressing enough. In fact, for many of us, our fibroids are probably one of the first things in our lives that we can't just take care of on our own.

Even without symptoms, having fibroids may make us feel damaged—and feelings of damage may lead to feelings of shame. Rose L. Levinson has written that shame is a familiar feeling to any of us who have ever said "I'm not enough"—not good enough, thin enough, young enough, sexy enough, smart enough—though I'm not sure too many of us ever ask, "enough" for what? Having fibroids may simply strike us as another confirmation that we don't measure up to some mythical, impossible standard.

ROBIN: *I started feeling like a hypochondriac because this became the focus of my life. Not feeling confident, not having the strength and energy to be a lover, a partner, to pursue my career—that really affected my self-esteem.*

WENDY: *I want somebody to make a decision for me. I've been saying to people recently that in a way, I wish my symptoms were worse, because if they were, then that would make me do something. The fact that they're not so bad leaves me to just dangle out there.*

KATE: *I wondered, why do I have this? Did I do something to create it? You know, [Dr.] Christiane Northrup says your creativity is blocked and I thought, well, I used to do art and music and I'm not doing that and I've got issues in my life that aren't resolved—so did I create this in my attitude and lifestyle? And regarding not having children and not finding a partner, if I lived my life differently, ate differently, had better relationships with men, maybe it wouldn't be like this. We all have our issues and relationship problems and eat things that aren't good for us. Did I eat more cheese than anyone else? I don't think so.*

Be Fruitful and Multiply?

If you don't have children, and fibroids threaten your ability to have them, you've lost something momentous: the ticket that other women have for immortality.

Even if you've been debating whether to have children or have decided that you're not going to, losing or reducing your ability to choose can take you out of the mainstream. Losing the fantasy that you could have children if you really wanted to is still a loss: of our self-determination; of the shadow self that we still might be; of our ability to connect, if only in our minds, with the generations before and the generations to come.

Not all of us struggle with the idea of genetic continuity, and of course, many women with fibroids already have children. But for those of us who don't have children, who delayed making the decision or haven't yet found the family situation we need to become mothers, the idea of not being able to have children is a little death. In a very real sense, the potential threat that fibroids pose to our fertility brings us face to face with our mortality. Who will look like us, ask to wear our good jewelry, go out into the world to fulfill some of the dreams that we've deferred?

JULIE: *I always thought I would have a career and travel and have fun, and then I'd settle down and have kids. That's just how I thought my life would go. And now, what if I can't have kids? How will the next act of my life go?*

LAURA: *I'm in a relationship now, and it's good, but I feel like my clock's ticking louder than any other 33-year-old. It's affected our relationship, and I've fought like hell for it not to, but I'm always kind of like, "So, we've been together for how long . . . ?" It's really not good; he feels the pressure.*

JENEANE: *When my doctor found the fibroids, he gave me an ultimatum—get pregnant or get a hysterectomy. That was very scary. I was also very bitter, because we hadn't put off having children on purpose.*

The years kind of flew by and there we were. We would have definitely moved things along sooner if I had known I was working on borrowed time as far as my uterus was concerned.

FELICE: *Pregnancy was in the hazy future, but the haze was thinning as I was aging and getting more comfortable with the idea. My mom was constantly pressuring me, and I feel society's pressures to be a mother. I do think stress might be a big factor in all of this. I just can't figure out how not to think about it when you are told you have to get pregnant now.*

Blood, Sweat, and Tears

What are the changes we confront when we have fibroids? How do we see ourselves? Are we different than we were before? Part of the answer depends on whether or not you're experiencing symptoms. Women who are bleeding heavily already have a changed idea of who they are—their lives have been thoroughly disrupted by fibroids.

It was Winston Churchill who said he had nothing to give but blood, toil, tears, and sweat. When you have fibroids, you may wind up giving more blood than you'd bargained for. Fibroid-related bleeding can make you sit out vacations, run out of a meeting, or leave the office. I've spoken to women who were bedridden for two weeks of every month; women who couldn't make travel plans because they could never, ever be more than a few feet away from a bathroom; and women who suddenly hemorrhaged at work, bleeding right through their clothes in a matter of seconds.

At the worst, bleeding can leave you debilitated, bedridden, and wearing adult diapers. But even the most day-to-day parts of life—like getting dressed in the morning—have a way of getting done with those unpredictable floods in mind.

BONNIE: *I was spending 10 days out of the month at home when I was having my period, unable to leave because of unpredictable flooding that couldn't be contained by any number of pads and tampons. I began wearing Depends adult diapers if I had to go to the store or run an errand.*

BARBARA: *The last two years were increasingly unbelievable. At work I went to the bathroom every hour—I freaked out at long meetings because the tampon only lasted one hour, the pad another hour.*

At home, I have white couches—I didn't sit on them when I had my period. I have a little stool I sat on. One day my period started while I was still asleep: I bled through the bedcovers and the duvet and spent the whole morning cleaning it up.

ELLEN: *I could've saved a lot of money on tampons if I'd had a hysterectomy sooner.*

So What's the Problem?

If your fibroids aren't causing any physical problems, or if they are, at least manageable ones, what's the problem? Fear of the unknown, for one; fear of having something wrong; even fear of cancer. Unfortunately, not all of our doctors are able to provide reassurance or information; finding that becomes our job.

Nora Coffey says that when women call her for guidance, "I do a lot of rhetorical questioning: 'If you hadn't gone to the doctor, would you have a problem?' Many weren't having a problem with their fibroids, and still don't. But now they're very focused on it because somebody told them they have a cantaloupe-sized tumor."

ANITA: *When I first found out I had fibroids, my initial reaction was shock and concern. I didn't know the implications or even what fibroids were. None of my previous gynecological exams had ever revealed that I had fibroids. I was a bit stunned and didn't know how to proceed. I'm typically very inquisitive, but despite being upset, I didn't take much action.*

FELICE: *During a regular annual exam, my primary-care provider discovered that my uterus was enlarged. She told me that it was probably due to fibroids and that it could affect my fertility. I had never heard of fibroids before. I felt sad and frightened. My husband said he could* *tell from my face the instant I came out of her office that something was wrong.*

JULIE: *I went for my yearly Pap smear, and we did a normal exam and when I was lying down on the table and he was feeling around, he said, What's that?! He immediately gave me a sonogram and said I had fibroids. He recommended me to this other lab to get a better, more thorough reading. I had a transvaginal sonogram and this woman seemed alarmed while doing it and said it was very large. She told me in centimeters and I'm terrible at math so I didn't understand what she was telling me.*

I was really nervous—I'd always been a really healthy person, and I was very scared. I'd heard about fibroids, and I knew that my sister had had an operation for them. My grandmother and my aunt both had hysterectomies at relatively young ages—they had fibroids as well. But somehow I didn't think it could be me.

Fibroids Are My New Hobby

Forget pottery. Forget learning Spanish, taking up modern dance, picking up that macramé project you stopped working on twenty years ago. Fibroids give you something brand-new to fill your time with: the search for good information, good doctors, choices about fibroid treatment, and people who'll respect those choices.

Once you manage to do all that, having fibroids may make you feel like a perpetual patient. I don't know if you watch *South Park,* the cartoon adventures of four round-headed eight-year-olds who seem to call the shots in their strange little world, but sometimes I imagine my fibroids are those kids—Stan, Kenny, Kyle, and Cartman (especially Cartman)—demanding to go to the doctor, go to the bathroom, get a heating pad, buy more sanitary pads. On bad days, I feel like I'm a well-designed sport utility vehicle for my fibroids, taking them where they want to go.

And then there comes a point for many of us when we have to make a decision about surgery. When doctors present fibroids as a cause for immediate concern, it's easy to feel confused, scared—a victim. Despite any urgency you may feel, or that your doctor may impart, there's almost always time to think about your options. But in the meantime, along with all your other responsibilities, goals, and expectations in life, you may have to spend time planning or at least discussing one or more future surgeries for fibroids.

TERRY: *I was 48 and I just did not want a hysterectomy. I did a lot of reading and went through a lot of stress. I presented my gynecologist at the time with the options I'd read about and she just dismissed them. And I was very distraught about the whole situation.*

I cried a lot. And then I pulled myself together and said, I know there are other options. I went to the medical school library and started looking up journal articles and reading books and magazine articles—everything I could get my hands on. I think I read seven books and about fifty journal articles, and I said, there are options out there and I just have to find a doctor who can do it, if my doctor won't.

LINDA: *I didn't want a hysterectomy, so I read as much as I could. I needed to find a doctor who would work with me, and I wanted to find a new doctor carefully. I decided to interview people and get someone who'd be a good fit. I asked friends; I asked doctors I know socially; I asked my kids' pediatrician about who his wife went to; I asked parents of my kids' friends.*

KATE: *When my doctor suggested surgery for my fibroids, I started calling people, asking do you know anybody who has fibroids, and I'd start calling them.*

I was scared, but I was sort of empowered, there's this whole world of information, it was exciting getting this information. I'd felt so alone—but when I found that there are so many people out there with this same thing, it was like a godsend.

You Are Who You Say You Are

How many cares one loses when one decides
not to be something but to be someone.
—COCO CHANEL

So how do your fibroids make you feel about yourself? Think about
it—maybe write down a list of your answers. Now think about the
woman you'd prefer to be. If you think of yourself as a woman with
fibroids, a woman who bleeds, a woman who can't have children, a
woman threatened by surgery, perhaps you can spend some time
thinking about all the other things you are. If you like, write those
things down next to your first list. You're not one or the other; you're
all those things, and probably more.

I think most women are fighters: As a gender, we're strong, sexual,
thoughtful, and competent. I also think that despite the gains made
by the feminist revolution, we still have to work harder on the job,
take care of more around the house, and be noisier about our health
care than men do.

Too often, I think, we put aside our business selves, our "yes-I-will-
lose-that-five-pounds" selves, the "who-are-you-to-tell-me-what-I-
should-think" selves, to be passive little girls in the doctor's office.
Despite a little self-deception among some members of the profession,
doctors aren't God. (And if for some reason you ever think they are,
it might be helpful to remember the 6,000-year-old Jewish tradition
that arguing with God is not only acceptable but necessary.)

Part of my own identification with my fibroids is how they define
my fears of the future—and reinforce negative body images I've had
since childhood. I have a bad back too, but I've never defined myself
as a woman with a herniated fourth lumbar. I have, however, said
that I'm a woman with fibroids. And now I have to ask myself, what
have I had to gain by this? What am I giving up if I change? What
am I afraid of?

Separation is one of the most fundamental human struggles; we
spend much of our lives figuring out when to hang on and when to
let go. If fibroids have been dominating your life emotionally, it may

be time to let go of your attachment and put them into perspective. If your fibroids are causing bleeding or pain, it may be time to look for the treatment that can help bring your life back to normal.

So perhaps you can let fibroids be your challenge: the next thing you'll handle, as you handle all the other issues that come up in your life. As the actress Cicely Tyson once said, "Challenges make you discover things about yourself that you never really knew. They're what make the instruments stretch—what make you go beyond the norm."

Having fibroids may force us to confront who we are as women, above and beyond biology. At an age before many of us are willing to confront mortality, menopause, or the loss of fertility, we need to look in the mirror and decide who we want to be when we grow up. Because when all is said and done, you're a lot more than the place your fibroids live.

~ 4 ~

Testing . . . Testing . . .

FINDING OUT ABOUT YOUR FIBROIDS

ONE OF THE most nerve-wracking things on any woman's calendar is the test trip. You write it down in your datebook, secure in the knowledge that you're a healthy, adult woman, someone who can handle your boss's panic attacks, pay the car insurance, and mop up a flooded basement. So you can certainly manage a visit to the doctor.

But as the day approaches, you might find yourself with some unexplainable butterflies in your stomach. Maybe you're irritable. Maybe you've been yelling at people who don't deserve it (or do, but for other reasons); maybe you feel like breaking into tears.

Personally, every time I walk into the doctor's office for a new procedure, I feel the way I did my first day of high school. My family had moved to a new town, and my mom dropped me off at the front door of a huge new brick building. I remember squaring my shoulders, clenching my jaw, and approaching the front door the way I imagined a knight would go into battle: ready for the worst. Even so, I've started to figure out that anticipating the worst isn't as helpful as bolstering my confidence and knowing I can handle what comes my way.

That said, the tests for fibroids are many of the same tests you've probably encountered for other conditions affecting your reproductive system. The differences lie in what you can expect to feel, *how* you can expect to feel, and the types of questions you might want to prepare to ask your doctor or radiologist.

Sometimes Less Is More

Many of us have access to medical tests that can help diagnose serious illnesses and determine treatment. But there's a downside. Tests take time and cost money, and they have a way of fueling anxiety both during the procedure and afterward, if you have to wait for results. When you're getting tested for fibroids, sometimes less is more.

According to Dr. Ricardo A. Yazigi, associate director of the Fertility Center at the Greater Baltimore Medical Center, an expensive and time-consuming regimen of tests is not necessarily an automatic next step once your doctor has felt fibroids in a pelvic exam. Says Dr. Yazigi, "There are several options for a first step. The first option is to do nothing—depending on the size and location of the fibroids, plus the symptoms and general history of the patient. In the vast majority of cases, if someone has no symptoms and no complaints of any sort, I probably won't do anything."

The most important thing you can do for yourself is to see your doctor at regular intervals, at least every six months. This visit is covered under the section coming up called "The Basics." It's the famous trip to the stirrups that every right-thinking woman resists, but that's your first and best line of defense for detecting any serious condition.

If you already have symptoms from your fibroids, your doctor will recommend at least one additional test; these tests are also described in depth later in the chapter.

What are some of the reasons your doctor may recommend diagnostic tests after your pelvic exam?

- If your doctor feels a lump in your uterus, or an enlarged uterus.
- If you have any symptoms, including abnormal uterine bleeding; pain in your lower back or radiating down your leg (possibly caused by a fibroid pressing on nerves near your spine); a change in how frequently you urinate, which would indicate pressure on your bladder; or other generalized abdominal pain.
- If you've been trying to get pregnant.
- If you have a history of problems in your reproductive system, such as fibroids, ovarian cysts, or endometriosis.

○ If you have a family history of ovarian, uterine, or other reproductive-system cancers.

This chapter is provided to help you ask the right questions. For instance:

○ If your doctor is recommending a test, what information does he or she expect to get?
○ What is the primary purpose of the test—and why is it appropriate for you?
○ How definitive is the recommended test in providing a diagnosis?
○ Can the test have a false-negative result, showing that you're healthy when there might be a problem? Or a false-positive result, showing a problem when you're actually fine? If the answer to either question is yes, how often does a false-positive or false-negative result occur?
○ If the test isn't definitive, what other procedures might be involved to get confirmation?
○ What will the test feel like? How does it work?
○ Does the test cause any pain, and if so, how can it be avoided or relieved?
○ Do you have to do anything—or avoid anything—in advance?
○ Are there any side effects after the test—or possible complications?
○ Will you have to go to the hospital? For how long? Will you need anesthesia?

Keep in mind that you want to schedule most tests, including your regular pelvic exam, when you're not menstruating (unless you're suffering from abnormally heavy bleeding); my doctors have routinely suggested scheduling appointments a week or so after the beginning of my period.

You might want to take a few minutes the night before your appointment to write down any questions you have. As my favorite high school history teacher once said, "There are no stupid questions." A caring doctor will respect any concerns you have and try to supply the information you need.

If you'd like a guideline to help chart your symptoms for discussion with your doctor, Dr. Susan M. Lark's *Fibroid Tumors & Endometriosis Self Help Book* includes twelve months' worth of charts you can fill in, logging twenty symptoms for each day of your cycle and grading them for severity.

The Buddy System

There's an important suggestion I'd like to make about your emotional well-being for those trips to the doctor, even the routine visits: Don't be embarrassed to bring a buddy with you to your appointment—a friend, relative, or significant other—who can act as your advocate at the doctor's office.

It's important to choose the right person to keep you company. No whiners, no moaners, nobody who is fidgeting about having to get back to the office (in that case, you might as well take along a three-year-old). You want someone supportive and upbeat, someone who has your emotional well-being in mind. It's hard to be your own best friend if you're nervous or anxious, feelings that can come up all too often during a medical test. Your advocate can help make sure you get all the information you need and help you process it in a balanced, thoughtful way.

The benefits of asking a friend or partner to keep you company extend beyond the test itself. If you're like me, your stress levels can climb to Mount McKinley heights the day or so before a doctor's appointment. Discussing your questions, fears, and feelings with your advocate will not only "prep" your friend or partner to help you get the information you need, but may also help you put any fears in perspective.

If you're comfortable with the idea and your doctor agrees, your advocate can even be present during your exam; he or she can certainly be with you when you speak with the doctor afterward.

If you have any reservations about asking someone to go with you, think of how you would respond if someone asked you for the same favor. Chances are, you'll realize that the person you ask will be glad to help, assuming her schedule permits.

JENEANE: *My husband went to EVERY doctor's appointment and ultra-sound with me. I am thankful he has his own business so he was able to get the time away. He wouldn't have had it any other way.*

HILLARY: *I think I would just take a tape recorder. I'm not sure if most doctors would allow you to tape record what they say, but that makes the most sense, because then you could listen to it when you were calmer.*

The Basics

Feet in the stirrups. A therapist I know tells me that this position was invented by Henry VIII, who wanted to see his child being born. And we all know how Henry felt about the women in *his* life.

You know the drill: You put on the little paper robe, scoot your bottom to the end of the table, and put your feet *there*.

Just before that awkward moment, before feeling my doctor's latex-covered fingers and the cold metal of the speculum, I try to keep my breaths even and deep, and imagine myself just about anywhere except where I am at that moment. (Try thinking about the warm sun on a secluded beach, floating in a quiet pool—or, if you don't mind having erotic ideas in odd places, you could even fantasize about being with a lover.)

You may feel some pain or tenderness as your doctor checks for any abnormalities. Most gynecologists can tell if you have one or more fibroids through the manual exam. For many of us, this may be the first time we've heard of fibroids—or known we had them.

If you do have one or more fibroids, your doctor can probably give you a rough idea of how large the largest one is: a golf ball, an orange, a grapefruit. You may also be told how your fibroids compare to the size of a fetus: 4 weeks, 12 weeks. (FYI, a 12-week-sized uterus, whether through pregnancy or fibroids, generally weighs about one pound.) Women who aren't actually pregnant can find this remarkably insensitive. Many women report being told that their fibroids are "dangerous" or "too large" at 12 to 16 weeks. (I don't like the idea of fibroids measured in weeks, either. However, since it's the current

Sports or Side Dish?

DOCTORS DO HAVE other terms for describing how big your fibroids are. But is it a lack of imagination or some kind of medical Rorschach test that leads them to use these same descriptions over and over?

> *Golf ball, baseball, pool ball, football, bowling ball*
> *Pea, walnut, lime, tomato, orange, grapefruit,*
> *cantaloupe, watermelon*

Can we get creative here? What about describing a fibroid as being the size of a full-blown rose, a small ice-cream sundae, a sequined purse—things we might not mind carrying around inside ourselves?

language, you'll see it used throughout the book. Over time, we can work on creating more acceptable terms.)

SANDY: *When my doctor measured my fibroids, he said "Oh, it's about seven weeks." I didn't know what he was talking about, and when he explained I was horrified. What a comparison! To say that a fibroid is the equivalent size of a fetus?! They would never use that to describe a growth in a man. What, just because it's my uterus, that's how you'd define a growth? It's really awful, partly because I've never had children and suddenly had to imagine that this thing, this thing I didn't want, was somehow a baby substitute. It's beyond insensitive.*

JULIE: *They described my fibroids—I had five—one was a grapefruit, one was an orange, and then there were three apricots. I started referring to it as my fruit bowl, and my friends would say, "When are you getting your fruit bowl taken care of?" People would say I had Carmen Miranda's hat in my stomach. But it was pretty horrifying that I had that much going on in there.*

Another test you are probably familiar with from basic office visits with your ob-gyn is the *Papanicolaou*, or *Pap*, test. Your doctor will use a small scraper or brush to collect some cells from your cervix and upper vagina; he or she will send the results to a lab to check for malignancy. The Pap test is designed to detect cervical cancer, but since it doesn't provide any information about the inside of your uterus, it won't show whether any uterine fibroids are malignant. Although this is unlikely in any case, other tests are available to determine the presence of cancer inside the body of the uterus (see the section "Ruling Out Cancer").

Average Size of the Uterus with Fibroids vs. Pregnancy

IF YOUR DOCTOR or radiologist describes your uterus in terms of a pregnancy, here's what he or she is talking about (you can come up with your own fruit analogies):

8-week pregnancy = 2 inches (5 centimeters)
12 weeks = 3 inches (7.6 centimeters)
16 weeks = 6 inches (15.2 centimeters)
40 weeks = 20 inches (50.8 centimeters)

Sonograms

Once your doctor has determined that you have a fibroid—or more than one—he or she will probably recommend that you get a *sonogram* to confirm the size, number, and placement in your uterus.

Sonograms, also called *ultrasounds,* create an image of your uterus and ovaries by bouncing high-frequency sound waves against your pelvis. The good thing about sonograms is that they're risk free:

The worse thing likely to happen is that you'll have to wipe cold, blue lubricating jelly off your tender skin with rough paper towels.

Sonograms are also the method of choice for checking up on a baby's progress in the course of a pregnancy. If you're trying to get pregnant or have suffered a miscarriage, I think it's especially important to bring a friend with you to the sonogram. It can feel very lonely sitting in a waiting room, wondering what might be going wrong with your body while seeing other women checking up on their (seemingly) successful pregnancies. Your friend doesn't have to join you in the exam room, but you'll do yourself a favor in terms of having a shoulder to cry on, should you need one.

Many gynecologists are able to perform an ultrasound right in the office, during your exam. If so, you probably won't even need to move from the table you're on. (By the way, even if you have a sonogram during your regular gynecological exam, many insurance companies consider it a separate procedure; depending on your insurance plan, be prepared for a separate—and sometimes expensive—charge over and above the office visit.)

If your doctor does not offer ultrasound, she'll refer you to a *radiologist*—a medical doctor with specialized training in performing visual tests like sonograms, X-rays, and MRIs. You'll have to make a separate appointment to see the radiologist; your doctor might be able to do that for you while you're sitting in her office. Once again, you'll be on that familiar table, feet propped up in stirrups. If you're having the sonogram in a radiologist's office, you'll generally only have to undress from the waist down. The doctor—or sometimes a trained nurse—will cover a probe with a latex sheath (similar to a condom), lubricate it, and insert it into your vagina. Unless you're very dry inside, or very nervous, the insertion shouldn't hurt at all. Your doctor may offer to let you insert the probe yourself, or, if you like this idea, you can ask to do it. Once the probe is inserted, the doctor will manipulate it; sometimes this can hurt, but the more you relax, the easier the manipulation can be. (Easier said than done? You bet.)

The probe is attached to a computer with a keyboard and screen.

As the doctor guides the probe, you'll begin to see blurry black and white images flickering on the screen: your uterus and ovaries, your fibroids, and any other interesting things that are in there. For instance, sonograms can detect the presence of polyps, which can be missed during a regular physical exam. Your doctor will explain what she's seeing, if you want to know.

The doctor will use the computer to measure the size of your fibroids in centimeters: Although this measurement can sound large, remember that 2.54 centimeters equals one inch. (For a quick visualization, take a look at your thumb: From the middle knuckle to the tip measures about one inch.)

You may want to ask questions during the test, or you may want to wait until all the data are collected. The great thing about a sonogram is that the results are immediate. If you're in your doctor's office, you can have a discussion about the results right away; if you see a radiologist, he or she won't provide a diagnosis or recommendation for next steps—that's your doctor's job—but can generally give you a report on the facts. Be sure to ask the radiologist for a copy of the report for your own files, as well as a copy of the images, if possible.

If you have sonograms done regularly, you can also find out whether the fibroids have grown since your last visit, and by how much. A tip:

When Is a Test Not Just a Test?

THERE ARE TWO kinds of tests for fibroids: the ones designed purely to show the size and location of fibroids, such as sonograms (ultrasounds) and hysterosalpingograms (HSG), and those that can sometimes help fix a problem. Thanks to microsurgery techniques, these procedures are two-for-one combos, diagnostic techniques that also allow your doctor to correct some problems right there and then. Examples of these two-for-one tests are hysteroscopy, laparoscopy, and dilation and curettage (better known as D&C). Tests in this latter group involve anesthesia and sometimes a trip to the hospital, usually on an outpatient basis.

Schedule your sonograms the same week of your cycle each time. Since fibroids may retain water, sonograms done the week before your period could show a larger uterus than at other times of the month. It doesn't matter which week of your cycle you schedule sonograms, as long as you're consistent.

If your fibroids become really large, your gynecologist or radiologist may do an abdominal sonogram. For this one, you have to fill your bladder, usually by drinking eight glasses of water—64 ounces!—and waiting until you feel "full," as the receptionist in my doctor's office gently puts it.

There are two problems with this, both of which involve your general level of comfort, or lack of it. First is the simple problem of wanting to let loose all that water. Be prepared to squirm a little between announcing you're ready and the test beginning. Second, drinking a lot of water in a short time can cool down your body temperature; since you might feel really chilly, it can pay off to plan time for a post-test coffee or a bowl of soup to warm up again.

The abdominal sonogram is simple. The radiologist slathers lubricant—and it's cold!—over your distended belly and runs the probe over your skin.

Doctors disagree about the benefits of the transvaginal, or endo-vaginal (where the probe is inside your vagina), versus the abdominal methods of doing a sonogram. The American College of Preventive Medicine gives vaginal ultrasound the edge over abdominal ultrasound for providing a higher level of detail. However, some doctors feel that views taken from the inside don't show the top of your uterus adequately, and certain types of fibroids can be missed.

In my case, when my radiologist doesn't feel he's gotten enough information on a vaginal scan, he sends me back out to the waiting room with a pitcher of water. Other doctors may start you off with an abdominal ultrasound (you'd come to the office with a full bladder); they can perform a vaginal scan afterwards, if need be.

If your doctor wants to visualize your fibroids more clearly, she may suggest a more advanced ultrasound, using either *fluid sonography* or three-dimensional imaging. Fluid sonography—more formally known as *sonohystography*—is similar in some ways to a

The Safety of Ultrasound

THE CONSUMER-PATIENT RADIATION HEALTH AND SAFETY ACT
of April 5, 1998, confirms the safety of the ultrasound procedure.
The act says that since the introduction of medical applications of
ultrasound in the 1940s, "Diagnostic ultrasound has proven to be
a valuable tool in medical practice. An excellent safety record exists
in that, after decades of clinical use, there is no known instance of
human injury as a result of exposure to diagnostic ultrasound."

traditional abdominal sonogram, except that instead of filling your
bladder, your doctor actually fills your uterus with saline solution in
order to stretch the walls of the uterus to get a more exact picture of
any fibroids.

You'll need to schedule an appointment for this procedure, partly
because you'll need to take a small amount of antibiotics, such as doxy-
cycline, an hour or two before. (If you're allergic to this or any other
form of medicine, of course, let your doctor know in advance.)

The doctor will insert a small tube into your vagina; one end of the
tube is attached to a bag of sterile saline solution, while the other end
extends into your uterus. The doctor will start filling your uterus with
the saline solution; this can create a strange, cold sensation.

With your uterus filled like a little water balloon, your doctor will
run the ultrasound probe over your abdomen. When the ultrasound
is complete, the doctor will remove the tube from your vagina, and
the saline solution will simply run out of your body. When you get
dressed, you will probably want to use a pad to soak up any extra fluid,
and absorb any spotting.

You may feel some pain when the doctor inserts the tube for the
saline; you may experience some cramping afterward. Talk to your doctor about whether you can take a pain reliever, such as acetaminophen,
an hour or so before the procedure to help ward off any pain.

You can probably go back to work after the procedure, if you choose,
but you may not feel at the top of your game. I suggest not scheduling

any important meetings if you can avoid it. In the evening, you'll take another small dose of antibiotics; you should wake up in the morning feeling no aftereffects at all. If you begin to run a fever, have heavy bleeding or severe cramps, be sure to call your doctor immediately.

A newer technique is slowly starting to replace fluid sonography as the "next step" in visualizing fibroids. Three-dimensional sonography provides a clearer picture than the two-dimensional imaging commonly in use. There's even something called four-dimensional sonography, but you won't need it for your fibroids. Why not? The big advance in "4D" is that it shows moving images; trust me, your fibroids would make a very boring movie.

While a sonogram is considered reliable in determining the presence, number, and size of fibroids, it cannot detect malignancy. Remember, most fibroids are benign. But if your fibroids are growing rapidly, your doctor will want to perform other tests to determine whether cancer might be present. See "Ruling Out Cancer" for information on these procedures.

How do you know if your fibroids are growing rapidly? According to Dr. Yazigi, fast growth "is really in the eye of the beholder. Not all fast-growing fibroids are created equal. If a 1-centimeter fibroid grows to 2 centimeters between office visits, that's 100 percent growth, but that's less significant than a 6-centimeter fibroid that grows 33 percent, to 8 centimeters. Regardless of the rate of growth, if a woman is urinating more frequently or having pain in her back or pain radiating

Sonogram Style

IF YOU HAVE to have sonograms often enough, you might want to start your day by dressing for a quick change—choosing a two-piece outfit instead of a dress; socks instead of pantyhose. My favorite outfit for sonogram day includes simple loose pants that go on and off easily, socks or knee-high stockings, and comfy shoes. I find it really helps to be able to leave quickly, with minimal fuss, when the test is over.

down her leg, or has abnormal uterine bleeding, even if the fibroid is not clinically significant, those would be causes for further study."

If your doctor wants to get a clearer look at your fibroids, there are several options. These "next step" tests range from MRIs, which take pictures from outside your body, to laparoscopic surgery, which is as up close and personal as possible.

Magnetic Resonance Imaging

Magnetic resonance imaging, or MRI, is another way that doctors can get a picture of your insides. It's not used as commonly for fibroids, partly because it's more expensive than a sonogram, but also because sonograms tend to be fairly accurate. When there's a question on a sonogram, however, MRI is another noninvasive way to get more information.

Magnetic resonance imaging relies on something that could be straight out of a science-fiction thriller: large, powerful magnets that energize subatomic particles in your body. For some women, MRIs are no big deal, but others find them unpleasant.

When you schedule the test, let the radiologist know if you are or might be pregnant. And since certain types of metal can interfere with the scan, be sure to mention if you have any metal in your body, from braces on your teeth to rods in your back . . . even shrapnel (hey, soldiers get fibroids too!). If you acquired any tattoos in your wild youth—20 years ago or more—you might want to mention that too, since older tattoos sometimes included metal flecks.

Beyond any normal test-taking anxiety you may have, the experience itself is a bit odd. You're led into a room with a large machine; a technician behind a glass wall will be in voice contact with you during the procedure. You're helped onto a sort of tray, which is then slid, with you on it, into a large tube. Surrounded by the cylinder at this point, you're a bit like the filling in a cannelloni.

The bigger the machine, the more expensive the magnets, so if you think the opening will be as small and narrow as possible, you're right. Sliding into the tube can bring up those astronaut fantasies

Top 10 Things You Resemble
While Taking an MRI

10. A banana in a banana split
 9. An astronaut in suspended animation
 8. One of those pretzels with cheese filling
 7. A tampon in a plastic inserter
 6. A poster in a mailing tube
 5. A cocktail frank in a wraparound biscuit (mmm, pigs in a blanket!)
 4. Someone trying out for the Olympic bobsled team
 3. The stars inside a kaleidoscope
 2. The moon inside a telescope
 1. A modern Sleeping Beauty, waiting for that magic kiss from you-know-who

you've been suppressing all these years; it can also cause feelings of claustrophobia, so meditating, chanting, or just closing your eyes and visualizing yourself someplace else can be a big help. Some people need more than imagery; if you're concerned about your reaction to being in an enclosed space, talk to your doctor about the possibility of having conscious sedation or even anesthesia. Both of these are used to help patients get through the test with as little discomfort as possible.

A new type of "open" MRI allows you to sit or stand during the test. There are two cautions, though: you'll still be positioned quite close to the magnets, so you may still feel a bit of claustrophobia. More important, open MRIs use less powerful magnets, which means that the exam can take up to twice as long . . . and the image might not be as accurate. For these reasons, some doctors think that open MRIs simply don't scan the uterus as well as the traditional tube.

An MRI is painless. But during the test, you'll hear bursts of horrific noise, like a jackhammer: This is the action of the magnets at work. If your reverie includes a beach, let this be the noise of a powerboat, arriving to take you somewhere fabulous. On a more practical note, you can ask for earplugs . . . or bring them with you.

Seriously, a relaxed attitude will be your best protection against the difficulties of this test: The worst hardship, assuming your insurance is covering the extremely high cost, are the fears the strange MRI environment can create.

Hysterosalpingography

Hysterosalpingography (HSG) is yet another way to take a picture of your uterus. Some doctors prefer the clearer picture it provides; some use it as a second opinion after you've had a sonogram.

The purpose of HSG, in our case, is to determine whether there are any abnormalities in the uterus. Specifically, it can help rule out fibroids as a cause of infertility. Unlike sonograms, HSG can help tell you whether your fallopian tubes are open or are blocked by fibroids.

When you schedule your HSG, remember that it's only a "snapshot" of what your body looks like. Since fibroids appear and grow on their own schedule, the test result is valid for only about a six-month period.

Although this test is a way to diagnose the reasons for infertility, it there's any chance that you're pregnant, you want to avoid this procedure since it could harm an embryo or fetus. To make sure that you're not pregnant, the Atlanta Reproductive Health Center recommends scheduling the test between days 7 and 10 from the first day of your period.

Dr. H. Winter Griffith, author of *The Complete Guide to Medical Tests,* recommends that you also avoid the test if you've got undiagnosed vaginal bleeding, if you have pelvic inflammatory disease, or if you're menstruating. You should tell your doctor if you know you're allergic to the dyes used for the X-ray, to iodine or seafood (because the dye contains iodine), or to any medications.

JENNIFER: *My HSG went very well. It was pretty painless, but a bit embarrassing, because it was a doctor who I did not know from Adam,*

and he took forever to get the tube inside my cervix because my uterus
was a bit misshapen and tilted. I was just uncomfortable with a doctor
I did not know doing this rather intimate test on me.

Here's what happens: You'll show up at your friendly radiologist's office. You'll undress either all the way or from the waist down and put on one of the little gowns you've come to know and love. (Well, to know.)

Before the test starts, some doctors will give you a nonsteroidal anti-inflammatory drug, such as Aleve or Motrin; some may give you a local anesthetic. If your radiologist doesn't, I suggest you ask, to reduce any potential pain.

You will lie on a very cold table, yes, feet in stirrups, and the doctor will clamp your cervix open with a special forceps (called a *tenaculum*). Next, using a syringe, the doctor will inject an opaque dye into your uterus. The dye creates a reverse picture of your uterus, fallopian tubes, and ovaries: they show up white on the X-ray film. Any abnormalities in the shape or lining of the uterus, as well as any obstructions, can be seen clearly.

According to Dr. Joseph Feste, retired associate clinical professor of obstetrics and gynecology at the Baylor College of Medicine and the University of Texas Health Science Center, "All intracavitary and submucous fibroids will create a distorted cavity on hysterosalpingograms, with the exception of very small tumors. If the radiologist injects the contrast medium very slowly, even the smallest tumors can be seen."

Cramps after the test are considered normal; if they continue for more than a day or so, call your doctor. Other complications can include bleeding, infection, or allergic reaction to the dye, which can show up as hives, itching, or low blood pressure.

By the way, I found this one so hard to pronounce I started singing it, like this: Hy-STER-o-sal-PING-o-gram, gram, gram. (Think of a Latin beat, or the Cream song "Sunshine of Your Love.") Try it; it makes remembering the name infinitely easier—and more fun.

Hysteroscopy

If you're old enough to remember *Fantastic Voyage,* this test may sound familiar. After you "assume the position" for the hysteroscopy, a tiny, thin, lighted telescope is inserted into your vagina, allowing your doctor and you to get an insider's view of your uterus, including the entrance to your fallopian tubes—a crucial area to check if you're trying to get pregnant. If other conditions are detected, such as polyps on the lining of your uterus, your doctor can do a *directed biopsy*—one that samples tissue right from the problem area. A hysteroscopy cannot diagnose fibroids in the wall itself or on the outer wall of the uterus.

Hysteroscopy is generally done with local anesthesia, but be warned: According to Dr. Fritz Wieser of the University Hospital of Vienna, Austria, an injection of a local anesthesia in the cervix "can be more painful than the hysteroscopy itself." In response to what some women call "intolerable pain," Dr. Wieser's team recommends the use of lidocaine spray to numb the cervix before the injection. In a study of 300 women, this two-step method made a significant difference, allowing for a pain-free experience.

There are three potential complications you should know about. One problem that can occur with any invasive procedure like this is perforation of the uterus. While the uterus usually heals quickly, scarring could be a potential problem if you're considering pregnancy.

The second complication is the possibility of fluid leaking into your bloodstream. Your doctor may use a saline solution or other fluid to enlarge your uterus to get a more precise view. Sometimes some of this fluid can leak into the blood vessels of the uterus: Too much fluid in your blood vessels can cause fluid on the lungs *(pulmonary edema)* or even seizures. As a rule, this is prevented by keeping track of the amount of fluid used during the procedure. For more about avoiding this particular complication, see the section on surgical hysteroscopy in Chapter 5.

Third, the procedure may cause bleeding. A little spotting afterwards is normal, but if you find you're bleeding a lot while you're recovering, make sure you call your doctor immediately.

LAURA: *The doctor who found the fibroid did a hysteroscopy in his office and it was easy. You're not completely knocked out but you're feeling good, and they just sort of penetrate with a scope and it's not traumatic at all. You just can't drive afterwards. He decided to attempt surgery through the hysteroscope, which not a lot of people do. But once he got in there, there was more than he realized. He got some of it out but he had to stop the surgery, so that wasn't a total success.*

Laparoscopy

Laparoscopy is a somewhat more invasive way for your doctor to get a firsthand look at you. By putting a tiny camera directly into your abdomen, your doctor can see the outside of your uterus as well as the surrounding pelvic structure. Laparoscopy can be combined with hysteroscopy to see what's happening inside your uterus, or with D&C to take a sample of the tissue inside your uterus.

This is surgery. Okay, it isn't a heart transplant, but it does require anesthesia and a surgical incision. Don't hesitate to ask your doctor questions about what you can expect to experience during and after the test. Don't feel that you have to take a laparoscopy lightly because it isn't "important" enough.

Laparoscopies are almost always done in a hospital, though on an outpatient basis, meaning you won't have to stay overnight. I always think I'm tough enough to go to a hospital by myself, and besides, I don't want to "bother" anybody by asking them to give up a few hours to be with me. Wrong, wrong, wrong. There is nothing nicer than having someone by your side when you walk into the hospital, no matter how routine the procedure.

You'll also have to arrange for someone to pick you up when you're ready to leave, since you won't be in much shape to drive. Some hospitals won't let you leave unless someone is there with you, even if, like me, you were only planning to get in the back seat of a taxi for the ride home.

The day before your laparoscopy, you won't be allowed to eat or drink anything for 12 hours; if you can schedule the test for the morning, you can minimize your fasting time. When you arrive at the hospital, you'll be given a locker for your clothing and handbag or other personal items. You'll change into a hospital gown, robe, and slippers, and you'll be issued a little plastic shower cap for the operating room. A nurse or physician's assistant will take your medical history and blood pressure. Laparoscopies can be performed with either local or general anesthesia; some doctors will start with a local and only move on to general anesthesia if they find a potential problem they need to explore more thoroughly.

If you decide to have general anesthesia, or the half-awake state known as "twilight," you'll need to have an informed conversation with your doctor beforehand about the possibility of doing further procedures while you're under. Depending on your condition, this may be a good, efficient option, but only you can decide if you are comfortable trusting your doctor's judgment during surgery, or if you want to have a further conversation before he or she does anything more than take a look inside.

If you're getting a local anesthetic, you'll be awake during the surgery, but you shouldn't feel anything after the injection. Remember, the injection can hurt—ask if the doctor will numb the area first. If you're having general anesthesia, you'll fall asleep almost instantly and not feel a thing until you wake up in the recovery room. The advantage of having local anesthesia means that you can stay up and chat with your doctor about what he or she sees and plans to do. If you're asleep, the advantage is, you're out! Of course, if you know of any allergies you have to anesthesia, be sure to tell your doctor, the hospital staff, and the anesthesiologist.

JANIS: *I'm a medically curious person. I probably should have been a doctor or nurse. At six, I asked to see my tonsils after they were removed, and the doc had them in a jar by my bed when I came to. So with that in mind, my gynecologist was happy to go with my wishes. I got to choose the music in the O.R.—Neil Diamond, 'cause the doc and I both liked him. They installed a mirror on the bed so I could watch what they were doing. They would not let me watch the initial cut, but after that I watched the whole thing.*

The surgical risks of laparoscopy include perforation of a blood vessel, the bowel, or the liver, though these last two complications are considered very rare. Your risk will be higher than normal if you suffer from obesity, heart disease, or lung disease; if you smoke; if you are in the late stages of pregnancy; or if you take certain medications, including antihypertensives, antiarrhythmics, diuretics, or beta-adrenergic blockers.

A laparoscopy won't leave you with any big souvenir scars. Once you're prepped for surgery, the procedure begins with two small cuts inside your bellybutton, about 1 to 2 centimeters long. The doctor will insert a needle through your abdomen to fill your uterus with gas—carbon dioxide, or CO_2—which distends your uterus and makes it taut. Carbon dioxide is easily absorbed by the blood, and as one study delicately says, "it does not support combustion." (So you can leave your fire extinguisher at home.) The most common effects of CO_2 on a young, or youngish, healthy woman include nausea and the uncomfortable feeling of being, well, full of gas.

The pressure in your abdomen also pushes against your diaphragm, which can limit your ability to breathe properly. And a really odd side effect noticed in surgery involving CO_2 is postoperative pain in your shoulders, possibly caused by the pressure of the gas throwing your body out of whack. In some cases, mostly involving older women, CO_2 can put pressure on your blood vessels and, therefore, on your heart. This means there's a slight danger of having a stroke.

A number of doctors have begun using *gasless laparoscopy*, a technique which eliminates any potential problems from CO_2. Instead of inflating the abdomen with gas, the surgeon simply lifts the abdominal wall with a special retractor. According to researchers at the University of Pennsylvania, gasless laparoscopy can be performed under local anesthetic with conscious sedation.

When the surgery is over, your doctor will close the incision with small sutures or staples and cover it with a small bandage. You'll rest in the hospital for a few hours to make sure your vital signs are all in order.

Your recovery should be pretty brief, probably no more than two days at home. One tip: If you have a laparoscopy with gas, don't drink anything carbonated—soda, seltzer, beer, champagne—for two days after surgery. The carbon dioxide still in your system can interact with these drinks, causing vomiting. Call your doctor immediately if you start showing signs of infection: headache, muscle pain, dizziness, or fever; if you start bleeding a lot from either the incision or your vagina; or if you have abdominal swelling or pain.

Ruling Out Cancer

DR. MITCH LEVINE: *I see a lot of women for a second opinion, who don't want to have a hysterectomy. A lot of times I hear the story, women go to the doctor, even for an asymptomatic fibroid, he examines her and says you've got a tumor and I'm scheduling you for a hysterectomy. It's very upsetting, they're scared, they heard the word "tumor" and they were scared into thinking they had cancer. They're often very relieved to hear that if they have asymptomatic fibroids, they don't necessarily have to do anything, and they don't have something that will kill them.*

CHERI: *The ultrasound tech told me I had fibroids. Once she assured me that they weren't cancerous and probably no treatment would be recommended, I relaxed.*

Fibroids are almost always benign. This is particularly important to remember since fibroids are often called fibroid tumors—a word with instant connotations of fast-growing malignant killers. The National Institutes of Health declares in no uncertain terms that "fibroids are **not** cancerous. Fibroids are not associated with cancer; they rarely develop into cancer (in less than 0.1 percent of cases). Having fibroids does not increase your risk for uterine cancer."

But don't some doctors tell us that fibroids can "turn into" cancer? The *Journal of Obstetrics & Gynecology* says that the answer to this question "remains uncertain." Dr. Victor Reyniak, clinical professor of ob-gyn and reproductive science at the Mount Sinai School of Medicine in New York, says that only 0.1 percent of fibroids become cancerous, "and usually in older age."

Other studies also estimate that between 0.1 percent and 1 percent of women with fibroids may get cancer. That equals 10 to 100 women out of every 10,000; statistically, women over 50 have a greater risk for uterine cancer than younger women.

Even on the low side, the risk for women with fibroids appears to be higher than the norm. According to the American Cancer Society, the rate of uterine cancer among women in general is about 0.02 percent, or 2 in every 10,000 women. Uterine cancer, which attacks the lining or walls of the uterus, is different from cervical cancer, which affects the round entrance to the uterus. Regular Pap smears have a good track record of detecting cervical cancer in the earliest stages, but they can't detect cancers deeper in the uterus.

Besides uterine cancer, the other concern that doctors sometimes raise is ovarian cancer. While this is not related medically to fibroids, some doctors express the fear that large fibroids could block their ability to feel ovarian cancer in a pelvic exam. However, a high-resolution ultrasound, MRI, or computerized axial tomographic (CAT) scan should be able to distinguish ovarian masses from uterine fibroids.

The odds are in your favor, but to play it safe, there are times when your doctor may want to test you for cancer. What are the traditional warning signs?

○ Rapidly growing fibroids (although bear in mind that as fibroids grow, they double themselves in size naturally)
○ A change in the consistency of a fibroid (something that also happens in a fibroid's natural "life cycle")
○ An enlarged uterus in a woman with no previous history of fibroids (regardless of whether she is pre- or postmenopausal)
○ Unusual bleeding at any age, before or after menopause: This is the most common symptom of uterine cancer. Bleeding of any kind after menopause is an especially strong indication of a potential problem.

If your doctor raises the specter of cancer along with a diagnosis of fibroids, how much do you need to worry? Researchers at the Johns Hopkins University School of Public Health discovered that among over a thousand women who had a hysterectomy for benign conditions like fibroids, almost 30 percent had "a lot" of fear that they'd develop cancer—and virtually every woman in the study had at least "a little" fear.

While a doctor might want to (and should) test you for cancer based on your symptoms and perhaps family history, that does not mean you *have* cancer. Before anybody gives you a diagnosis, they must be able to rule out the benign possibilities. If you are found to have cancer, hysterectomy is considered absolutely necessary.

Unfortunately, some doctors recommend hysterectomy as a way to prevent future cancers. There's no question that a woman without a uterus can't get uterine cancer, but as you've seen, your risk is statistically low. Unless your family history or other factors suggest you're at risk, you should think long and hard about this type of "preventive," or prophylactic, surgery: For most women, the risk involved in surgery is greater than that of getting cancer.

On the other end of the spectrum, some women with both cancer and fibroids report that their original doctors never tested for cancer, assuming that their unusual bleeding was due to their fibroids. For this reason, women who have gynecological cancers strongly recommend seeing a gynecological oncologist (a doctor who specializes in women's cancers) to rule out cancer. If you're bleeding in any unusual way and your fibroids are in the uterine wall (intramural) or on the outer wall (subserous), or if you're past menopause, insist on a biopsy; if you have cancer, with luck, a biopsy will catch it early.

In general, your best offense against cancer is a good defense: Regular pelvic exams by a thoughtful, caring, and knowledgeable doctor can spell the difference between early detection and—however small the chances—an unpleasant surprise.

A range of methods can be used to test for cancer, from the relatively simple blood test called a CA-125 to an outpatient visit to the hospital for a D&C.

IRIS: *My ob-gyn and I discussed several options to stop the bleeding. He suggested a vaginal hysterectomy. I countered with other options, but he felt those procedures would not be appropriate in my case, basically because of the numerous fibroids in my uterus. I finally agreed to the vaginal hysterectomy.*

I had a follow-up appointment with my doctor three weeks after the surgery and could hardly wait to be released to work. When I went to that appointment my doctor told me that he had sent a harmless-looking polyp from my uterine lining to the lab for biopsy. It was a low-grade endometrial sarcoma, a very rare cancer, and I was being referred to a specialist. In fact he had already scheduled an appointment for me. He had no information to give me on the cancer. That is how I started my research into medical and health issues, trying to find out about my cancer. It is a "hobby" I still continue to this day. In fact I now work in the healthcare field.

CA-125

A CA-125 is a simple blood test that is most often used to diagnose ovarian cancer; a doctor may recommend it if he or she is concerned that your fibroids prevent checking your ovaries in a manual exam. Less often, CA-125 can be used to detect a form of uterine cancer.

The entire test consists of your doctor drawing blood from your arm, just as he or she would in any normal blood test. The procedure will be over in seconds. The blood is then sent to a lab for analysis.

The lab will look for something in your blood called a *biochemical tumor marker.* Higher levels of this marker in your blood may indicate the presence of cancer cells; then again, it may not. Readings under 35 generally mean you're fine, although the range varies, so that even a reading of 45 can be considered safe.

But here's the rub: Fibroids can sometimes cause false-positive results on a CA-125 test. Other noncancerous conditions that can cause elevated levels are advanced endometriosis, recovery from surgery, and even pregnancy. You have no idea how much I wish I'd known this when I got back my own elevated results—three times in a row.

According to the Abramson Cancer Center of the University of Pennsylvania, elevated CA-125 levels can be found in 1 to 2 percent of healthy individuals and in patients with nonmalignant conditions— even women who are menstruating.

Uterine Cancer

THREE TYPES OF cancer affect the uterus. The most common is *endometrial* or *uterine cancer,* which begins in the lining of the uterus, or endometrium. The second type, called *uterine sarcoma* (leiomyosarcoma), starts in the muscles of the uterus. The National Cancer Institute defines uterine sarcoma as "a very rare kind of cancer . . . in which cancer (malignant) cells start growing in the muscles or other supporting tissues of the uterus." Uterine sarcoma is the cancer most likely to mimic fibroids, although again, it is considered quite rare. The third type of cancer affecting the uterus is *cervical cancer.* This can be most commonly detected with an annual Pap smear.

The risk for endometrial cancer most often begins for women in their thirties; the risk of uterine sarcoma (leiomyosarcoma) begins more often in a woman's forties. After menopause, the first sign is unusual bleeding, which may be a "watery, blood-streaked flow that gradually contains more blood." The minimum treatment for all types of uterine cancer is hysterectomy.

If uterine cancers are detected early, five-year survival rates are over 90 percent.

If you are getting your first CA-125 (or CA-125II or LPA, two newer—somewhat more accurate—versions), remember that this is your baseline reading. If the values seem elevated to your doctor, more tests will be needed to confirm a diagnosis. Even though these procedures are time-consuming and potentially invasive, they can help detect a real malignancy—or, more likely, put your mind at ease that your condition is benign.

TINA: *My doctor said "cancer" and that's when my brain stopped functioning normally. I was so upset; I left her office and went across the street for a glass of wine. It was only two in the afternoon, but I needed a drink. Actually, the first thing I did was call my mother, and then I got a drink. Although my test reading was high, something like 55, it was not defini-*

tive. But all I heard was cancer. Not "maybe" not "it's possible" not any of the ten other things I'm sure my doctor said to put the test in perspective.

To make a long story short, I didn't have cancer. But I spent a frightening few weeks while other tests bore out the final diagnosis.

Knowing more now than I did then, I'd try to postpone panic until after a confirming procedure, like a biopsy or D&C.

DOPPLER SCAN

One of the coolest tests I've ever taken was a Doppler scan. The technical term for the test is *transvaginal Doppler velocimetry*. Basically, it can tell how fast the blood in your uterine arteries and related blood vessels is flowing toward your fibroid. This could be another next step, short of biopsy, that your doctor may suggest to determine the possibility of cancer: A cancerous growth sucks blood toward it at a faster than normal rate, even faster, as a rule, than fibroids.

The test is generally performed by a radiologist. Much of the procedure is similar to a sonogram: The doctor will cover a probe with a latex sheath, lubricate it, and insert it into your vagina. Again, unless you're very dry inside or very nervous, it shouldn't hurt at all. The doctor will manipulate the probe; you'll hear the sound of your own blood rushing through your veins.

This is the cool part. Listening to your blood is like listening to the ocean, only knowing all that power and energy is harnessed inside you. I have to confess, I found the experience surprisingly erotic and extremely relaxing—not the normal trip to the stirrups. It also helped that I got a clean bill of blood flow!

BIOPSY

This is what your doctor may do to check for possible cancer cells, especially if a sonogram shows abnormal growth. *Biopsy* is simply the term used for taking a sample of tissue from your body and analyzing it under a microscope.

If your doctor is concerned about fibroids in the wall or on the outside of your uterus, getting a biopsy requires laparoscopic surgery, which, as we discussed earlier, is a procedure that requires checking into a hospital. If your fibroids are in the uterine lining, there are several different options, including hysteroscopy, endometrial biopsy, or D&C.

An endometrial biopsy is quick and requires only a local anesthetic. Once you're prepped for surgery, your doctor will insert a flexible tube in your uterus. The tube has a plunger on one end; the doctor applies a little pressure to remove a sample of tissue from the lining of your uterus. According to the *Harvard Women's Health Watch*, "endometrial biopsy is 90 percent accurate in identifying abnormal endometrial tissue"; when it's done in addition to a sonogram, accuracy goes up to almost 100 percent.

D & C

Dilation and curettage, or D&C, has been common for years, although newer technology like hysteroscopy is starting to make it less common. Simply, the procedure involves scraping the lining of your uterus. The tissue sample is sent to a pathology lab to check for cancerous cells.

D&C is primarily diagnostic, although it's sometimes used to try to control very heavy bleeding. Like all the tests, it's used to check up on a variety of conditions, including endometriosis and abnormal uterine bleeding. Although it can help your doctor identify fibroids in the uterine cavity or those just under the lining, it can't diagnose fibroids in the wall or those that are attached to the outer wall of your uterus.

Although a D&C doesn't take very long, it generally has to be done in the hospital, using either local or general anesthesia. It's almost always an outpatient procedure: See the section on laparoscopy for a discussion on outpatient surgery and decisions about anesthesia, and combining several procedures at once. In fact, if your doctor detects any problems during D&C, he or she may want to explore further by doing laparoscopy.

MY MOTHER: *Fifteen years ago, when I had my first D&C, I was in the hospital for four days. The next time it was three. This time I was in by 6 a.m. and out by noon, and I felt well enough to have lunch in a restaurant. Times have changed!*

LEONIE: *The D&C was uneventful, and after surgery the gynecologist told me that he'd found and removed several polyps as well, and that everything else looked fine.*

Dilation—opening your cervix—is a kind of mechanical process. Your doctor will use a series of small metal rods, each one slightly larger than the next, to widen the entrance to your uterus. A slower but more "natural" alternative is Laminaria tents, small tubes made from Japanese seaweed. When they're inserted, the seaweed absorbs moisture from your body and expands, eventually widening your cervix.

Curettage comes from the word "curette," which is the name of the small spoon your doctor inserts into your dilated cervix to gently scrape the lining of the uterus.

After having a D&C, you may have cramps, light bleeding, fatigue, or discomfort that can last anywhere from a few days to a couple of weeks. Since your cervix and uterus will be irritated for a while, you should let everything rest for three or four weeks after the procedure: This means avoiding intercourse (or any sex play that involves inserting anything into your vagina) and using sanitary pads instead of tampons.

Complications from D&Cs can occur in up to 3 percent of patients. The risks include infection, injury to the cervix, and puncture of the uterus. For this reason, many doctors prefer the more technologically advanced techniques we've already discussed, such as hysteroscopy.

Since these new technologies are less invasive, take less time, and—because most don't involve a hospital stay—are less expensive, ask your doctor if there are any alternatives to having a D&C. Bear in mind, D&Cs have been the standard for a number of years: It may simply be the technique with which your doctor is most comfortable.

BARBARA: *My D&C pinched, but it didn't hurt. He cleaned me out in his office really quick—it cost $600 for 10 minutes' work—but I was completely and totally wiped out from it. I don't know how I drove myself home. I was supposed to cook dinner that night, but instead I spent two days in bed.*

IRIS: *I had no fear about the D&C, as my mother had one or two herself and we discussed them prior to mine. The D&C was done in my doctor's office with his assistant, a dear woman who has been with him for years and still is. I remember that the D&C was uncomfortable, no severe or sharp pain, just very uncomfortable. I broke out in a sweat, and his assistant placed a cool damp cloth on my forehead and held my hand. I saw the container which contained some of what he removed—it looked like raw liver pieces, just like the clots I had been passing.*

WAVE OF THE FUTURE

A relatively new test, developed at Thomas Jefferson University in Philadelphia, is apparently able to distinguish benign fibroids from malignant tumors.

The test, called *reverse transcriptase polymerase chain reaction (RT-PCR)*, is able to identify a specific gene—the gamma-smooth isoactin gene—that indicates whether a tumor is malignant or benign. If the gene is found, the tumor is benign. Researchers working on the test consider it definitive, leaving no "gray zone" of uncertainty about whether a tumor is cancerous or not.

If the experiments with this new technology are successful, it should be able to give many more women the comfort of knowing for sure that their tumors are benign—and help eliminate the need for both biopsies and so-called "cautionary" surgeries, that is, hysterectomies done when a doctor suspects cancer or wants to prevent future occurrences.

Taking "Bloods"

"You've got anemia," a doctor said to me.

"How do you know?" I asked.

"All women have it," he said. "You have it too. I really think you should consider a myomectomy."

This was not quite scientific enough for me, so I scheduled a series of blood tests—which medical professionals shorten to "bloods"—with another doctor. I actually expected that I did have anemia: After all, most women are supposed to get too little iron in their diets, my periods had been much heavier in the past few months, and I was much more tired than usual. Surprise, surprise: My blood tests were 100 percent normal. I felt better immediately.

What the second doctor had ordered was a complete blood count, or CBC. This took about five minutes while a nurse drew three vials of blood from my arm. A week after the test, I phoned the doctor's office for my results: After they told me everything was normal, I asked them to fax me a copy of the report, which showed my hemoglobin values, hematocrit, and a number of other measurements, compared to the norms. I was able to see for myself that all of my stats fell comfortably within the boundaries of good health. Of course, if there is anything that stands out on a blood report, you and your doctor should have a conversation about it. A first line of defense against anemia, for example, may be iron pills, rather than a surgical procedure.

A word about "normal" results: According to Dr. Wassim H. Shaheen of the University of Kansas, "5 percent of healthy people have abnormal test results." Getting an experienced second opinion is critical before proceeding with any radical treatment based on a lab test.

If you're having heavy bleeding or are scheduled for any kind of surgery, the other blood test that you and your doctor might consider is a coagulation profile. This can rule out von Willebrand's disease, a condition we discussed in Chapter 2.

After the Testing . . . Now What?

Now that you've been poked, prodded, and photographed (at least from the inside), what do you do with the information you get from your tests? For starters, take a look and see which of these descriptions best applies to you:

○ Your fibroids are stable, not causing any pain or abnormal bleeding, and you're not trying to get pregnant.

○ You're experiencing painful symptoms or lots of bleeding.
○ You're worried about possible infertility.
○ Your doctor is concerned that your symptoms might indicate cancer.

Depending on which of these describes you, you have a lot of choices for what you decide to do next.

- **YOUR FIBROIDS ARE STABLE, NOT CAUSING ANY PAIN OR ABNORMAL BLEEDING, AND YOU'RE NOT TRYING TO GET PREGNANT.**

Whew—you can feel good that you're one of the many women who can live and let live as far as your fibroids are concerned. You should schedule regular checkups with your doctor every six months. (Some doctors prefer seeing you every three months, for up to a year, depending on your age and general health, so talk to your doctor to set up a schedule that works for you individually.)

If your fibroids aren't bothering you, you don't have to do anything beyond getting your checkups. But in the meantime, you may want to explore some lifestyle options, such as reducing stress or making some changes in your diet. If you're concerned about the presence of fibroids in your body, you may want to look into some of the potential remedies offered by Chinese medicine, including acupuncture, or learn more about homeopathic and naturopathic remedies. See Chapters 6, 8, and 12 for more about these topics.

- **YOU'RE EXPERIENCING PAINFUL SYMPTOMS OR LOTS OF BLEEDING.**

You're the best judge of how bad your symptoms are. There are several possibilities for relief, but some women find that a "cure" is elusive.

You should certainly make sure your doctor rules out the possibility of cancer, especially if you might be approaching or have gone through menopause.

Surgery is a distinct possibility, ranging from hysterectomy on one extreme to newer techniques that can help leave your uterus intact (though some of these may cause infertility). Your doctor may suggest trying the drugs called gonadotropin-releasing hormone (GnRH) agonists, which have been shown to shrink fibroids and help reduce bleeding. You can learn more about surgical techniques and drug therapy in Chapter 5.

Diet, exercise, and lifestyle can also play a part in improving your overall health. Although these alone probably won't "cure" you, some women feel that changes they've made significantly reduced their symptoms. You can read more about changing your lifestyle in Chapter 8.

Acupuncture, herbs, and naturopathic and holistic remedies have also given many women relief. Although for some of us, using anything outside of Western medicine requires making a leap of faith, you may want to learn more about these areas before making a decision to use—or reject—them. See Chapter 6 for an introduction to these non-Western areas of specialization.

Lastly, if you're hurting, you may want to open channels of communication with the people you love—family, friends, or your partner. Emotional support and a sympathetic ear can help alleviate some of the anxiety that pain and bleeding can cause. For a discussion on reaching out and accepting support, turn to Chapter 11.

• YOU'RE WORRIED ABOUT POSSIBLE INFERTILITY.

Fibroids can prevent conception, lead to miscarriage, and be the cause of enormous frustration and dashed hopes. But many, many women with fibroids conceive and carry to term beautiful, healthy babies.

If ultrasound, HSG, hysteroscopy, or laparoscopy have indicated that fibroids might be the cause of your infertility, you too might be a candidate for surgery. In your case, though, the options are much more specific, since keeping your uterus healthy and functioning is the primary goal. Turn to Chapter 5 to see which surgical techniques might work for you.

If you've achieved the first step of your goal and have become pregnant, congratulations! Now the objective is to have a healthy, successful delivery. See Chapter 10 to learn more about how fibroids can affect the course of your pregnancy, and get tips from some of the women who've been there.

- **YOUR DOCTOR IS CONCERNED THAT YOUR SYMPTOMS MIGHT INDICATE CANCER.**

Remember, less than 1 percent of women with fibroids actually get cancer of the uterus. But if it happens that you receive a diagnosis of cancer, try to remember the following steps:

o If the diagnosis was made on the basis of one test, keep in mind that you need a biopsy to confirm the presence of cancer; ask your doctor to determine the stage of your cancer (I, II, III, or IV).

o Go for a second opinion (or a third, or a fourth if necessary) to make sure you are informed of all possible treatment options.

o Call the Cancer Information Service at 1–800–4-CANCER to find out about cancer centers and programs supported by the National Cancer Institute and to receive their helpful booklets on cancer of the uterus, uterine sarcoma, and cervical cancer.

While discussing uterine cancer in any meaningful depth is outside the scope of this book, the Resources chapter lists several organizations you can contact for more information.

∽ 5 ∾

Best of the West

WHAT OPTIONS DOES conventional medicine offer us? More than it used to. Although invasive surgery, and particularly hysterectomy, continue to be regarded by many physicians as standard treatment for fibroids, some doctors have long used less invasive techniques. Others are experimenting with new treatments designed to cut down time in the operating room, as well as the wear and tear on our bodies, and in general provide a wider range of choices. There are six treatment paths you can explore—we'll cover them in depth in this chapter.

For each path there are a number of issues and questions to consider, including finding the right doctor, understanding how to match up a therapy that your doctor may suggest with your own life goals, and getting a clear picture of the pros and cons of all the medical marvels at our disposal. And don't forget to read Chapter 6, which talks about some alternative ways to handle troubling fibroid symptoms.

Finding Dr. Right

Finding a doctor to treat your fibroids can be a tricky business. Trying to find the "right" doctor when you're wondering if there's something wrong can be a challenge to your schedule, pocketbook, and anxiety

level. Not every doctor performs, or is equally skilled in, every procedure ... and unfortunately, not every doctor will be on your health
plan. So what are some of the things you might want to consider?

For any procedure, be sure to ask your doctor about his or her experience. Find out how long your doctor has been performing the kind
of treatment he or she is recommending, and how many procedures
he or she has actually done.

Ironically, you also have to make sure that doctors who are
specialists—even famous—for certain fibroid treatments will give
you a complete rundown of your options. In this case, it's important
for you to stay objective, weighing what the doctor is good at versus
what you might actually want for yourself.

DR. VICTOR REYNIAK: *I think women should be informed. There
are many books written by physicians that are basically sales gimmicks.
Everybody has their schtick.*

WENDY: *I think the problem with going to these guys who specialize in
one particular thing is that they're targeting one market, which is great
if you fit, but if the shoe doesn't fit, you're out of luck.*

And then there's the delicate question of gender: Can a male doctor
understand a woman's body and emotional concerns? For years, I was
adamantly opposed to going to male gynecologists, owing to some early
unpleasant experiences. Since then, I've come to agree with Dr. Judith
Reichman, author of *I'm Too Young to Get Old*, who tells us, "A good,
compassionate doctor is a good, compassionate doctor, no matter what
their gender." While statistics show that male gynecologists are still more
likely to recommend hysterectomies, younger doctors of both genders
are more likely to talk to you about a range of treatment options.

One important resource for assessing your potential doctor is his
or her other patients. Feel free to ask for a list of women you can talk
to—and then call a few of them for a heart-to-heart. While the women
on a list like this have most likely had positive experiences, you'll
still be able to pick up a lot of clues about the procedure, the doctor's
bedside manner, and recovery time.

Here is a list of questions you might want to ask of—or about—your doctor. Not every question will apply to you, but they may help you organize your thoughts.

Does the doctor have the right accreditation? Your doctor should be Board-certified and have advanced training in specialties such as laparoscopy, hysteroscopy, or interventional radiology, depending on the procedure he or she is offering you.

Does your doctor support your goals? Some doctors will only do hysterectomies; others will do everything they can to preserve your uterus. And some just don't get it: They can't understand why you would want to preserve your uterus—or have it taken out. For me, trusting that my doctor and I share the same goals is as important as his or her technical skill.

Does your doctor talk to you in a way that you like? Doctors are not uniformly known for their communication skills, but most of us want our doctors to have a caring attitude in addition to a high level of expertise. Be wary of doctors who try to scare you or intimidate you, and don't accept a diagnosis—for anemia, infertility, even bleeding—without test results to back it up.

Does the doctor have any malpractice actions against him or her? A call to your state's Department of Health, or a visit to their Web site, should help you determine if your doctor has been involved in legal action. A trip to the New York State Department of Health's Web site confirmed that a well-known doctor lost her license to practice in New York due to a number of serious charges.

Does your doctor work in a managed care organization? If so, he or she may need a lot of pressure from you to manage your case as aggressively as necessary. It should be no surprise to learn that, according to a study in the *New England Journal of Medicine*, doctors working for managed care organizations feel they need to increase the number of patients they see every day; more than half of the doctors polled said

Basic Questions to Discuss with Your Doctor

o How many fibroids do I have?

o What size is each fibroid and how big is my uterus?

o Where are each of my fibroids located?

o How will I know if the fibroids are getting larger? How often should I get a sonogram?

o Could my fibroids be the reason for my symptoms (if any)? What other problems can fibroids cause?

o Could any other condition be causing my symptoms (if any?). If so, how can we isolate the causes and treat each one appropriately?

o What are my treatment options (watchful waiting, hormone treatment, surgery, or other alternative)?

o Which treatment would you recommend for me? Why?

o Are there alternative treatments? Can you explain them? Can you recommend any of them?

o Is there anything I can do on my own to help relieve my symptoms?

they were discouraged from referring patients to specialists, which in some cases led to reduced quality of care.

KACI: *I've requested information from the hospital where I had my last surgery. They're sending me a packet with stats on their gynecologists . . . This is kind of like bobbing for apples blindfolded, but I can't really go by word of mouth because none of the women I know have had problems similar to mine. But I will find someone right for me, even if I have to see fifty different doctors.*

ANGELA: *Unlike many doctors and certainly unlike my first doctor, she was very sensitive to how I felt. She never pushed me to have a hysterectomy, but she said I could wait as long as I wanted. She never told me what I should do. When I asked her what she thought, she always answered what she would do herself, and I found that to be very useful.*

Measure Twice, Cut Once

This old advice for woodworkers applies equally well to making certain you're making the right decision on how best to treat your fibroids.

Unless your symptoms are life threatening, you usually have time to think about your treatment choices, do your homework, and talk to women who've had the procedure(s) you're investigating. But remember, you're unique: No one else has your physical, emotional, or sexual concerns. No one else has your specific lifestyle situation or goals. It's important to take the time to think about who you are, what you want, and the impact of any treatments you're considering.

Tools and Techniques

Have you ever heard about "laser surgery?" I'm betting you have—it's written about all the time. But here's a misconception: "Laser" is not a type of surgery. It's one of many tools a doctor can use to perform various types of surgery.

And Now, a Word from Our Sponsor

Much of what we hear about new "breakthroughs" comes from the folks who produce drugs and devices. Large pharmaceutical companies and equipment manufacturers have three targets for their advertising and publicity. The two biggest targets are doctors and hospitals, since they're the ones who'll be placing the orders and spending the money. But guess who the third target is? You got it: It's us. The idea is, if we get excited about a product, we'll clamor for it, forcing our doctors into making a purchase or giving us a prescription. (It's the same theory that drives Saturday-morning kiddie-oriented advertising.) Given the lack of 100 percent acceptable treatments for fibroids, these companies are trading on a vulnerable and eager audience, but the truth of the claims is rarely as simple as those first press releases can make them seem.

Lasers can be used in myolysis, myomectomy, or hysterectomy; they can be used in abdominal surgery with a large incision or in laparoscopic surgery with a tiny incision. Doctors use many tools besides lasers for fibroid surgery. Harmonic scalpels, for instance, use high-frequency sound waves to cut tissue, much as lasers use high-frequency beams of concentrated light. Other tools use electricity to create heat or cold. And, of course, many doctors still like to use the traditional instruments, or what my doctor calls a "cold knife."

At times, there may be reports in the press or on TV about a new "type of surgery" that really is about a different, possibly better tool for performing fibroid surgery. Sometimes these "breakthroughs" get a lot of positive publicity before they've proven themselves. One rueful doctor writes that "with any new medical device, the initial enthusiasm [is] tempered by actual clinical experience."

WHAT'S THE "LEAST INVASIVE" PROCEDURE?

Most of us, I think, if we absolutely have to have fibroid treatment, want the quickest, easiest kind, one that will give us the fastest recovery, cause the fewest problems, and leave the smallest scar.

But there are two ways to define "least invasive." Doctors often define "least invasive surgery" as the one that is easiest in the operating room, but it might also be defined as the surgery that leaves your body most intact. Keep in mind that an easier day in the operating room is not always the best measure for long-term success.

HILLARY: *My current gynecologist—a woman—wants me to have a hysterectomy if I ever have to do something about my fibroids, because it's easier—for her.*

If you do opt for surgery, your doctor should let you know this: Any procedure may have to be turned into something more "invasive" unless you specifically forbid it ahead of time. For instance, laparoscopy (microsurgery) may need to become a laparotomy (open abdominal surgery) if the surgeon finds more problems than anticipated. If you have specific instructions, put them in writing for your doctor and

Your Body, Your Choices

How do you match up which treatment path, if any, fits your ideas about your body, your lifestyle, and your long-term concerns? Take a look at the following chart to start seeing how your current and future lifestyle choices can help focus your medical options.

There's no right or wrong: The path that's best for you may depend as much on your lifestyle and state of mind as it does on your symptoms.

If You Say	Talk to Your Doctor about
I want to keep my uterus and I'd like to keep open the option of getting pregnant	watch and wait; myomectomy, including hysteroscopy; or (perhaps) embolization
I want to keep my uterus but I don't want to have any (or any more) children	watch and wait; myomectomy; embolization; focused ultrasound, myolysis; or cryomyolysis
I'm open to losing my uterus, if need be, but I want to keep my ovaries so I won't need hormone replacement therapy (HRT)	total hysterectomy, which removes your uterus, including the cervix, but leaves your ovaries and fallopian tubes in place
I'm open to losing my uterus but I'm concerned about vaginal prolapse—and my future sex life!	supracervical hysterectomy, which removes just the top part of your uterus, leaving your cervix, ovaries, and fallopian tubes
I only want to have one (more) surgery in my life; I'm concerned about cancer in my future	total abdominal hysterectomy, which removes your uterus, the cervix, ovaries, and fallopian tubes

the hospital; it could also be helpful to have a family member or good friend available during surgery who can confer with your doctor on your behalf, if necessary.

JENEANE: *Either my husband or my mother stayed with me each night. We believe this as a fundamental family value—you NEVER spend time*

alone in a hospital because someone ALWAYS needs to be looking out
for you and your rights.

The Six Treatment Paths

We do have choices. While all the options have pluses and minuses, Western medicine offers women with fibroids six treatment paths:

- Watch and wait
- Drug therapy (alone or in combination with surgery)
- Uterine Artery Embolization (UAE), which cuts down the blood supply feeding the tumors
- Focused Ultrasound Surgery (FUS), which destroys fibroids with heat—and without surgery
- Surgical procedures that remove or neutralize the fibroids and keep your uterus intact (myomectomy, myolysis, and cryomyolysis)
- Hysterectomy, which removes your uterus, and perhaps other parts of your reproductive system

The First Path: Watch and Wait

The fact is, many of us don't have to do anything about our fibroids. As we've seen, millions of women have fibroids—and at least half don't know they have them. Many women live with their fibroids for years, with and without symptoms.

You probably know that in emergencies like fires, the people with the coolest heads are the ones who are most likely to come out safely. The same idea applies to treating fibroids: It's important to resist any temptation you may have to panic or make decisions in a hurry. Choosing whether to treat your fibroids should be based on any current symptoms and not the idea that your fibroids will cause a problem "someday."

Your doctor can be an important influence. If your doctor is calm, compassionate, and matter-of-fact, it's less likely you'll feel pressure to do anything in a hurry. If your doctor says you don't need to do

Should I Get a Second Opinion?

GETTING A SECOND opinion from another doctor is a good way to make sure that a treatment is the right option for you. Many health insurance plans actually require that you get a second opinion before you have any surgery: Check to see if your insurance company will pay for a second opinion. In order to get the most value out of a second—or third—opinion, be sure to keep your own file of medical records, including any test results, sonogram reports, and prescriptions, to bring with you. It is also helpful to keep a log of your symptoms. Be sure both doctors explain their opinions clearly to you.

anything, don't assume he or she doesn't care about you. Dr. Mitch Levine, a gynecologist in Cambridge, Massachusetts, emphasizes that "Just because you have a fibroid, you don't have to do anything. You can still get pregnant, you can still live your life. And you don't have to have a hysterectomy, it doesn't matter how big the fibroids are, or where they are."

Here are some questions to ask yourself:

○ Are my fibroids interfering with my way of life?
○ Is my period getting heavier than normal—or am I bleeding heavily at other times of the month?
○ Is there pain or pressure on other organs (kidneys, ureters, bladder, or rectum)?
○ Could my fibroids be the reason I haven't been able to conceive or carry to term?
○ Does simply knowing I have fibroids disturb me enough to do something about them?

If the answer to any of these questions is yes, you'll want to read on to find out what your options can be. On the other hand, if you and your fibroids have made a mutual nonaggression pact, you might not need to do anything more than have a checkup and sonogram every three to six months, depending on your doctor's advice. Do take a look at the chapters in this book about diet, stress, and estrogen for tips to help keep yourself healthy. You may never need treatment for your fibroids at all.

BARBARA: *I don't think you should do anything until your body tells you to.*

KIM: *I went to my general practitioner and she says unless you absolutely, for medical reasons, have to have them out, don't. Because, she says surgery can be worse than whatever minor symptoms you're having from the fibroids. And I kind of agree with her. If you don't need surgery, don't have it.*

HILLARY: *My doctor sat me down and said three things cause you to have surgery: excessive bleeding, pain, and urinary dysfunction. And she said, if you don't have these things, you do not need surgery, no matter how big the fibroid is. If you don't have symptoms, you don't have to do anything. A fibroid is part of your body—it's made up of the same things that are already inside you. It's not a foreign object like a piece of glass that you swallow. She made me feel so much more comfortable. Because what a male doctor had said is that I had this toxic thing in my body and I had to get it out.*

LEONIE: *I first found out I had fibroids in my early to mid-thirties. My gynecologist—a woman—told me I could look forward to a hysterectomy by about 38 or 39! I was devastated. I was single and had never had a strong desire to have children, but even so, to be told that my options were just about over was traumatic.*

    After a few days, I pulled myself together and started doing some research. A friend at work told me about her doctor. She was marvelous. She sent me for an ultrasound, which my first doctor had never mentioned, and told me that there was no need for me to have a hysterectomy, that we could just wait and see if the fibroids were actually growing. And that's what I did, for the next 17 years!

The Second Path: Drug Therapy

Before trying surgery to relieve fibroid symptoms, there are a few types of drugs your doctor might recommend, ranging from items you probably already have in your bathroom medicine cabinet to professional-strength, do-not-try-this-at home monthly injections. Here's a look at what's out there.

NSAIDs

NSAID, pronounced "em-sed" or "en-sayd," stands for nonsteroidal anti-inflammatory drug. It's something you already have right at home, maybe even in your purse: yes, the ever-popular aspirin, as well as over-the-counter drugs known (generically) as ibuprofen, acetaminophen, and naproxen. NSAIDs can help control cramps sometimes and even bleeding—by slowing down the production of prostaglandins; acetaminophen may actually lower estrogen levels. Doctors recommend that you don't take any of these drugs—as harmless as they may

Stamp Out Cramps

IF YOU'D LIKE to try remedies that don't come from the drugstore, you might like to try one or more of these ideas to put your cramps to rest:

- Place a heating pad or hot water bottle on your abdomen or lower back
- Take frequent hot baths, at least 10 minutes each
- Have a cup of hot tea—try ginger, cinnamon, or peppermint
- Use pads instead of tampons
- Do moderate exercise—even a slow walk around the block can help
- Relax—stress can heighten pain
- Have an orgasm—alone or with your partner

seem—for more than 10 days, or more frequently than recommended on the label. Since aspirin thins the blood, it is not recommended at all if you are bleeding or prone to heavy periods. Of course, if you have very painful cramps or heavy bleeding, don't tough it out—talk to your doctor.

KACI: *I was able to control the bleeding of my last period somewhat with ibuprofen. The key is to start taking it a couple of days before it comes.*

FELICE: *One doctor told me to take double doses of Advil for my painful periods, which seemed to help for a while, but eventually the pain got worse. I was then given a prescription for naproxen, which is now sold over the counter as Aleve.*

THE PILL

Occasionally doctors will prescribe the birth control pill to control fibroids, especially if you have troubling symptoms. The low estrogen levels in low-dose pills may stop fibroids from growing; some doctors think the Pill can also be helpful in treating excessive bleeding or cramps. A study of over 800 women showed that the risk of fibroids actually decreased the longer women were on the Pill.

On the other hand, the Pill may make existing fibroids grow more—but regular monitoring by your doctor can help you detect significant changes. The clinical information for Ortho, a popular brand of birth control, states that women with fibroids "should be carefully observed. Sudden enlargement, pain or tenderness requires discontinuation of the use of oral contraceptives."

In the Harvard Nurses' Health Study, the only relationship researchers found between the Pill and fibroids was "a significantly elevated risk among women who first used oral contraceptives at ages 13–16 years." This relates to some findings about the effect of estrogen on younger women and girls: We'll discuss that more in Chapter 7, "A Question of Estrogen."

Obviously, taking the Pill has a number of benefits, not least of which is birth control. So if you're on the Pill, or are considering it, you may want to talk to your doctor about the low-estrogen options and monitoring your fibroids on a regular basis.

WENDY: *I went on the Pill, and in fact it helped with my bleeding. After six months, I had a sonogram and the fibroids had grown a lot. So my gynecologist said, I think you'd better go off the Pill.*

BONNIE: *I began to gush blood toward the tail end of my period. I went for an evaluation by midwives and was given a large dose of birth control pills to see if that would control the bleeding. Although the flooding stopped, I was now bleeding every day. My next period was extremely heavy with some flooding. My hemoglobin was very low and I was tired a lot.*

I had an ultrasound, which revealed a large fibroid, measuring 6.7 centimeters. I stopped taking the estrogen, as fibroids are thought to be caused by too much estrogen.

GnRH Agonists

About 35 years ago, doctors discovered a class of drugs called *gonadotropin-releasing hormone (GnRH) agonists.* One of the most commonly used brand-name GnRH agonists is Lupron (leuprolide acetate); it's approved by the U.S. Food and Drug Administration (FDA) primarily for treating endometriosis and prostate cancer. Using GnRH agonist therapy for fibroids is one of the most controversial choices women have, next to hysterectomy.

What are GnRH agonists, exactly? GnRH appears in your body naturally; it's a messenger hormone that tells your body to make estrogen. GnRH agonists are bigger and stronger than your own GnRH but have a similar chemical structure, so they can block out your natural hormones and keep your body from producing estrogen. The technical term for this, and I'm not kidding, is *chemical castration.*

Since fibroids need estrogen, among other things, to grow, cutting off the supply often makes fibroids shrink. But cutting off your estrogen has a lot of other consequences: When the estrogen fuel tank in your body reads "empty," your body begins to react to the changed conditions.

What Happens to My Body Without Estrogen?

Unfortunately, science has not yet devised a way to cut off estrogen only to your fibroids. If you take a GnRH agonist, your body is deprived of estrogen for as long as you take the drug. The effect this can have on you is very individual: Your reaction might be mild or very severe. The most common side effects of low estrogen include:

o hot flashes
o lower sex drive
o vaginal dryness
o loss of bone mineral
o weight gain and bloating
o depression
o possible increase in cholesterol levels
o possible increased risk of coronary artery disease
o possible severe pain, resulting from the rapid shrinking of fibroids

One of the more serious side effects is the loss of bone mineral, since this can lead to osteoporosis. Some doctors worry that the decrease might not be reversible; in some studies, bone mineral loss continued for as long as a year after the treatment had stopped. As a result, the FDA generally limits any use of GnRH agonists to six months. Before putting me on GnRH agonists, my doctor suggested I could help counter any loss of bone density by taking 1500 milligrams of calcium every day and doing weight-bearing exercise.

While it's not a solution to bone loss, you can get a bone scan (a *bone mass indicator*, or BMI) to measure your bone density before and after GnRH agonist treatment. Doing the test before your treatment will give you a baseline measurement, and doing it afterward will help you see if in fact you suffered any bone loss. Unfortunately, I only had a bone scan after my treatment, and while the reading was low, I have no way of knowing if I was affected by the GnRH agonist treatment or if, as is possible given my family history, my bone density was already low.

Your doctor can refer you to a radiologist for a bone scan. It's quick and simple: The whole procedure takes about five minutes, and you don't even have to change out of your street clothes.

So Why Use GnRH Agonists?

There are times when GnRH agonists may be the lesser of two evils. Some doctors like to use them instead of surgery if fibroids seem to be preventing pregnancy. The advantage is that even a temporary shrinkage of your fibroids may give you a "window" to try conceiving again, without having to recover from surgery and without the potentially weakened uterus that surgery can leave behind.

If you're perimenopausal and experiencing painful or uncomfortable symptoms relating to fibroids, a course of GnRH agonists may give you relief before the natural effects of menopause take over to reduce the estrogen in your body.

More controversial is the use of GnRH agonists before surgery. The idea is that your fibroids will be smaller by the time you have the operation and, theoretically, easier to remove. Since GnRH agonist treatment can also cut down bleeding, some doctors prescribe them

Drugs Your Doctor May Mention

GNRH AGONISTS COME in a variety of brand names, including Lupron and Lupron Depot, Synarel (nafarelin acetate), and Zoladex (goserelin acetate). They're not identical—Lupron is the strongest—and they get taken differently, either as an injection, a nasal spray, or monthly implants. Ask your doctor not just about recommended doses, but about minimum doses, which can sometimes be equally effective in reducing the size of fibroids.

Danocrine (danazol) is not a GnRH agonist but an androgen, a drug that's chemically similar to the male sex hormone testosterone: It may also be prescribed to stop heavy menstrual bleeding caused by a fibroid. The side effects aren't pleasant: They include an increase in male characteristics, such as facial hair and a deeper voice.

to make surgery shorter and easier, with less blood loss and less possibility of transfusion. Shrinking your fibroids before surgery may also mean that you can choose a procedure that's easier on your body, with a smaller scar and a shorter stay in the hospital.

However, not every doctor recommends using GnRH agonists before surgery. In some cases, this is because of the number of women who find the side effects extremely difficult to handle. Also, while fibroids in their "natural" state are in a sort of shell, making them relatively easy to identify and scoop out of your uterus, GnRH agonists make fibroids soft and harder to remove. Using GnRH agonists can also be one of the reasons fibroids "grow back" after myomectomy: In fact, they may make some fibroids so small that they're missed during surgery, only to grow again later.

DR. VICTOR REYNIAK: *I hate Lupron with a passion because my patients hate it. Patients are absolutely miserable on it. Mood shifts, depressions, hot flashes, vaginal dryness, insomnia. As a surgeon I don't like Lupron too much, because when you go in, the fibroids are mushy, they degenerate. It's like scooping chocolate pudding out of the uterus. Ugly.*

But I will use it in three instances. Number one, if the patient is extremely anemic and I have to arrest the bleeding and rebuild her hemoglobin. Number two, I sometimes see fibroids that are humongous, actually beyond the scope of standard myomectomy: I want to decrease them if they're more than 24 weeks in size. The third instance is when I have a woman who really wants to preserve her beauty and she says look, I don't want to have a big scar. So I will use Lupron to decrease the size of her fibroid and facilitate the cosmetic removal.

KACI: *I had one injection of Lupron, which was a disaster. I had it during my period and I bled heavily for 21 straight days. The doctor finally had to give me Provera to stop the bleeding. I had become anemic, my blood count was 8 point something . . . I later went on Synarel, which is nasally administered, for six months to get the fibroids down to a manageable size to make a myo more possible. It worked, but I had occasional breakthrough bleeding.*

This Is Your Brain on Drugs

I can tell you, speaking for myself, that taking Synarel, a brand name for the GnRH agonist nafarelin acetate, was not a fun experience. I experienced huge fluctuations in body temperature, feeling ice cold one minute, burning hot the next; the hot flashes were exactly like the feeling I once had when I ate a whole red chili pepper by mistake. During these flashes, I sweated profusely: I needed to shower as often as three times a day and got into the habit of carrying a bottle of deodorant around town with me.

My sleep was disrupted, my appetite was unpredictable, and most disturbing of all, I became depressed in a way I'd never experienced in my life. If I saw a large puddle, I would consider the possibilities of drowning. I called my doctor and told her I wanted to throw myself under the wheels of the Madison Avenue bus.

"Hang in there," she said. "Call me every day, or every hour if you need to, but remember, this is only chemical." She emphasized those words again: *only chemical.*

Eventually I realized that's just what human beings are: a mass of chemicals. And, in fact, one of the areas that GnRH agonists affect is the *hypothalamus,* a tiny little portion of your brain that—surprise!—regulates functions like hunger, sleep, libido, and body temperature.

So if you take a GnRH agonist, don't be surprised if you're "not yourself" while you're on it. You're not.

MARY: *In June my doctor suggested I try a new treatment that would put me into menopause and possibly shrink the fibroids. This was a nasal spray called Synarel. I was on this, complete with hot flashes and wild bad moods, for about six months. I was very bitchy. I would blast off to anyone, usually my husband. Fortunately my ob-gyn talked with my husband a lot about the effects of the hormone changes.*

I was scheduled for a myomectomy to remove the fibroids in November. The Synarel apparently didn't shrink the fibroids but did seem to minimize the blood loss during surgery.

CAROLYN: *I felt rotten—hot flashes, major headaches, face flushing, emotional, zero sex drive, extremely dry vaginal tissues. It was a miserable three months. It was a good thing that they were shots and not pills, 'cause there were days that there was no way I could have forced myself to take a pill to make me so miserable.*

DR. GARY BERGER: *I employ GnRH agonists, but not routinely. I usually discuss the option with patients, the benefits, the disadvantages. I'll usually recommend it for a patient who has a pretty bad bleeding problem, particularly if they're anemic. You have to correct the anemia before scheduling surgery. Or if they're having a lot of pain, I'll recommend getting them on that preoperatively. I would say for most patients, they elect, if given the choice, not to take the GnRH agonist because of the side effects.*

But Hey, It's Temporary

The good news about GnRH agonist therapy is that it's temporary. The bad news . . . is that it's temporary.

As soon as you stop taking the drugs, you should feel more like your old self with every passing day. I can tell you that the first weekend that I knew my estrogen was kicking in again, I couldn't stop giggling.

On the other hand, as soon as your estrogen is flowing, your fibroids will most likely start growing again. Most studies report that fibroids and uterus regain their pretreatment size within three to six months after ending GnRH agonist therapy. One study did show a permanent effect: In the Netherlands, where doctors followed a group of patients after GnRH agonist treatment, 40 percent of the women remained symptom free up to five years later.

A big, controversial, unanswered question is this: Are the side effects of GnRH agonists also temporary? Many doctors seem to think so. For instance, consider this rather glowing review: "This biochemical castration induced by GnRH agonist administration is . . . safe, effective, complete, and reversible." But is it?

Dr. Linda Abend, founder of the National Lupron Victims' Network (NLVN) believes that the side effects of GnRH agonists have been minimized by the medical establishment. Participants in the NLVN claim a variety of frightening, permanent side effects, from memory loss to debilitating, lasting bone pain.

I asked several doctors about the points raised by the NLVN. Most felt that the women involved were probably blaming other illnesses on their GnRH agonist treatment. However, it's worth remembering the lessons of thalidomide and DES, two "safe" drugs that, years later, proved to be anything but. Don't take any drugs without finding out the likelihood of side effects—and weighing the pros and cons yourself.

DR. BRIAN WALSH: *Do I use Lupron? For some patients, I do. I view it as a necessary evil. I only use it when it's important to get the estrogen level really low, and when I really need to shrink a fibroid, for instance, when I want to remove it using a hysteroscope, I think you'll get more shrinkage with Lupron versus Synarel.*

The Progesterone Parallel

ALONG WITH ESTROGEN, progesterone may be a big player in helping fibroids grow. Studies of *antiprogesterone* drugs are showing real promise in treating fibroids.

At the University of California, San Diego, doctors experimented with an antiprogesterone called mifepristone (also known as RU-486, the so-called "abortion pill"). After 12 weeks, the drug reduced fibroids by almost 50 percent—without depriving the women treated of their natural estrogen. Mifepristone was significantly more effective than Lupron in reducing both uterine artery blood flow and uterine volume.

In February 2003, doctors at the University of Rochester Medical Center in Rochester, NY, published results of a pilot study showing that low doses of mifepristone shrank fibroids by more than 50 percent, on average. The results of both six-month and one-year studies, according to the studies' co-leader, Dr. Steven Eisinger, were "dramatic." A larger study was launched in 2004; results were not available as of this writing.

The FDA actually approved mifepristone under the trade name Mifeprex on September 28, 2000, for use in chemical abortion, limiting distribution to doctors (the drug is not available in pharmacies), and requiring three office visits. The side effects of the drug when taken for chemical abortion are numerous and unpleasant. In contrast, the women in the Rochester test, according to Dr. Eisinger, "felt much better."

Asoprisnil, another antiprogesterone drug, is also showing promise. Preliminary tests among women with fibroids showed that asoprisnil reduced the "intensity and duration "of uterine bleeding, and shrank larger fibroids as much as 50 percent—without any signs of estrogen deprivation. As of this writing, asoprisnil is in late-stage clinical trials.

Researchers are also investigating drugs that may suppress other fibroid growth factors: these include pirfenidone and interferon alpha.

The Third Path:
Uterine Artery Embolization

In the early 1990s, Dr. Jacques-Henri Ravina noticed something strange happening in his Paris, France, ob-gyn practice: Women scheduled for fibroid surgery started calling to cancel their operations.

All of these women had undergone a procedure called uterine artery embolization (UAE). This technique has been used since the late 1970s to stop hemorrhaging after childbirth and pelvic surgeries; in a crucial twist, Ravina began suggesting UAE to patients before their fibroid operations to help minimize bleeding during surgery. When the women reported that embolization alone had relieved their symptoms, Ravina realized he might be onto a whole new way to manage fibroid-related bleeding.

Embolization works by injecting material into specific arteries to reduce the blood flow to target organs; diseased tissue is killed while healthy tissue is left alone. The procedure is done by a specialist called an *interventional radiologist (IR)*. As of year-end 2004, about 50,000 women worldwide have been treated with UAE; in the United States, about 13,000–14,000 women get UAE for their fibroids every year. (UAE is also called UFE, for Uterine Fibroid Embolization, by some specialists; it is the same procedure.)

The technique works on fibroids because, like little vampires, fibroids need blood to grow. When the blood supply is cut off, the fibroids shrink, and in some cases, die. If you remember our discussion of degeneration in Chapter 2, you'll remember that sometimes this happens naturally. UAE, in effect, makes all your fibroids degenerate at the same time.

Dr. James Spies, Chairman and Chief of Service at Georgetown University Medical Center's Department of Radiology, says that some fibroids may be better candidates for UAE than others. He says that "submucosal and intramural fibroids appear to have greater shrinkage and greater symptom control than subserosal fibroids," possibly because subserosal fibroids, the kind growing on the outer wall of the uterus, have figured out how to draw their blood supply from other places in the pelvis that UAE wouldn't affect.

There is no age limit for UAE and no limit as to how large your fibroids can be, although fibroids over 20 weeks in size will tend to shrink less than smaller ones. One very large fibroid will also tend to shrink less than several smaller fibroids.

Caveat emptor: UAEs take surgical procedures, and income, away from gynecologists—a problem pervasive enough to have made the front page of the *Wall Street Journal*. If your gynecologist doesn't recommend UAE, ask why—and then do your own homework. Some insurance companies, though not all, have denied coverage, saying that UAE is experimental; your IR may be able to help you deal with this.

GAIL: *I went to a doctor who told me she'd put me on Lupron for three months and then do a myomectomy. I discovered inadvertently walking home from a dinner party that a friend of a friend had had this new procedure, and that's how I was introduced to UAE—I thought that was really the wrong way to be introduced to it.*

I didn't want to put Lupron in my body. It puts you in an artificial

*menopause and changes your biochemistry, and I wasn't willing to do
that. But I would have done it if I hadn't heard about UAE, because I
had no other options offered to me.*

CAN YOU GET PREGNANT AFTER HAVING UAE?

UAE hasn't been around long enough in the United States for long-term
studies on pregnancy; as a result, the American College of Obstetricians and Gynecologists (ACOG), recommends myomectomy for
women with fibroids who both need some kind of treatment and hope
to maintain their fertility.

Still, there is evidence that some women, at least, are able to get
pregnant and deliver healthy babies after having UAE (you cannot
have UAE while you're pregnant). In a follow-up of 555 women between
the ages of 27 and 42 who'd had UAE, Canadian researchers found
that 21 of the women (4 percent) had gotten pregnant—three of them
twice; 18 delivered their babies, mostly at term. Three of the women
had complications involving the placenta, requiring close monitoring in the last weeks of the pregnancy. A French study of 454 patients
reported 30 pregnancies, with three of those requiring surgery.

ACOG reports a total of 50 pregnancies after UAE, but again, with
a certain number of complications: Almost 60 percent of the women
delivered by cesarean (some electively); 28 percent delivered early; 13
percent had extremely heavy bleeding after delivery.

DR. JAMES SPIES: *A good third of the women we see are interested in
the possibility of fertility, and what we tell them is if there s a medical
alternative, they ought to have that first. There are no guarantees about
pregnancy at this stage.*

WHO IS THE "BEST" CANDIDATE FOR UAE?

Condoleezza Rice had UAE in November 2004, but you don't have to
be the Secretary of State to be eligible. While UAE is technically available to any woman with fibroids, doctors identify the ideal candidate
as someone who:

○ is past childbearing, or is willing to take a risk of infertility;

○ has significant symptoms;

○ is being told that she requires a myomectomy or a hysterectomy; or

○ wants to maintain her fertility but has been told by a qualified obstetrician/gynecologist that the size, position, and/or number of fibroids mean that a myomectomy will probably not be successful.

There are also a few reasons why you might *not* be a candidate for UAE:

○ If you have any kind of active infection, especially a pelvic infection

○ If you're pregnant

○ If you have a life-threatening allergy to contrast dyes

○ If you have endometriosis or adenomyosis

○ If you have pedunculated fibroids

○ If you have cancer

○ If your fibroids aren't giving you any trouble

Before you have UAE, you should have a complete gynecologic exam, as well as a sonogram and/or an MRI to make sure you're a good candidate for the procedure. You should have a normal Pap smear within the last twelve months. If you're bleeding profusely, especially between periods, you should have a complete blood count (CBC) and an endometrial biopsy to rule out endometrial cancer. If any other tests are suggested, ask about the risks, as well as what the doctor plans to learn.

In addition to your general medical history, you should discuss any medications you're taking with your IR. There are reports that synthetic progesterone, found in some birth control pills and other medications, can contribute to UAE failure.

Tell your doctor and the radiologist if you smoke, if your blood doesn't clot properly (see the section on von Willebrand's disease in Chapter 2), if you're allergic to contrast materials, taking GnRH agonists, or have any kidney problems. As with any invasive procedure, do have a frank discussion with your IR about his or her experience . . . and don't be afraid to go to another doctor if you're not comfortable.

WHAT'S IT LIKE TO HAVE UAE?

While you are under conscious sedation, a catheter—a slender tube, no wider than a piece of spaghetti—is inserted into the large artery near your groin. The puncture mark is about where the elastic on the bottom of your underwear hits your leg. You're injected with a special dye, which can make you feel warm. The dye shows up on an X-ray machine, which the doctor uses to guide his movements.

When the catheter is in your uterine artery, the doctor releases tiny particles called *PVA (polyvinyl alcohol)*, no larger than grains of salt. The flow of your blood directs the particles to their destination, where they lodge and slow down the flow of blood to your uterus. This reduced blood flow causes your fibroids to degenerate. Then, since most of us have two uterine arteries, the catheter is guided to the other artery and additional PVA is released. Typically, the procedure lasts about 60 to 90 minutes.

Dr. Robert Worthington-Kirsch of Philadelphia, Pennsylvania, a leading practitioner of UAE, says, "There's an emphasis on minimal invasion of the body. Most IR procedures are done under local anesthesia or a local with conscious sedation. There is less distortion to the body, so there's less recovery time and less time in the hospital."

PVA vs. Gelfoam

THERE ARE THREE materials doctors can use for blocking your uterine arteries: PVA, gelatin microspheres, and gelfoam. PVA is permanent: You're injected with about a teaspoon's worth of tiny plastic particles that lodge in your arteries to reduce blood flow. Gelatin, on the other hand, is temporary: It's absorbed by the body after 10 or 20 days. Gelatin microspheres are specifically approved by the FDA for UAE.

LEONIE: *I went through the whole UAE without any sedation or anesthesia other than the local injection to numb the incision site. I had no pain at any point during the procedure.*

BONNIE: *The ultrasound they did before the UAE showed my fibroids were 17 centimeters! I was awake, watched the procedure on a screen, and was fascinated. The only downside was the after-pain. I was given morphine and I felt like I was in heavy labor for three days after the procedure. Then I was fine. My bleeding vanished immediately, and since then, my periods are lighter than they ever were in my life. I feel great, have no residual symptoms, and lead a normal life. I can't say enough about this procedure!*

ROBIN: *My ob-gyn was pleased to confirm my feeling that the fibroid and my uterus have shrunk substantially after the UAE. I no longer feel a tennis-ball-sized lump. The fibroid is present but much smaller, and I don't experience any discomfort or bladder pressure. I have had two periods since the procedure, though in the first six weeks afterward, I didn't have a period. No complaints about that!*

How Successful Is UAE at Relieving Fibroid Symptoms?

Various doctors report up to 90 percent improvement in heavy bleeding, and up to 95 percent improvement of pain and pressure symptoms; over 90 percent of women surveyed say they're satisfied with their results.

In the United States, doctors and researchers have been tracking about 2,500 women a year—roughly 20 percent of all the women in this country having UAE—through The FIBROID Registry (short for the Uterine Artery Embolization (UAE) Fibroid Registry for Outcomes Data). Launched in August 2000, The FIBROID Registry was created "to assess the procedure's durability, impact on fertility and quality-of-life, and to obtain data which will allow researchers to compare UAE to other fibroid therapies."

The study's first results, based on the experiences of more than 3,000 women, showed that in the first 30 days after UAE:

- More than 99 percent left the hospital without any serious incidents.
- Less than 5 percent experienced severe problems—mostly involving pain—after going home.
- About 1 percent needed additional surgery; a tiny fraction (0.1 percent) of these were hysterectomies.
- There were no deaths.

In Ontario, Canada, doctors following the results of more than 500 women found that, three months after the procedure, over 90 percent of the women reported a big improvement in their quality of life:

- On average, the fibroids shrank to one-third to one-half their former size.
- About 80 percent of the women reported less bleeding, fewer cramps, and/or less need to urinate frequently.

The Fine Print

EVERY PROCEDURE—EVEN NONPROCEDURES like watch and wait—has its own set of risks and benefits. As you read about the possible complications of UAE and the other treatments discussed throughout the book, please remember that the intention is neither to scare you or influence your decision in any particular direction, but to provide the information you need to make your own informed decision.

COMPLICATIONS AND SIDE EFFECTS

After the procedure, you can expect to feel fairly bad cramps. As a result, most women stay in the hospital overnight for pain management, although some are able to go home the same day. You can help manage this decision depending on your own comfort level. For this or any other procedure, make sure you have a way to contact your doctor for at least twenty-four hours after you go home. In the Ontario study, the majority of the women (almost 80 percent) stayed in the hospital for one night, with most requiring some pain relief; the rest stayed two nights or longer.

The average recovery time for UAE is about two weeks. It's not unusual to feel nauseous or exhausted for a day or more; you may also continue to have some pain. Your doctor should give you prescriptions to help mitigate these problems before you go home. Longer-term, you may have a pink or brown discharge (the remnants of degenerating fibroids) for a few weeks or even months after the procedure.

About half of the women who have UAE develop something called *postembolization syndrome,* which generally feels like a fever but can resemble menopause, complete with hot flashes, mood swings, nausea, and cramping. It typically begins within 5 days of having UAE, and lasts for one or two days. If your symptoms are serious, don't hesitate to go back to the hospital to make sure you don't have any other complications.

You may also not get your period back right away: It can take as long as five months for your body to return to normal. However, various studies report that anywhere from 2 to 15 percent of women go into menopause following UAE; for women over 45, that number climbs as high as 43 percent. Dr. Scott Goodwin, the first IR in the United States to perform UAE for fibroids, suggests that this may be the result of some of the PVA particles blocking blood flow to the ovaries, causing *ovarian failure.* Another possibility is that some women's ovaries may depend on blood flow from the uterine artery.

The possibility of ovarian failure is one reason IRs are very cautious about recommending UAE to women who are still interested in having children. Even if you're no longer interested in having children, women in their 40s and older need to consider the possibility of going into menopause early.

It doesn't happen often, but some serious side effects of UAE can show up as long as a year after the procedure. Call your doctor immediately if you develop a high fever, pelvic cramps, heavy vaginal bleeding, pain anywhere below the waist (including your abdomen, legs, buttocks, and vagina), or incontinence.

AFTER YOU HAVE UAE, CAN YOUR FIBROIDS COME BACK?

In 2002, Dr. Michael Broder published the results of a five-year study of women who'd had UAE. One of his findings was that 25 percent needed "further invasive treatment" for their fibroids.

As Broder writes, this is "biologically plausible" since only the main uterine arteries are blocked during UAE; smaller blood vessels continue to supply the uterus, allowing it to survive. The fibroids themselves are not removed. As a result, fibroids that shrank but didn't completely "die" can start to grow again.

Studies indicate that anywhere from 1.5 to 10 percent of women undergoing UAE will have a hysterectomy at some later time.

The Fourth Path:
Focused Ultrasound Surgery (FUS)

In October 2004, the FDA approved Focused Ultrasound Surgery (FUS) as the latest weapon in the war on fibroids. Other names you may hear for this process include "MR-guided FUS" (MRgFUS), or "ExAblate 2000," which is the brand name of the machine used.

The process combines ultra-sensitive MRI technology with high-intensity ultrasound—up to ten thousand times more powerful than the ultrasound in your doctor's office. There are no knives, needles, or any other sharp objects involved. You are not cut open; there is no scar. So how does it work? After the MRI locates your fibroids, the ultrasound waves are literally beamed directly onto your fibroids. (Does this remind anybody besides me of Dr. McCoy's sickbay on *Star Trek*?)

All that power creates temperatures of up to about 194° Fahrenheit, enough to destroy fibroid tissue. What's even more startling is that the MRI component of the procedure can target fibroids so well, there's little or no damage to the surrounding areas. Your body helps too: The extra collagen in fibroids seems to absorb heat more than normal tissue—while all the arteries and veins around the uterus help cool down healthy areas.

If you decide to have FUS, you'd begin by getting a diagnostic MRI, just as you would for UAE, to confirm the size and location of your fibroids. The day of the procedure, you'd go to the hospital, where you'd be sedated, largely to help you keep still while you're being treated. The ExAblate 2000 resembles an MRI; the ultrasound equipment is beneath it. You'd lie in the machine for three to four hours, depending on how many fibroids you have and how big they are, while the doctor aims the ultrasound beams at your fibroids. After resting in the hospital, you'd go home the same day.

So far, doctors have seen serious side effects in 2 percent of the women having FUS, versus 13 percent having hysterectomy. In a published statement, Dr. Elizabeth Stewart, Clinical Director of the Center for Uterine Fibroids at Brigham and Women's Hospital in Boston, and one of the lead researchers of the technique, said, "We found that overall, women tolerated this treatment extremely well. All women who underwent the procedure were treated as outpatients and only one required continued observation. Additionally, no patients were seen for complaints between the treatment and follow-up period, and, most encouraging, 75 percent rated pain as mild."

Early results show that between 70 and 80 percent of women treated with FUS report that their symptoms—and quality of life—had improved, although the fibroids didn't necessarily shrink very much. (This is similar to overall results for UAE.) On the downside, 20 percent of the women tested needed surgery of some kind within a year. Researchers are continuing a three-year study to determine how well FUS works in a broader group of women.

Now the caveat: Because it's new, we don't yet know the long-term effects of FUS. In addition, FUS is currently (a) limited to just a few locations in the United States, (b) expensive, and (c) probably not covered by your insurance company. Given the potential, these obstacles should be overcome with time.

FUS is not recommended—yet—for women whose fibroids are bigger than 10 centimeters, or whose uterus is larger than 20 centimeters (about 18 weeks), or when fibroids are close to the bowel or bladder.

You can't have FUS if you've already had UAE, have certain abdominal scars in the area, or want to get pregnant.

The Fifth Path:
Surgery That Saves Your Uterus

Here's where we start getting into the more familiar ground of surgical techniques. All of these procedures keep your uterus intact while either killing off your fibroids or removing them. Although the procedures we'll cover here are not done by the majority of gynecologists, you can find surgeons throughout the country who are well-respected experts in these operations.

MYOLYSIS AND CRYOMYOLYSIS

Myolysis and cryomyolysis are two related techniques that, like UAE, kill off your fibroids while leaving them inside the uterus. Both involve a two-stage process, first shrinking fibroids with GnRH agonists, then applying either extreme heat or cold to kill the fibroids. They both require a small amount of surgery, but they can provide relief for your fibroid-related symptoms while allowing you to keep your uterus.

Myolysis, also known as myoma coagulation, uses heat to kill the fibroid and its blood supply. It's been around for just under 10 years, though it's practiced on a limited basis. According to Dr. David Olive, Chief of Reproductive Endocrinology and Infertility at the University of Wisconsin-Madison Medical School, it was developed to offer women a less invasive alternative to myomectomy and to provide doctors with a surgical technique that is relatively easy and fast to perform.

First, your doctor will put you on GnRH agonists for three months. Next, using laparoscopic surgery, your doctor will pierce your fibroids with a laser or electrified needle, destroying the blood vessels that feed the fibroids. The fibroid itself is not removed, nor is the uterus opened.

The downside: The needle affects only a very tiny area (5 millimeters) at a time. If your fibroids are large, it will take quite a few insertions to kill them, potentially causing several adhesions (internal scars). This is why doctors recommend taking GnRH agonists for three months before myolysis to shrink the fibroid before the procedure. After myolysis, fibroids generally stay at their smaller, post-GnRH-agonist-therapy size.

Cryomyolysis is still fairly experimental. In this technique, after two or three months of GnRH agonist treatment, the doctor uses a needle to freeze your fibroids rather than burn them. One insertion of a freezing needle can affect 4 to 6 centimeters at a time, a far greater area than can be reached at once using myolysis. Two small studies show that cryomyolysis may have long-term promise. Doctors at Yale University School of Medicine found that cryomyolysis seemed to make fibroids stay at their new, smaller size after GnRH agonist therapy ended; an Italian study of 63 women who had cryomyolysis showed that 80 percent remained symptom free a year after the procedure.

One reason myolysis may not have caught on is that it doesn't actually remove the fibroids. It also makes the uterus too weak to carry a developing baby, and therefore for all intents and purposes, leaves you unable to have a child. However, you're still able to conceive after either myolysis or cryomyolysis—you'll need to use birth control after either procedure.

What about Endometrial Ablation?

The early headlines gave a lot of women the impression that endometrial ablation could help make hysterectomy a thing of the past. Lost in the hoopla was the next-to-last paragraph of the FDA's first press release, which said that ablation was not effective in treating fibroids. So, not surprisingly, the whole topic has created some confusion. Here's what endometrial ablation is—and what it isn't.

What *ablation* can do is help stop dysfunctional uterine bleeding (bleeding without an obvious physical cause), one of the top reasons, after fibroids, that women get hysterectomies. Ablation works by burning or even freezing the inside of the uterine lining (the endometrium), where new blood vessels grow every month before menopause. Like myolysis, ablation has the curious effect of leaving you technically able to conceive but probably unable to have a baby, so it's not appropriate if you still want children—though you'll still have to use birth control to avoid a tubal pregnancy.

But here's the thing: If fibroids are the reason you're bleeding, ablation alone won't help too much. Why not? While ablation destroys the lining of the uterus, it doesn't affect any fibroids you may have. In fact, according to Dr. Joseph Feste, "It is of utmost importance that there are no other pathologies, such as polyps or sub-mucous fibroids" that could be causing your bleeding. Dr. Brian Walsh says simply: "I wouldn't do an ablation for fibroids." However, a recent study indicates that ablation done with a myomectomy can reduce bleeding more than myomectomy alone, depending on where your fibroids are located. (We'll discuss myomectomy in more detail later on.)

Another area of confusion is Uterine Balloon Therapy. This is a brand name for a device that doctors can use to perform an ablation. It's a nifty little number that uses a water balloon—really—attached to the end of a catheter. The balloon is blown up inside your uterus and heated, cooking your lining. Not exactly Betty Crocker territory. This is one of several devices used for ablation, and they simply aren't effective for women with fibroids. Dr. Walsh noted the publicity about the technique a little sadly: "I've gotten phone calls from hundreds of women with fibroids who want the balloon treatment, and things don't quite line up that way."

LEONIE: *I went to the Internet and started looking up balloon ablation and other uterine ablation procedures. I was a little disturbed when I realized that ablation would permanently destroy the uterine lining—which could make early detection of uterine or cervical cancer more difficult. After reading about the procedure, I realized it would do nothing at all for the fibroids—they could continue to grow, especially if they were within the uterine wall or on the outside of the uterus. I wasn't thrilled about how much damage the procedure would do for such little return—my interest lay in getting rid of the fibroids, not just in stopping the heavy bleeding.*

Myomectomy

Myomectomy presents one of the great mysteries of fibroid care. While it preserves the uterus and has been around for a generation or longer, relatively few doctors have taken the time to learn it or offer it to their patients.

You can think of *myomectomy* as a "fibroidectomy": It removes your fibroids and leaves the rest of your uterus intact, or includes additional surgery to repair the walls of the uterus. Although the surgery is less destructive than hysterectomy, at most only one myomectomy is performed in the United States for every five hysterectomies done for fibroids. Estimates of the number of myomectomies performed each year range from about 20,000 to 44,000, versus more than 200,000 fibroid-related hysterectomies.

Part of the reason for this is the traditional medical point of view, which says that you only need your uterus if you still plan on having children. Therefore, the logic goes, only women still interested in having a child qualify for a myomectomy.

But what if you simply want to keep your uterus because you like it? Because you were born with it? Because you get great uterine orgasms? Take heart: Dr. Francis L. Hutchins, author of *The Fibroid Book*, writes that myomectomy can be a reasonable treatment for any woman, "regardless of future childbearing options." In other words, you can have a myomectomy at any age and regardless of your family status.

When would you want to consider a myomectomy? Dr. Stanley West told me there are four reasons that he believes a woman should get a myomectomy: "She wants to get pregnant, and can't sustain it; she's bleeding heavily, massively; she's in a lot of pain; or the fibroid's so big that it's interfering with other organ functions."

WENDY: *My doctor said, you know, I think you should consider having a hysterectomy. I asked her, how about myomectomy, and she said, only on TV. Only on TV. She really pooh-poohed that. And she also said, for myomectomies, people are usually younger: At your age—42—people would recommend a hysterectomy. It was a very short conversation, that was kind of it. So I decided I'd better get some other opinions.*

HILLARY: *My gynecologist took one look at my fibroid and said, take it out, take it out now, and while you're at it, you might as well have a hysterectomy because you don't want kids anyway. I was 40. It took me six months to recover from the trauma of that; it became my life. No matter who I was talking to on the phone, they would say, how are you, and I would say, I think I have to have surgery.*

Why Won't a Doctor Recommend a Myomectomy?

Doctors often want to minimize the number of invasive surgeries you may have in your lifetime; the logic is that once an organ is removed, it can't cause problems later in life. No uterus, for instance, means no chance of uterine cancer. In my opinion, this is a little like saying we should all get frontal lobotomies now, before we all go crazy.

What you need to focus on is the end result: Do you want to keep your uterus and other reproductive organs, or are you comfortable with the idea of being without them?

This is not a judgmental question: While many women have strong feelings associated with their reproductive organs, others firmly place their femininity in their heads and in their hearts. There is no right or wrong answer, as long as it's *your* answer and not just your doctor's.

Here are some of the arguments offered against myomectomies, and some answers to help you make an informed decision.

○ *Hysterectomy eliminates a woman's lifetime risk of uterine cancer (2 to 3 percent) and cervical cancer (1 percent). Myomectomy does not.*

True, but hysterectomy removes your uterus forever. Not only does a myomectomy help you maintain your fertility, if that is a goal, it does not result in any of the risks or discomforts that can arise from removing an entire organ. Sensible check-ups, ultrasounds, and Pap smears can help detect uterine and cervical cancers early.

○ *Hysterectomy has a 100 percent cure rate for heavy bleeding and pelvic pressure due to fibroids. Myomectomy does not.*

True. In a review of over 40 studies, the Agency for Healthcare Research and Quality (AHRQ), found that myomectomy stopped or reduced heavy bleeding from 80 to 100 percent of the time, and improved pain anywhere from 50 to 90 percent of the time. They conclude that there is "a 90 percent likelihood" that women having a myomectomy will feel substantially better for at least two years.

○ *Your fibroids can grow back and require repeated surgery.*

True, but once again, the latest information suggests that this happens about 10 percent of the time—meaning that there is a 90 percent chance that you will remain fibroid free. Even when fibroids grow back, there is generally a five- to ten-year window of relief from symptoms. And new fibroids may not give you any problems at all.

○ *Myomectomy is harder to perform than hysterectomy.*

True. But a doctor skilled in myomectomy will not have a problem doing the surgery. Dr. Francis L. Hutchins writes, "I find abdominal myomectomy in general to be a procedure quite comparable with other major pelvic procedures, such as hysterectomy."

○ *More women need transfusions during myomectomies than during hysterectomies.*

Maybe. While many sources report that myomectomies include a somewhat greater risk of bleeding and need for transfusion, this may have more to do with the skill of the doctor performing the surgery. A five-year study of women who had either myomectomy or hysterectomy revealed that there was less blood loss in myomectomy than hysterectomy, and there was no difference in transfusion rates between the two groups. In a 2002 article in *Obstetrics & Gynecology*, Dr. Michael Broder reports that "myomectomy and hysterectomy have similar blood loss . . . and complication rates."

○ *Myomectomies can scar your uterus, which would lower your chances of getting pregnant.*

True. This is why many doctors will suggest you try to get pregnant before seeing if you need surgery. However, if you can't conceive or maintain a pregnancy, and fibroids are the reason, a myomectomy will often improve your chances.

DR. STANLEY WEST: *I went through medical school, never saw a myo-*
mectomy. I went through internship and residence training in gynecology,
never saw a myomectomy. It is more difficult, takes longer, and it takes
more skill So most doctors shy away from it, they don't know how to do
it, they don't know how to control the bleeding, and it's a frightening
experience to them. So they're frequently doing hysterectomies, taking
things out.

Myomectomy operations are actually similar to hysterectomies in
terms of the basic techniques. Like hysterectomies, they may be done
one of three ways:

o Vaginally, on an outpatient basis
o Using laparoscopy, also on an outpatient basis, but with a longer
   recovery period
o Through abdominal surgery

The kind of myomectomy that could be best for you depends on
the number, size, and location of your fibroids, your surgeon's experience and skill, and your preferences. Bear in mind that even with the
best intentions, a myomectomy may turn into a hysterectomy in the
operating room because of medical need.

Vaginal Myomectomy

Most often called *hysteroscopic resection,* or simply *resection,* vaginal
myomectomy can be done only if you have relatively small fibroids inside
the cavity of your uterus. It's most effective for pedunculated fibroids, the
kind that grow on a stalk. These are also the fibroids most likely to cause
symptoms of heavy menstrual bleeding or to prevent conception.
    The way it works is this: Using the hysteroscope, as we saw in Chap-
ter 4 ("Testing . . . Testing . . ."), your doctor will insert a miniature
camera via your vagina; your uterus will be filled with saline solution
to expand the walls. Then, using another tool, your doctor will shave
your fibroids away bit by bit, until they're at the same level as the wall
of the uterus.

Resection won't work if you have fibroids anywhere but the uterine cavity or the uterine lining. Why not? Only the part of your fibroid that is inside the cavity of your uterus can be shaved away; anything inside the wall or on the outer wall will still be there, siphoning blood and interrupting the normal working of your uterus.

Your doctor can use various tools for hysteroscopic resection, including laser, a cutting electrode, or a vaporizer. Most of the time the procedure is done without making any cuts in either your skin or inside your uterus, but some doctors prefer inserting a laparoscope in a tiny incision near your bellybutton; this improves their vision inside the uterus and can help prevent the risk of perforation. Some doctors will recommend that you take a GnRH agonist for a month or two to shrink the fibroids or to reduce the possibility of bleeding.

NANCY: *A month before the procedure, my doctor persuaded me to take one shot of Lupron to keep bleeding during the surgery to a minimum. He was able to operate through my vagina, so I had no incisions or scars.*

The surgery takes about 30 minutes and can be done on an outpatient basis. Although a diagnostic hysteroscopy can be done in your doctor's office, you should only have surgical hysteroscopy in a medical facility that has the latest fluid management equipment.

What's so important about fluid management? Fluid overload is one of the most frequent—and most dangerous—risks of hysteroscopic resection. The problem is that your body can absorb the saline solution that's pumped into your uterus during surgery; extreme amounts of this extra saline can be fatal.

Traditionally, a nurse has had to stand by and measure the amount of fluid coming out to make sure it's close to the amount that went in. Much safer are new machines that include automated fluid management systems, which not only measure fluid going in and coming out but set off an alarm if your fluid intake is too high. Dr. David Olive advises that you "should insist upon it" when you have your surgery.

Hysteroscopic resection is a deceptive procedure: Despite being quick and requiring no repair work (often not even stitches), it requires a lot of experience. Only about 10 percent of ob-gyn physicians actually perform resections; another 20 percent have been trained but don't perform the procedure because even they lack the necessary expertise. Your doctor should have advanced certification from the Accreditation Council for Gynecologic Endoscopy to perform hysteroscopy.

Laparoscopic Myomectomy

Laparoscopy is microsurgery; it can be used for a wide variety of surgeries, such as myolysis, cryomyolysis, myomectomy, and hysterectomy, including supracervical hysterectomy. Also called endoscopy, videolaseroscopy, and videolaparoscopy, laparoscopic surgery can be easier on your body than traditional open abdominal surgery *(laparotomy)*. Most women getting laparoscopy lose less blood, spend less time in the hospital, have a smaller scar, and recover more quickly.

In Chapter 4, we talked about a "test" laparoscopy, where a mini-camera is lowered into your abdomen. The difference in a surgical procedure is that in addition to the camera, the doctor makes one or more small cuts lower down on your belly, near the bikini line; each of these cuts might be no larger than the size of a short fingernail.

An amazing amount of activity can take place through these tiny incisions; instruments are inserted that can cut, grasp, remove, repair. The assortment of tools can include retractors, lasers—even sterile plastic baggies.

The operation is performed using hand-eye coordination. A video monitor shows a view of your insides; the surgeon and operating room staff move the instruments while they watch what's happening on the monitor. In fact, they're able to see much of what makes your body tick: liver, appendix, the top layer of intestines, bladder and kidney tubes (ureters), as well as your uterus, ovaries, fallopian tubes, rectum, and the bottom part of the cervix (the opening to the uterus), called the "cul-de-sac."

The doctor will remove the fibroids in very small pieces, generally with the help of a mechanical device called a *morcellator* (which chops your fibroids up into "morsels"). If your fibroids are too large to remove laparoscopically, your doctor might elect to perform what's called a laparoscopically assisted procedure. In this case, the cut near your bikini line might have to be enlarged to several inches.

LAURA: *My doctor did a laparoscopy and looked around—he didn't like what he saw, so he made a bigger incision. He wanted to save my uterus, but he might have been afraid he would nick my uterus so I couldn't conceive, and that would be the worst thing. I woke up and he said good results, we got everything . . . I had the surgery a few days before my thirtieth birthday and I thought, I can't believe it, I'm going to go into my thirties healthy. I was so happy, it felt like a new era.*

If you still want to have children, you need to proceed carefully when it comes to laparoscopic myomectomy. Some doctors feel that the sutures—the stitches or staples used to repair your uterus—may be more secure in an abdominal myomectomy, allowing your uterus to safely hold several pounds of developing baby. One of your jobs, if you decide you want laparoscopic surgery, is to find a very skilled, very experienced surgeon with specialized training. These surgeons can perform the complicated suturing technique to repair your uterus firmly enough to carry children, should that be your goal. A 2005 article in *Fertility and Sterility* says that "meticulous repair . . . is essential for women considering pregnancy after laparoscopic myomectomy to minimize the risk of uterine rupture."

However, if your fibroids are in the wall of your uterus (intramural), even the most experienced surgeon may not be able to repair your uterus so that it's strong enough to carry a child. In a 1996 article, Dr. Camran Nezhat, one of the most respected and experienced laparoscopic surgeons, wrote, "Women of childbearing age who require a myomectomy for an intramural fibroid should undergo either an abdominal myomectomy or a modified laparoscopic procedure to ensure proper closure."

DR. GARY BERGER: *For intramural and subserosal fibroids of any significant size, I do an open incision. The benefit of the open surgery is the control, absence of blood loss, precise suturing.*

Many laparoscopies are done on an outpatient basis, though some doctors will keep you for a 23-hour "day," which lets medical staff observe you overnight. Like hysteroscopy, some physicians offer "office laparoscopy," where the doctor actually operates on you in the office while you're under light sedation. This is not common practice; use common sense and caution before agreeing to have surgery anywhere but a hospital or fully equipped outpatient surgical center.

Your doctor may also recommend that you take a GnRH agonist starting three to four months before the procedure, especially if your uterus is very large or you've become anemic. Why? A smaller uterus helps make the surgery easier and safer; the reduced blood flow to the uterus leads to less blood loss during surgery and less need for a possible transfusion. One potential problem, however, is that some fibroids may become too small for the surgeon to see and remove—meaning that they could begin to grow again after surgery. If your doctor recommends taking GnRH agonists, consider the benefits and risks of these drugs—and consider the possibility of surgery that uses a larger incision, without drug treatment.

Complications among healthy women undergoing laparoscopy are rare, but there are some potential problems you should know about. Among the most common are urinary tract injuries. They're no small matter: Recovery time for ureter and bladder injuries after surgery can be as long as three to four months, and then you might need additional surgery. Other potential complications from laparoscopy include damage to the intestines, infection, nicked blood vessels, damage to the bladder or kidney tubes, and damage or scarring of the gynecologic organs, which may create fertility problems in the future.

Abdominal Myomectomy

Many doctors prefer performing abdominal surgery for both hysterectomies and myomectomies, as opposed to the newer methods of laparoscopy and hysteroscopy. How come? Because

○ the technique is traditional and comfortable.
○ abdominal surgery allows the surgeon the greatest field of vision, an

important consideration for removing fibroids and other growths that may not have appeared on an ultrasound.

o it's easier for the surgeon to make sure all blood vessels have been tied off and the surgery is "clean" before he or she is finished.

In her book *Having Your Baby: A Guide for African-American Women,* Dr. Hilda Hutcherson advises that if surgery becomes necessary,

Myomectomy or UAE?

MANY DOCTORS SAY that for most women, the choice of surgery is a matter of personal preference. But there are some early reports comparing UAE with abdominal myomectomy (although not hysteroscopic or laparoscopic myos). Here's what they found.

UAE is gentler on the body: after UAE, women tend to use pain medication for about 3 to 4 days (on average), versus about 7 days after a myomectomy. Women having UAE tend to have fewer complications, and return to work or other activities 2 to 4 weeks sooner than women having abdominal myomectomies (recovery time for less invasive myomectomies is shorter).

The two procedures may actually work best on different symptoms. A study at Stanford University determined that both UAE and abdominal myomectomy were "equally effective in controlling pain." However, UAE was better at reducing heavy bleeding, and abdominal myomectomies were more effective in reducing the size of the uterus, and relieving feelings of pressure.

In the long run, some of the women who have either procedure will need follow-up surgery of some kind. For women who didn't need further surgery, one comparison concludes, "satisfaction and relief of symptoms was similar."

If you're planning to get pregnant, myomectomy is still the standard recommendation. Early indications are that pregnancy is possible after UAE, but just how possible is not yet known. We'll talk more about your options before pregnancy in Chapter 10.

"abdominal myomectomy is probably better than the new laparoscopic surgery. Studies have shown that laparoscopic surgery may not be as effective in removing all the fibroids, may cause more adhesions to form, and may carry more risks to future pregnancies."

A SEVEN-STEP CHECKLIST FOR PAIN MANAGEMENT

Surgery is a powerful disruption to your body, and abdominal myo-mectomy has the most potential for pain, along with a longer recovery time, than the other types of surgery we've discussed so far. But some doctors use techniques during surgery that help minimize or eliminate the causes of pain. Advanced pain management techniques can mean fewer days in the hospital, quicker recovery, and less disruption to your body and your life. While every doctor has his or her own "standard operating plan," Dr. Brian Walsh shared his strategy for minimizing disruption to the body during fibroid surgery:

Small incisions: The smaller the incision, the shorter the recovery.

Horizontal incisions: Horizontal incisions go in the same general direction as your muscles. Vertical incisions are under more tension, so they're going to hurt more.

Nerve block on the skin: Even with general anesthesia, a nerve block on the skin before the incision numbs the nerve fibers, keeping the pain pathway from ever getting started.

Intravenous pain reliever during surgery: A high-potency Motrin-type drug, an antiprostaglandin called *ketorolac,* is delivered through the IV, preventing the prostaglandins that can generate pain from ever getting off the ground.

No retractors: Retractors bruise muscle. Instead, the doctor may use his or her hands, or just raise the uterus up outside the incision.

No abdominal packs: These irritate the intestine, which can slow down the return of bowel function.

Tourniquet or Pitressin to minimize bleeding: A tourniquet on the uterus shuts off the blood supply to minimize blood loss: It's like shutting off the water main to your house before you work on the sink. If there's any additional bleeding with the tourniquet in place, an additional option is to inject a drug called Pitressin.

After surgery, ask your doctor about *transcutaneous nerve stimulation,* or TENS. This is a little battery-operated device that you can use to send mild electric pulses to the area around your surgical incision; the stimulation helps release endorphins and block the sensation of pain.

WHAT ABOUT SCARRING?

If you're considering an abdominal procedure, there are two types of scarring that you should discuss with your doctor.

The external scar, which is the one most of us worry about, is minimal in laparoscopic surgery and nonexistent in vaginal surgery. In abdominal surgery, a six- to eight-inch incision is made in the lower abdomen: either the horizontal "bikini" cut, popularized by none other than Jacqueline Kennedy, or a vertical cut, running from your navel to just above the pubic bone. The advantage of the bikini cut, of course, is that it's harder to see after it heals; it also may heal more quickly. The vertical cut may be necessary if your uterus is very large (over 24 weeks).

Internal scars, also called *adhesions,* are one of the leading causes of postsurgical complications from both abdominal and laparoscopic surgeries. After any kind of surgical trauma—whether it's an incision, cauterizing, or suturing—internal tissues can get joined together, causing scar tissue to form. Adhesions can also result from tissues being touched or simply exposed to the air.

Adhesions generally form within the first few days following surgery; while they normally don't cause problems, they're associated with up to 20 percent of female infertility cases and are found in up to half of patients experiencing chronic pelvic pain. A type of plastic film is available that may help keep adhesions from forming; ask your doctor about the possibility of using this or a similar product if you need surgery.

RECOVERING FROM SURGERY

There are some interesting new ideas about recovery that may change the picture for abdominal surgeries. True, most of the time, traditional abdominal myomectomy requires a three- to five-day hospital stay and a recovery period of about six weeks. But some patients and doctors report dramatically different experiences.

According to Dr. Brian Walsh, before you can go home from the hospital after surgery, you need to be walking, eating, passing gas, urinating, and have a normal body temperature. "Typically," Dr. Walsh says, "that happens in two days, 48 hours."

BARBARA: *You have gas, and until you pass it they won't let you leave the hospital. I remember walking around at 4 a.m. around the nurses' station because I was very uncomfortable.*

But there are some things you can do that could hasten your recovery time. If you believe you're going to recover quickly, for instance, you may heal faster after surgery. Dr. Walsh confirms that women who

Don't Worry, Be Happy

YOUR ATTITUDE TOWARD having surgery—and about your whole life—can make a big difference in how well and how fast you recover. Doctors think there's a link between your emotions and your immune system, which in turn affects how your body heals.

You don't have to be overjoyed that you're providing an exciting career opportunity for your friendly local surgeon. But if your life makes you happy—if you enjoy your friends, family, work, hobbies—surgery will be a bump in the road. If you've done your homework about your fibroids and know you're making a good decision for yourself, so much the better..

bring relaxation tapes with them into the operating room seem to sail through surgery.

"You see them the next morning, they've won," he says. "They've taken their shower, they've put on their clothes, they're smiling, and they're having their breakfast. And I don't know if the patient who uses a relaxation program is the type of person who would do well anyway, or if the program itself enabled them to do better, but I know it's a good sign. When I hear that somebody wants to use a program like that, I know she's going to want to go home the night after her surgery, not that very night, but the night after. It's great—those patients always do well, always."

Dr. Victor Reyniak actually has his patients prepare for surgery. "Have you ever tried running a marathon without training?" Dr. Reyniak asks. "If you prepare yourself and train for surgery, and your body is ready for that insult, which it is, the body recovers fantastically, much better."

Dr. Reyniak recommends a regimen of aerobic exercise for 45 minutes three times a week, iron and folic acid, and a good mental attitude. "Come in with a good attitude," he says, "I'll get you out of the hospital in a jiffy." Dr. Reyniak's myomectomy patients are in the hospital for an average of three days and, as a rule, are ready to go back to work in two weeks.

JULIE: *I did a lot of exercise every day before the surgery to help get myself strong and I think that helped. I really bounced back, so I think it's really important to be in good shape.*

If you have a hysteroscopic or laparoscopic myomectomy, you can probably go home the same day. In my own experience, I was in the hospital for four days following an abdominal myomectomy, but back home within hours after having a hysteroscopic procedure. My recovery times were different too, reflecting the different levels of invasiveness of the two procedures: I needed about a month to fully recover after abdominal surgery, but only a day or two to feel completely myself after hysteroscopy. Remember, though, that not every type of surgery is appropriate for every type of fibroid.

KATHY: *I was 48 when I had an outpatient myomectomy, and I did go home the same day; the surgery started at 9:30 that morning and I was home in my bed by 3:30 that afternoon. I took a shower the next morning, and about four days later I was actually driving back to work.*

The Sixth Path: Hysterectomy

Like any surgery, hysterectomy can relieve troubling or disabling symptoms; like any surgery, it can also create new difficulties. The problem with hysterectomy is not that it exists or is an option for women who have fibroids. The problem is that many, many doctors will recommend a hysterectomy and not tell you about your other options.

Rx: Have One Hysterectomy and Call Me in the Morning

From a medical point of view, a hysterectomy is a neat, one-time way of curing you—not only of your fibroids but also of any possible future problems.

When is a hysterectomy medically necessary? Doctors agree that in cases of cancer, it's mandatory: This accounts for about 10 percent of the hysterectomies done in the United States every year. Hysterectomies are vital for women whose lives are at stake because of emergency bleeding or complications during pregnancy or delivery, and there are women who've researched their options and feel that hysterectomy is the choice they prefer. But that leaves a large number of surgeries that may be unnecessary.

Would a doctor really recommend an unnecessary operation? A panel of physicians studying almost 500 hysterectomies found that a whopping 76 percent did not meet the standards established by the American College of Obstetricians and Gynecologists (ACOG). Lapses included not providing women with information about all of their other options, and not conducting tests to determine the root cause of pain or bleeding.

A number of troubling statistics underline the question of how

Do We Have Too Many Hysterectomies?

IN THE UNITED STATES ...

○ Almost 1,700 hysterectomies are performed every day: that's about one every minute, 24/7.

○ Hysterectomy is the second most common operation for women of reproductive age, after C-sections.

○ Fifty-two percent of all hysterectomies are performed on women younger than 44.

○ One in nine woman between the ages of 35 and 45 has a hysterectomy.

○ As of 2005, about 22 million women have had a hysterectomy— roughly 20 percent of the adult female population.

○ Hysterectomy rates for women age 45 to 54 are increasing more than for any other age group; by the time we reach 60, one out of every three of us is likely to have had a hysterectomy.

○ American women have more hysterectomies than women in any other Western country.

○ Estimated hospital costs for all hysterectomies are *at least* $5 billion a year. At that rate, the hysterectomy "business" could earn a place on *Fortune* magazine's list of America's 500 biggest companies, right up there with Southwest Airlines, Mattel, and Unisys.

many hysterectomies happen for nonmedical reasons. According to the CDC, between 1994 and 1999, over 1.3 million women in the United States had hysterectomies for fibroids—which equals 38 percent of all hysterectomies in the United States during that time. In fact, the number of hysterectomies for fibroids is rising, and fast: between 1993 and 1999, there were 11 percent more hysterectomies for fibroids, while hysterectomies for cancer went down by more than 20 percent.

Race seems to play a part. A Maryland study of more than 53,000 women confirmed that black women had more fibroids and more symptoms than white women. Even taking this into account, they were 25 percent more likely to have a hysterectomy than their white counterparts. They were also more likely to have surgical complications and a longer hospitalization. Most frightening, the black women in the study were more than three times as likely to die in the hospital. The CDC's latest data show that black women between the ages of 40 and 44 are 60 percent more likely to have a hysterectomy than white women in the same age group.

Do social factors make a difference? In Denmark, doctors followed almost two thousand women over eight years. Which women in the study were most at risk for having a hysterectomy? Would you guess, women with alarming medical conditions? Well, guess again. Women with less education, fewer friends, and a less supportive family were more than twice as likely to have a hysterectomy than women with more education and a wider social network.

Being informed can also make a difference. A public education campaign in one part of Switzerland resulted in a sharp drop in hysterectomies, compared with the rest of the country. Hysterectomy rates among American women drop by as much as 30 percent when they get better information about their options.

Maybe you'll share my conclusion when I read these studies: Until doctors are better educated across the board about the problems of hysterectomies, all of us need to stay well informed about our treatment

Four Reasons You Don't Need to Have a Hysterectomy (No Matter What Anyone Tells You)

1. You're not going to have any (more) children.
2. You're over 35.
3. You "might" get cancer (though you have no family history and are otherwise healthy).
4. Your mother (or grandmother, or sister, or best friend) had one.

options, surround ourselves with supportive family members and friends, be willing to stand up for what we want and need, and find doctors who listen and share our goals.

ANGELA: *There's no bad surgery; there are just decisions you don't make yourself.*

Perhaps you're considering a hysterectomy to take care of your fibroids, but you still aren't sure it's the right answer for you. Assuming that your doctor hasn't given you a diagnosis of cancer, how many of these other conditions apply to you?

○ You have chronic severe pain and/or heavy menstrual bleeding due to one or more large fibroids.
○ You do not want to have any (more) children.
○ You've explored the surgical options, including myomectomy, with your doctor or even better, a specialist who does myomectomies routinely.
○ You've explored UAE or FUS with an experienced interventional radiologist.
○ You're comfortable with the idea of your sexual and feminine identity with or without your uterus.
○ You've discussed the possible side effects of hysterectomy with your doctor and your partner or a close friend.
○ You've gotten a second, third, even fourth opinion.

Unless you can say "Yes" to all, or even most of these points, you may want to consider some of your other options.

MARY: *I love and adore my children and urge all women to seek another opinion. If I had listened to the first ob-gyn, I would have had a hysterectomy and never have had my two children.*

KACI: *Fifteen years ago, doctors were pushing hysterectomy even more than now, and I had to take charge and see several different ones before I could find one who finally did a myomectomy on me at age 34.*

LINDA: *When my doctor said I needed an immediate hysterectomy, I said, no, we're not going that route. I was asymptomatic, so I thought, there's no rush.*

HYSTERECTOMY FOR TROUBLING SYMPTOMS

But don't you need a hysterectomy if you've got symptoms? Not necessarily. As we saw in the earlier sections, even severe bleeding can often be controlled with methods less drastic than hysterectomy. Regular checkups and monitoring are important, as is being well-informed about your options. For instance, a sudden onset of bleeding, as frightening as it is, is not an automatic ticket to surgery.

Similarly, if you experience the sudden, awful pain of degenerating fibroids, you or your doctor may also be tempted to cut everything out. The pain of a degenerating fibroid, as bad as it can be, is temporary. The same is true of the awful feeling of bleeding completely through your clothes. Even if you decide you want a hysterectomy afterward, you can think about it calmly after you feel better (in a day or two), making sure you make a decision you're happy with in the long run.

If you have a partner or friend who might take you to the hospital in an emergency, let them know your wishes about having a hysterectomy. Add this to the emergency information you carry in your wallet, along with your blood type, allergies (especially to medications), and whom to call in case of emergency.

MAYBE, BABY

Most hysterectomies are performed
on reproductive-aged women.
—CENTERS FOR DISEASE CONTROL

Another common reason for hysterectomy is how you answer your doctor when he or she asks, "Do you want any (more) children?" Traditionally, if you said no, many doctors would—and still will—suggest that you might as well get a hysterectomy. But as we discussed in the section about myomectomy, if a new baby is not in your future plans, does that mean your uterus should come out? Many women don't think so.

LINDA: *I'm not planning to breastfeed again, but I'm not planning to cut off my nipples!*

Despite this, you might be surprised to learn, as I was, that most hysterectomies are performed on women who are still in their reproductive years. Between 1994 and 1999, 52 percent of all hysterectomies were done on women younger than 45.

DR. MITCH LEVINE: *A young woman came to me from New York—I'm in Boston—and I was her thirteenth opinion. She had seen twelve other doctors who'd all told her she needed to have a hysterectomy. Her fibroids were quite large, about six months, but she was quite young and hadn't had children yet, so I said, why don't we try just taking out the fibroids and leaving the uterus in? And this beaming smile came over her face. We did the surgery and she had a very short recovery—the endorphins or whatever, she was probably so euphoric, she felt so great—and she subsequently did have children.*

OH, OH, OVARIES

I was taught in medical school that at menopause
the ovaries stop functioning, shrivel and dry
up. (In fact, I was taught that that was what
happened to postmenopausal women as well.)
—DR. SUSAN LOVE, WRITING IN
THE NEW YORK TIMES

According to the CDC, more than half of all women having hysterectomies lose both ovaries. So this is important: Removing your ovaries is not indicated when you have surgery for fibroids.

In July 2005, a UCLA study published in *Obstetrics & Gynecology* revealed that keeping your ovaries reduces the risk of heart disease, stroke, osteoporosis, and Alzheimer's disease. This is because, as

Dr. Susan Love writes, the ovaries produce hormones "before, during, and after menopause." These include *androgens,* which keep your libido going and play a part in keeping both your heart and bones strong after menopause.

When you lose both ovaries (not just one), you go into what's called *surgical menopause,* which is more sudden and often more severe than natural menopause. (Unfortunately, there's evidence that your ovaries need your uterus to function: About 30 percent of women have a loss of ovarian function—menopause—after hysterectomy.)

Dr. Christiane Northrup, in her book *Women's Bodies, Women's Wisdom,* tells us that part of the ovary becomes active only as we approach "midlife." Northrup cites numerous studies showing that the ovaries keep producing hormones even after menopause; she adds the perspective of Taoist cultures, in which, in her words, "the ovaries are thought to contain large amounts of the life-force that constantly produces sexual energy." Even if Taoism is not part of your cultural belief system, the respect shown for a woman's body is markedly different from that of our throwaway society.

For women willing and able to take hormone replacement therapy (HRT) after their ovaries are removed, it's important to know that these drugs don't bring your hormone levels back to where they were before surgery. Dr. Stanley West, in *The Hysterectomy Hoax,* is emphatic: "There is no substitute for natural hormones . . . You need your ovaries."

But as we know, every decision is individual.

ANGELA: *I'm awfully happy not to have ovaries anymore. Whenever I hear about ovarian cancer I say to myself, oh, thank God I don't have to worry about that one. And I feel just great.*

NANCY: *My sister needed to have a hysterectomy, and the hospital where she was scheduled for surgery insisted that it was their standard protocol to remove both ovaries. She didn't want to lose any healthy body parts, and after she raised a huge fuss, her doctor was able to find another hospital that would let her have the hysterectomy but keep her ovaries.*

Risks of Hysterectomy . . .

Obviously, hysterectomy means you'll never be able to get pregnant or have a period again. (For some women, these aren't risks, but relief.)

Keep in mind that removing your uterus can create a whole new set of problems. Talk with your doctor about the possible physical complications of hysterectomy, including the risks of bladder or bowel injury, intestinal scarring, infection, blood clots, and pelvic pain. According to Dr. Nelson Stringer, "30 percent of all injuries to ureters and bladders in the United States occur during hysterectomy." Other side effects of hysterectomy are similar to the side effects for similar types of surgery.

Of course, pointing out a risk doesn't mean it's definitely going to happen: If you're satisfied that the benefits of having a hysterectomy outweigh the risks, and it feels like the right decision, then you're likely to be happy with the outcome.

. . . and the Emotional Fallout

For some women, losing their uterus represents a loss of femininity. There's also a danger of a change in how you respond to sex. Hormone changes make some women lose their interest, some experience pain or dryness, and others miss the sensations in their uterus during orgasm—or even lose their ability to have an orgasm. We'll discuss this topic in more detail in Chapter 9, "Sex and the Single Fibroid."

Does hysterectomy cause depression? Changes in hormones, self-image, and postsurgical problems, if any, can certainly contribute to depression after hysterectomy. To complicate things a little more, up to 25 percent of all women get seriously depressed at some point in their lives, regardless of whether they've had a hysterectomy. Studies suggest you might be more likely to experience depression after a hysterectomy if:

○ you weren't offered any other options for treatment;
○ you have a history of depression;

o the surgery wasn't needed to treat a life-threatening condition;
o you're unhappy in your marriage or relationship; or
o you still want to have children.

If any of these are true of you, you might want to consider how a hysterectomy will affect your feelings. If you absolutely need or desire a hysterectomy and you think depression might be an issue, you can help prepare yourself. For instance, counseling can be a helpful outlet to talk about fears of losing your femininity, not being able to enjoy sex, or even how the operation may affect your spouse or partner.

ROBIN: *The sonogram showed a fibroid at about 16 weeks in the wall, intramural, in the back, in the lower part. My doctor said, "You need a hysterectomy, you're not going to have any more children, and we can't do a myo because of the danger of bleeding." But he's a cutter, that's his business. I absolutely refused . . . I didn't want a hysterectomy because I have a history of depression and I didn't feel up to the emotional and physical stress of a hysterectomy.*

Natalie Angier, in her fiercely written book *Woman: An Intimate Geography*, reminds us, if we needed to hear it, that "the womb does not define a woman, philosophically, biologically or even etymologically. A woman does not need to be born with a uterus to be a woman, nor does she have to keep her uterus to remain a woman."

Some women experience separation from their uterus as a blessing, a necessary clearing away of an organ that's outlived its usefulness or that simply causes far too many problems. For other women, losing the uterus is a passage requiring recognition, respect, and a period of mourning. There's no right and no wrong: only a question of understanding how you feel and accepting what you need.

DR. BRIAN WALSH: *I have a number of patients who say their hysterectomy is the best thing they ever did. I think this highlights the fact that psychologically they were well prepared before their surgery. For the women who felt like they really didn't have an option except hysterectomy and made a decision against their better instincts, it's almost predestined they're going to have a horrible recovery. They'll have lots of minor complications and they'll regret their decision.*

I've had some patients for whom I've done a myomectomy—they knew their fibroids could grow back, and five years later, when the fibroids have recurred, they'll come in and say, "I wanted a myomectomy then, but I want a hysterectomy now." They'll do great after surgery. But had they had a hysterectomy the first time through, they wouldn't have.

BARBARA: *The myomectomy I had eight years ago worked for a while, but after I started bleeding so heavily again, I just wanted it to go away and never come back. The hysterectomy is absolutely what I wanted. I have never felt better. I recommend it to anyone in my situation.*

JANIS: *I have never felt less of a woman after my hysterectomy. I used those organs to produce two amazing children, but my femininity, sexual attractiveness, and sexual desire are between my ears, not in my female organs!*

IF YOU'RE CONSIDERING HYSTERECTOMY . . .

There are three basic types of hysterectomy; the key difference is in how much of your reproductive system is removed. The different names these operations go by are described below, but essentially, hysterectomy involves the loss of either:

○ part of the uterus *(supracervical hysterectomy)*;
○ the entire uterus *(total hysterectomy)*; or
○ all reproductive organs *(total abdominal hysterectomy)*.

Supracervical Hysterectomy

This technique is a great example of "everything old is new again." Until the 1950s, it was the hysterectomy of choice, but when cervical cancer was discovered as a major killer, the procedure fell out of favor. Now that Pap smears can detect cervical cancer with a fairly high degree of accuracy, assuming that you get them done on a regular basis, supracervical hysterectomies are becoming an option again.

Supracervical hysterectomy leaves you more intact than any other type of hysterectomy; your doctor takes out only the top portion of your uterus, leaving the cervix attached to the vagina and surrounding ligaments. The advantages are that your bladder function and sexual response are preserved better than in any other hysterectomy; you may also have less risk of surgical and postoperative pain and complications. A comparison of supracervical and total abdominal hysterectomies revealed no difference in either complications during surgery, or the success of the outcome during two years of follow-up.

The surgery is most often done using laparoscopy. Dr. Joseph Feste explains, "If a woman doesn't have prolapse of the cervix, cervical dysplasia, or cancer, we can use laparoscopy to remove the top portion of the uterus where fibroids usually are, leaving the cervix in. We can do this with women who have fibroids up to a 16-week size, sometimes even a little bigger. Using a special instrument, we can cut the uterus into small pieces and suction out the pieces, leaving the cervix attached and overall offering a much less invasive surgery."

Dr. Mark Perloe, medical director at Georgia Reproductive Specialists, in Atlanta, says, "Leaving the cervix in place is a great procedure. Patients almost always go home with better pelvic support and better sexual response."

Total Hysterectomy (TAH)

Just as with myomectomy, there are three types of surgery that doctors use for total or total abdominal hysterectomies (TAH): Which one is best depends largely on the size of your uterus and your doctor's experience with each technique. For more information on laparoscopic and abdominal surgery and a discussion of pain management, take a look at the preceding section on myomectomy and surgery basics.

Vaginal Hysterectomy

A typical cut-off for vaginal surgery is a uterus smaller than a 12- to 14-week size due to fibroids, though some doctors have been able to remove a uterus as large as 20 weeks in size.

The benefits of vaginal hysterectomy are that it tends to take less time in the operating room (though surgery can last over two hours, depending on the difficulty of the operation), leaves no visible scar, and probably creates no internal scarring. Since you don't have to heal from an incision, your recovery time should be quicker than it would be for abdominal surgery.

How Many Ways Can You Say "Hysterectomy"?

Supracervical Hysterectomy
Also known as: subtotal hysterectomy, partial hysterectomy
Removal of: the back portion of the uterus only. You keep your cervix, ovaries, and fallopian tubes.

Total Hysterectomy
Also known as: simple hysterectomy, partial hysterectomy, complete hysterectomy
Removal of: the uterus and cervix. You keep both ovaries and fallopian tubes.

Total Abdominal Hysterectomy (TAH)
Also known as: hysterectomy (or total hysterectomy) with bilateral salpingo-oophorectomy (THBSO), hysterectomy with bilateral oophorectomy
Removal of: the uterus, cervix, both ovaries and fallopian tubes, ("Salpingo" refers to your fallopian tubes; "oophorectomy" refers to your ovaries.) A "radical hysterectomy," done in the case of cancer, also includes removing supporting ligaments, tissue, the upper portion of the vagina, and possibly the pelvic lymph nodes.

On the other hand, since your doctor isn't able to see inside your entire abdominal cavity, there is greater potential for damage to the bladder and rectum.

One thing to be aware of is that vaginal hysterectomies are so easy—for your doctor—that some may be tempted to suggest it as a quick and simple solution for your fibroids. Dr. Herbert Goldfarb, in his book *The No-Hysterectomy Option: Your Body—Your Choice,* warns against vaginal surgery that is too quick and seems too easy: "If your doctor tells you that he or she can 'get your uterus out in thirty minutes,' you should seriously consider why it is being removed . . . The 'thirty-minute' vaginal hysterectomies that doctors boast of performing are often procedures that don't have to be done in the first place!"

Laparoscopically Assisted Vaginal Hysterectomy

If your fibroids are too large for a vaginal hysterectomy, your gynecologist may recommend a laparoscopically assisted vaginal hysterectomy (LAVH), adding the element of laparoscopy to a vaginal procedure. If it's appropriate, LAVH can be much easier on your body, and promote a quicker recovery, than traditional abdominal surgery. But remember, LAVH becomes technically impossible if your fibroids are too big.

What's the benefit of LAVH? It can help avoid an abdominal hysterectomy. However, it's still more invasive than a "regular" vaginal hysterectomy, if that is indeed an option for you.

Abdominal Surgery

As we said when we discussed myomectomy, many doctors prefer performing abdominal surgery for both hysterectomies and myomectomies. Abdominal hysterectomy is the simplest of all the surgeries you could be offered and is standard training for all gynecologists. Your hospital stay will usually last for three to five days; total recovery generally takes four to six weeks.

CHERI: *My surgery was scheduled for 7:30 a.m. I was out of surgery by 9:30 and woke up in my room feeling great. No pain. My IV wasn't even hooked up. I had visitors and had a great time! I felt great! The next morning, my doctor asked me if I'd like to go home that day. I was astounded. "TODAY?" He said, "Sure—we're not doing anything for you here that you can't do at home. This place is for sick people!"*

ANGELA: *After my hysterectomy, I did feel like things were weird in there a little bit. I have a very, very close friend from childhood, I mean literally from nursery school, who had a hysterectomy a year ago, and it was very helpful to talk to her because my doctor, who's wonderful and supportive, feels that as long as everything is OUT, it's fixed. But my friend said to me, don't be concerned if it doesn't feel right at three months, even though your doctor will say it's cured, it's over, it's completely healed. She said that three months isn't enough, and she was so right. It's been about nine months now, and I do feel much better. I still feel occasionally a funny pulling or a funny numbness, but I'm not conscious of it anymore in any way that disturbs me, and I understand now that over time even that will recede.*

JANIS: *I wanted the surgery, I was not one bit apprehensive. I was actually excited the day of the surgery. My recuperation was normal . . . in the hospital for four days, home resting for a week, up and out for a couple of hours a day the second week, and back to work after four weeks, feeling terrific.*

Decisions, Decisions

Once you've considered all your options, take a quiet moment. Go out for a walk. Lie on the couch and look at the ceiling. And ask yourself these three questions:

○ Am I totally comfortable that I've made the best decision for myself?

○ Have I gotten enough information?
○ Does the decision feel right on a gut level?

If you answered "yes" to all these questions, and your decision is to proceed with treatment, go back to your quiet thinking mode for another moment and ask yourself these questions:

○ Am I confident that my doctor is acting in my best interests?
○ Do I trust him or her?
○ Do I feel good that he or she will take a minimalist approach and still get the job done?

DR. BRIAN WALSH: *A patient should make the best decision that feels right for her. Very often patients will come into the office and they'll have a chart of the pluses and minuses, the pros and cons, but I think when it comes to decision-making in life, the most important decisions are not made on an intellectual basis. They're made on a very emotional, visceral level. So when a patient says to me, I just don't know what to do, I say, well, forget your list—how do you really feel? Deep down, what feels right to you? And I'll say, that's what you should do.*

DR. JAMES SPIES: *If a woman comes in to find out about UAE and she walks out and says forget this, I'm having a hysterectomy, in a way it's a victory—that's a decision she's been brought to by receiving the information. I try not to bias people one way or the other because I do think it's a very personal decision, and for five women you might get five different decisions.*

If you're not sure, if you have doubts, if you just don't know whether you should have a hysterectomy—or any elective procedure for fibroids—it's okay. Unless you're bleeding badly enough that your life is in danger, the good news is that you can wait. Another month of getting additional medical opinions, of talking to your family and friends, doing research, thinking, meditating, praying, or relaxing will not hurt you. And it may help.

Remember, the least educated women can be at the highest risk for hysterectomy, as are the women with the least emotional support. The women who go into any kind of surgery content and relaxed have the best recoveries. No matter what you decide, make sure you feel educated, and emotionally supported by at least one key person in your life. And if you go into surgery, know that you're making the best possible decision for your body and your quality of life.

↶ 6 ↷

But Wait, There's More

FIBROIDS AND ALTERNATIVE MEDICINE

UNTIL ABOUT 100 years ago, most women only had access to what we now think of as "alternative" remedies. In the twentieth century, medical science built a superhighway, bypassing the "slow road" of therapies like herbs, homeopathy, and traditional Chinese medicine. But that road kept meandering along, and in the last few years more and more of us have turned onto it. While doctors such as Andrew Weil and Christiane Northrup promote the intelligent use of both alternative and medical therapies, other medical doctors remain skeptical of any treatments that haven't gone through controlled lab testing and peer-reviewed studies. Of course, numerous alternative-therapy practitioners provide help to at least some of the millions of people who search them out every year.

There are dozens—if not hundreds—of types of alternative therapy. Dr. David Eisenberg, Director of the Division for Research and Education in Complementary and Integrative Medical Therapies at Harvard Medical School's Osher Institute, defines alternative medicine as including chiropractic, acupuncture, massage therapy, biofeedback, megavitamins, homeopathy, relaxation techniques, guided imagery, prayer, spiritual healing, self-help, commercial diets, folk remedies, hypnosis, vegetarianism, macrobiotics, herbal remedies, and forms of "energy" healing that involve touch, magnets, or other devices. The National Center for Complementary and Alternative Medicine (NCCAM), a government office, also includes Ayurveda, Native American medicine, and mind-body techniques such as yoga, music therapy, and others.

While some alternative therapies offer the possibility of eliminating your fibroids, most seem to offer more hope for relieving fibroid-related symptoms, like bleeding, cramps, and fatigue.

Enough evidence exists about certain therapies that you can examine some of the pros and cons and make a reasonable decision about whether you want to try them. Some other treatments have been mentioned either to me personally or once or twice in the literature I've been able to find; these are more questionable but still may appeal to you. As we'll discuss in Chapter 12, belief may play a part in how well any treatment works, whether conventional or alternative.

The alternative therapies that seem to have success dealing with fibroids are based on the theory of homeostasis—the body's ability to heal itself when it is in balance. The different therapies have a number of elements in common, all intended to bring your body back to its balanced, healthful state. These include cleansing the liver, reducing excess estrogen or bringing estrogen into balance, improving circulation, improving digestion, and reducing stress.

Common sense confirms much of the wisdom of these approaches. For example, estrogens in our environment can throw our systems out of balance, and certain foods contribute to extra estrogen in the system. The liver, in charge of eliminating toxins as well as extra estrogen, can get overburdened and not eliminate estrogen as efficiently as it should. Improved circulation may help direct blood flow away from our fibroids, and anything that relieves stress may help keep our fibroids from growing—and keep us from focusing on them more than we need to.

One caution: Some women prefer to use alternative remedies exclusively, even when their fibroid symptoms get worse. Use your own common sense to know when something is improving your health or not.

Alternative Medicine Feels Good

What can alternative medicine offer us that conventional medicine can't?

As we've seen, standard medical techniques for fibroids can be, in the abstract, somewhat primitive. You can cut fibroids out, burn them, freeze them, starve them. By contrast, alternative practices are more subtle. In theory, they aim to alter the source of the problem by manipulating your energy flow and gently redirecting your body to heal itself.

Alternative medicine is often called "holistic," because most alternative therapies treat us "as a whole." Think of your body as a garden: Conventional medicine will find a weed and bring in weed killers or gardening tools; alternative practitioners will evaluate the ecosystem to find out why the weeds are growing in the first place.

Rina Nissim, author of *Natural Healing in Gynecology,* writes, "The natural healing approach . . . is a holistic one which recognizes the emotional, social and environmental factors in disease, and which treats the person as a whole being."

Many times, alternative therapies are delivered in peaceful, soothing surroundings: My acupuncturist turns on soft music and lights a candle as I lie on the table; contrast this with the harsh light and cold instruments of a doctor's office.

And then there are the therapists themselves, often people who feel a warmth and connection to others as healers. Unlike many doctors, who these days are not only more rushed than ever (often against their wishes) but trained to look for specific symptoms, alternative therapists talk to you about your life, your work, your problems. It can be a more comforting, nurturing experience than many of us are able to get with our doctors, and that alone may explain why we're going to alternative therapists in record numbers.

But Will It Work?

We know that Western medicine works a certain percentage of the time: For most fibroid treatments, doctors can tell you with a fair degree of certainty what you can expect and when. And Western medicine is, for better or worse, fast. Like many aspects of our society, Western therapies for fibroids offer a certain amount of instant gratification, satisfying to those of us who don't feel we have the time or patience for anything but an instant "fix."

Alternative medicine moves at a different pace. Treatments are often slow; the course of treatment may be months or years instead of literally hours, as in the case of surgery. While surgery may have a recovery period of several weeks, some types of alternative treatments, such as homeopathy, may actually make your symptoms worse for several weeks before they get better. And unlike conventional medicine, alternative therapies can't make any guarantees. Your fibroids may shrink, or they may not.

In terms of reporting which alternative therapies may work on your fibroids and which won't, analyzing alternative practices is tricky. Unlike Western medicine, which has a series of standards and governing authorities (such as the U.S. Food and Drug Administration, or FDA), alternative medicine has no such regulation. Furthermore, scientists are just beginning to study alternative medicine in a way that's consistent with conventional treatment.

For instance, when it comes to herbal preparations for fibroids, I've found dozens of individual herbs and herbal recipes purported to shrink fibroids, minimize bleeding, or cure cramps. There are no large studies that tell us which of these are effective, or for whom, or under what conditions. We'll discuss the limitations of herbs—along with the possibilities—later in the chapter.

Acupuncture, on the other hand, is an "alternative" that is quickly becoming mainstream in our culture. It is coming under more scientific scrutiny, both on its own and in combination with other alternative remedies, as a way to provide relief for fibroid symptoms and, occasionally, to eliminate the fibroids themselves.

Healing methods such as homeopathy actually defy Western medical thought. According to the *New England Journal of Medicine*, this and other therapies not only have no objective proof that they're effective but are based on principles that "violate fundamental scientific laws."

Best of Both Worlds

BOTH WESTERN MEDICINE and alternative remedies have a lot
to offer—and a lot to be cautious about. What's interesting is how
much the two approaches can potentially complement each other
in your total health care. The chart below starts to sort out some
of the things alternative medicine can do better than conventional
medicine, and vice versa.

Alternative Therapy	Conventional Medicine
Evaluates and treats your fibroids as part of a larger system	Evaluates and treats your fibroids as a local, specific problem
Herbal, homeopathic, and naturopathic remedies are tailored specifically to you	Surgery and drug therapies are "one size fits all"
Often a calm, relaxing office or treatment environment	Often a sterile, cold office or treatment environment
Treatment does not usually include serious side effects during or after the procedure	Treatment may include serious side effects either during or after the procedure
Works on the theory of homeostasis, that the body can heal itself	Works on eliminating the problem
May work best on symptoms like bleeding and cramps	Offers few options for treating symptoms without invasive procedures
Seems to work best on smaller fibroids	Treatments available for fibroids of all sizes
Generally takes some time to work	Generally works quickly or immediately
Needs to be part of an ongoing routine; stops working when you stop treatment	Generally works after a single intervention (such as surgery or UAE); only requires follow-up visits for checkups

Alternative Therapy	Conventional Medicine
Comparative studies and large-scale trials are starting to become available for certain remedies	Numerous articles, studies, and trials about fibroids (though not all are conclusive)
No proven standards for treating fibroids	Generally accepted standards for results of drug and surgical therapy
No pharmaceutical regulation for herbs or creams; potency can vary widely	Drugs and surgical equipment are regulated by the U.S. Food and Drug Administration
Most treatments not covered by insurance	Treatments often covered by insurance

A number of doctors, I think rightly, suggest that many of us are inconsistent when it comes to our medical choices. We'll scrutinize every last journal article on myomectomy, for instance, but take the word of a single claim for an herbal remedy as gospel. However, history is littered with examples showing us that science isn't always right—and health care for women probably has more examples of that being true than many other areas. One sensible approach is to explore alternative therapies with a qualified practitioner, without neglecting what Western medicine has to offer.

Western Herbalism

Of all the different kinds of alternative treatments, the most common is herbal medicine. Since many herbs contain natural plant estrogens (also called *phytoestrogens*), how they work may depend on your stage of life. If your fibroids are giving you problems and you haven't yet reached menopause, herbal remedies may be able to help by suppressing some of your natural estrogen. On the other hand, if you've already reached menopause, moderate amounts of herbs or other sources of phytoestrogens may relieve some of your symptoms, while large amounts may make your fibroids grow or cause bleeding. If you're on hormone replacement therapy (HRT) or birth control, certain phytoestrogens can block the effects of those drugs.

There's a lot of controversy about whether herbs can be good medicine. Part of the problem is that herbal supplements aren't regulated; the U.S. Congress actually exempted these products from FDA regulation in 1994. As a result—just in case you haven't been in a grocery store, drug store, or health food store recently—the supplement market is now very big business.

Without regulation, of course, there's no standard of quality; the pills or tonics you buy might contain the herbs shown on the label, in the amount that's listed, or they might not. In California, researchers who bought 25 different ginseng preparations from a single health food store found that some brands were dozens of times more powerful than others—but there was no way to tell without chemical testing.

Since supplements don't deliver a consistent amount of herbs, it's easy to take too much. And since we tend to equate "natural" with "safe," it's easy to forget that herbs can interact with prescription or over-the-counter medicines, just like "regular" medicine. According to Patricia Eagon, an herb researcher, this can lead to dangerous drug interactions or overdoses.

A FIBROID HERBAL

So herbs are a tricky business. Some can affect your body like estrogen, others mimic progesterone. Remember that fibroids may get bigger and bleed more as a result of either estrogen or progesterone, so be prepared to watch your symptoms carefully.

Researchers have found that several different herbs can make uterine cells divide or grow. Since a fibroid starts from just a single uterine cell, giving those cells the wrong growth message is not something a woman with fibroids wants to encourage.

Then there are herbs that may help reduce bleeding, ease cramps, cleanse your system, and perhaps even shrink your fibroids. These are often prescribed as teas or in capsule form. Often, a practitioner will recommend a mixture of several herbs to accomplish your goals. Just like prescription medicine, consistency is important; your practitioner will help you work out a schedule and starting dosages.

A number of herbs can cause bad reactions, especially if you're pregnant, have a systemic disease like lupus or HIV, or are taking prescription medicines. It's prudent to consult a qualified herbalist before trying herbal therapy; you should also tell your doctor about any herbs you plan to take.

You'll also need some patience: It can take weeks or months for herbal remedies to have an effect. Some practitioners recommend that dosages should start small and be built up, and that you should take a one- or two-day break every ten days to give your body a rest.

Controversial Remedies for Women with Fibroids

The herbs in the following list are popular traditional remedies for fibroids, bleeding, or cramps that simply may not be good for your fibroids or may have risky side effects. Even this information is not definitive, so use your judgment. If your herbalist recommends one or more of these treatments, discuss these issues with him or her, and keep an eye on your symptoms.

- **Black cohosh** is a highly studied herb, especially in Germany, where it's a popular form of HRT (sold under the brand name Remifemin), though it's limited to six months' use. Research has shown black cohosh can make uterine cells divide, as well as make bleeding and cramps worse.
- **Blue cohosh** is a traditional Native North American remedy for cramps; in research, blue cohosh did not promote uterine growth. However, blue cohosh can raise blood pressure and constrict the blood vessels leading to the heart.
- **Chaste tree berry**, or Vitex agnus-castus, is a very well-known remedy, long used to regulate heavy bleeding and shrink fibroids; it's also said to be calming and relaxing. Like black cohosh,

though, chaste tree can make uterine cells divide. In addition, if you're taking birth control pills, chaste tree may make them ineffective.

○ **Dong quai** *(also called angelica or dang gui)* is well known as an almost all-purpose "woman's remedy." Its benefits include regulating menstruation and relieving cramps, stabilizing blood sugar levels, and enhancing the function of the immune system. Research has shown that dong quai increased uterine weight; according to Dr. Susan Love, you should avoid dong quai if you have heavy menstrual bleeding or fibroids.

○ **Licorice** (the herb, not the candy) is a phytoestrogen that in tests did not promote uterine growth. However, it can raise your blood pressure, moreso if you're on the Pill, and can only be safely used for four to six weeks.

○ **Motherwort**, recommended by some sources as a beneficial uterine tonic, may make bleeding worse.

○ **Red clover** and **cramp bark**, two remedies for reducing cramps, raise estrogen levels significantly.

Herbs That May Help

The following chart shows a number of different herbs and the symptoms they may help relieve. This list doesn't include every possible herb for every symptom, but reflects information from several sources, including *Healing Fibroids* by Dr. Allan Warshowsky and Elena Oumano, *Natural Healing in Gynecology* by Rina Nissim, *The Complete Woman's Herbal* by Anne McIntyre, and the *Encyclopedia of Healing Therapies* by Anne Woodham and Dr. David Peters.

Dr. Warshowsky says that although there are more and more studies being done, the trick to using herbs safely for the time being is to rely on as much anecdotal information as possible, and to work with an experienced physician, or licensed healer, testing dosages very cautiously, to ensure they have no ill effects on you. Using herbal and homeopathic products from reputable companies also reduces risks.

Herbs That May ...	Shrink Fibroids	Detoxify	Control Cramps	Control Bleeding
Beth Root				•
Black Haw			•	
Blue Flag		•		
Borage		•	•	
Cinnamon				•
Cramp Bark			•	•
Dandelion		•		
Echinacea	•			
False Unicorn Root				•
Garlic	•	•	•	•
Ginger			•	
Hops			•	
Lady's Mantle				•
Nettle				•
Partridgeberry			•	•
Raspberry Leaves			•	
Red Raspberry			•	•
Sequoia Buds	•			
Shepherd's Purse				•
Skullcap		•	•	
White Ash	•			
Wild Yam				•
Yarrow	•		•	•

I Yam What I Yam

The use of natural progesterone, made from wild yam, is one of the more aggressively marketed alternative remedies available for women with fibroids.

Search for "natural progesterone cream" on Google and you'll receive pages and pages of results . . . all from commercial suppliers. Manufacturers claim amazing benefits from their products, including relief of PMS, infertility, fibroids, and a host of other conditions. The FDA, for one, isn't happy about this at all. A strongly worded letter from the FDA notified the chairman/CEO of one leading manufacturer that such "medical" claims were against the law, and furthermore, his products hadn't been tested properly.

Unfortunately, the FDA doesn't actually regulate natural progesterone creams (short of sending warning letters), so like herbs, there is no guarantee of how much—or how little—progesterone you get in each dose. A study of one popular brand of natural progesterone found that there wasn't enough progesterone in the product to counter the effects of estrogen—even in postmenopausal women—and that the cream wasn't well absorbed through the skin. In a separate study, researchers concluded that the amounts of progesterone were appropriate, but "in light of the potential risks associated with long-term progesterone use, the authors question whether topical progesterone products should be available OTC [over-the-counter]."

The Canadian government banned the sale of progesterone creams in 1997, since manufacturers could not offer enough proof that their products worked as claimed. In the United States, the FDA has only approved progesterone for oral consumption.

DR. VICTOR REYNIAK: *Using progesterone cream to reduce fibroids is worthless. Progestins work only if there is a dysfunction, if there's a deficiency of progesterone because a woman is anovulatory. And women with fibroids ovulate normally. So using progestins really serve no purpose at all. These doctors who sell creams to put on your belly, it's a scam, it's a money-making machine.*

On the other hand, some women do find relief using natural progesterone cream, especially from symptoms like heavy bleeding and severe PMS. Is it a placebo effect or the real thing? Could it be that progesterone cream helps women whose estrogen levels are surging while their own progesterone levels are going down? Part of the confusion is how progesterone affects fibroids. There's reason to believe that progesterone can make fibroids grow; as we discussed in Chapter 5, *antiprogesterone* drugs like RU-486 have been shown to make fibroids shrink.

Traditional Chinese Medicine

Chinese philosophy tells us that *qi* (pronounced "chee") is the life force. Qi flows all around us, and travels through the body via 12 specific meridians (channels) that connect all the major organs. According to traditional Chinese medicine (TCM), each of these organs is in charge of different functions in our bodies; problems occur when the flow of qi to or from the organ is blocked.

Fibroids are said to be the result of blocked energy in the liver and gall bladder; according to TCM, these are the organs in charge of regulating all growth, wanted or unwanted. (Since qi is responsible for moving the blood, this block is also called blood stasis, or blood stagnation.)

How can this kind of block occur? According to TCM, growth that's either stifled or out of control—including spiritual and emotional growth—blocks the energy of the liver; in response, the liver creates an "overgrowth" somewhere in the body, such as fibroids.

The purpose of TCM, which includes acupuncture, Chinese herbalism, and other techniques, is to help the body heal itself by allowing the qi to flow freely.

Qi is made up of two equal but opposite forces called *yin* and *yang*; these need to be in balance for perfect health. Yang is associated with heat, dryness, light, action, and expansion. Yin is cold, damp, dark, and quiet; it's associated with the earth, interior, and deficiency. The liver, which regulates fibroids, is a yin organ.

Fibroids are a symptom of disharmony between yin and yang. Clearing an imbalance might mean clearing away accumulated heat (yang) or reducing too much cold (yin). A TCM practitioner will work with you to create homeostasis—the balance of yin and yang—to treat your fibroids.

Your TCM practitioner will evaluate your symptoms, check your pulse, and inspect your tongue to diagnose your energy. The two primary treatments, acupuncture and herbs, are most often used together, but in order to examine how each one works, let's take a look at them one by one.

ACUPUNCTURE

Does acupuncture shrink fibroids? The answer is maybe—though your chances are much better if your fibroids are small. A researcher at a major university told me that women typically use acupuncture as a last resort, when their fibroids are too big, or their symptoms too severe, to benefit.

It's possible that acupuncture can slow the growth of fibroids. Some practitioners think that there are points on the body that control and prevent the growth of cells. Stimulating these points may keep fibroid cells from growing.

Acupuncture may be more consistently successful in treating pain or bleeding from fibroids. The World Health Organization recognizes acupuncture as an accepted therapy to reduce the pain of menstrual cramps and regulate menstrual bleeding, among numerous other conditions. This type of treatment isn't necessarily quick. Finding relief may take up to six months.

NORA COFFEY: *Acupuncture seems to help a fair number of women reduce heavy bleeding. I think there are more women that have had success in reducing bleeding with acupuncture than not.*

DR. BRIAN WALSH: *I'm open-minded about alternative medicine, but it depends on what the problem is. For instance, I'm sure there are many factors that influence pain, and for patients with pelvic pain who want to work with an acupuncturist, I'll support that decision. All I care about is the bottom line: Does she still experience pain? I don't care how she got there, but if she doesn't experience pain anymore, that's a success.*

Acupuncture doesn't hurt, but you might feel pinpricks when the needles go in. Some therapists apply a low electric current to the needles to stimulate the acupoints even more. I've also found this to be painless. Your therapist may combine acupuncture with other techniques to strengthen the healing process, such as pressure *(acupressure)*, burning herbs *(moxibustion)*, or Chinese herbs in pill or tea form.

In China, an acupuncturist has to complete extensive training in Western medicine, acupuncture, and Chinese herbalism. Acupuncturists in the United States are licensed by state; this means the requirements vary. Both Western physicians and traditional acupuncturists generally caution patients to consult their primary physician about all treatments.

FELICE: *I found a local acupuncturist and Chinese medicine practitioner and began seeing her once a week and committing myself to three or four months with her. She felt that the fibroid was probably too big to shrink but that she could stabilize the growth, help with my menstrual pain and PMS, and lessen the bleeding. So far none of those things have happened after three months. The sessions were relaxing except when the needles were initially put in. She would put lots of needles around my uterus, two in my forehead, a few in my legs and then later, some on my back. It was relaxing to lie on the table with the pleasant music, and the moxibustion felt nice. Moxibustion is where she heats up some herb that smelled like sage and puts the burning herb near the different points.*

KIM: *There was a practice that the acupuncturist gave me and I did for a long time every time I took a shower, focusing healing light on my fibroids and having the light burn them away. But that was to be done in conjunction with all the other things she told me to do, the diet, the vitamins, the progesterone, and all that stuff. And she was realistic that it's a very difficult thing to do, and I wasn't committed to making those changes.*

CHINESE HERBALISM

Chinese herbalism is the second major component of TCM. Herbalism is also practiced according to the balancing principles of yin and yang. Since the liver in its healthy state is "cold" or yin, some practitioners may diagnose your fibroids as being the result of too much heat, and prescribe herbs accordingly. On the other hand, certain foods are considered too "yin," which can also encourage fibroids by causing an excess of cold. The secret is determining and treating the cause of disharmony.

So can herbs treat fibroids? Several studies done in China and Japan show encouraging results, but just like Western herbal remedies, there isn't yet a consistent standard of reporting. Of course, this doesn't mean these remedies aren't effective. Here are some of the findings:

In a study of 110 women, a traditional Chinese remedy called *kuei-chih-fu-ling-wan* (also known as *keisha-bukuryo-gan* in Japanese) improved bleeding 90 percent of the time and shrank fibroids 60 percent of the time.

Another study of 223 women with fibroids reported that individualized herbal treatment helped reduce heavy menstrual bleeding for at least half the women, reduced the size of fibroids significantly for about a third of the women, and helped fibroids disappear for a small group. Overall, the treatment helped over 85 percent of the women in the study.

More recently, doctors in Tokyo found that a traditional Japanese (Kampo) medicine called *Toki-shakuyaku-san* improved heavy bleeding, cramps, and other symptoms associated with heavy bleeding, such as dizziness and feeling cold.

In Shanghai, researchers reported success in shrinking fibroids with an extract from a vine called *Tripterygium wilfordii Hook. f.*, or as the locals call it, thunder god vine (U.S. researchers, not half as poetically, call the same substance T2, and for ease of pronunciation, not to mention typing, so will I). Used incorrectly, T2 can be highly toxic.

> ## *Chinese Herbs and Formulas*
>
> HERE ARE SOME other Chinese herbs and formulas said to help fibroids or their symptoms:
>
> **Cinnamon and Hoelen F.** *(gui zhi fu ling wan)***:** for painful fibroids or cramps
> **Cinnamon and Persica:** for fibroids
> **Cinnamon and Bulrush C.** *(shoo fu zhu yu tang)***:** for fibroids or heavy bleeding
> **Blue Citrus:** for fibroids
> **Yun Nan Bai Yao:** to control bleeding
> **Chih-ko and Curcuma C.:** for fibroids and other tumors

In the T2 experiment, fibroids shrank in up to 70 percent of the women treated. The remedy took time: on average, fibroids shrank by about half after six months, when treatment stopped. About a third of the women also stopped having their periods during the treatment. The researchers discovered that T2 helped reduce estrogen and progesterone levels; what we don't know is whether fibroids grew back after treatment ended.

On the other hand, a survey of women who said they'd tried Chinese herbal remedies, combined with changes in diet, found that only 7 percent got relief from their fibroid-related symptoms. Apart from whether the remedies themselves worked or not, it's possible that some women in the study just gave up too soon: Making teas or decoctions with Chinese herbs tends to be time-consuming—and they taste terrible. One possible solution is to ask your TCM practitioner to prescribe freeze-dried herbs, which can be taken in capsule form. Of course, if you're taking any medications or have any health conditions, consult with your TCM practitioner and doctor about any possible interactions.

FELICE: *My acupuncturist put me on a Chinese herbal formula that was made up of cinnamon, poris, red peony, moutan, persica, rhubarb, dong quai, bulrush, sparganium, and lurcitna zedoria. I was to swallow a heaping teaspoon of this dirtlike substance three times a day with meals. It was supposed to strengthen my uterus, regulate my hormones, decrease the bleeding, shrink the fibroid. I felt no effects.*

JEANNE: *I heard about an Asian preparation that helped reduce fibroids and I said, you know, I think I'd rather try that before I try surgery. I talked to my gynecologist about it and she had no problem, so I went to a woman who's both an MD and a Chinese medicine person, who wore a lot of crystals and had a little shrine. She gave me the equivalent of a prescription of premeasured, preprocessed Chinese herbs; one is called Crampbark Plus and the other is Bupleurum Entangled Qi Formula. They're freeze-dried, so you don't have to make teas, and I started taking them and had diminished symptoms. When I went back to my gynecologist for my checkup, my fibroids had shrunk from over 10 centimeters to below 9, and she said, you're getting to the size now where we wouldn't operate unless they're causing you trouble.*

PUTTING IT ALL TOGETHER

Most TCM practitioners will use several complementary therapies to treat your fibroids. Dr. Warshowsky, for instance, evaluates what he terms "the imbalances" of each patient's physical and emotional states, and creates a course of treatment based on the results—often including some combination of herbs, diet, exercise, meditation, even talk therapy. "This is not new," Warshowsky says. "Hippocrates said, 'We treat the person, not the disease.' This is the oath that every doctor swears to."

In order to test how well combined therapies work to reduce or eliminate fibroids, Dr. Lewis Mehl-Madrona, a physician at both the University of Pittsburgh Medical School and the University of Arizona College of Medicine, and author of *Coyote Medicine*, put together a study of over 70 women, including a control group, to monitor the results of a combination of alternative treatments versus conventional care. The women in the test portion of the study went through a weekly regimen of acupuncture, Chinese herbal treatment, nutritional therapy, guided visual imagery, self-hypnosis, and bodywork. At the end of six months, over 80 percent of the women in the test group had some success in reducing or stopping the growth of their fibroids. The success rate for the women who sought out conventional treatment was 32 percent.

According to Dr. Mehl-Madrona, "The most important aspect of this study is the demonstration that the growth rate and the size of uterine fibroids can be affected by complementary medicine intervention."

For the women in the test who were happy with their results, the biggest downside was the price tag. On average, the program cost $3,800 per person, and the expense was not covered by insurance. (Some insurance companies are starting to offer limited coverage for alternative therapies; check with your provider.)

However, Dr. Mehl-Madrona, not surprisingly, reports that "patient satisfaction is greater with complementary medicine treatment than with surgery, at least among the subset of patients who sought this form of therapy."

Buyer Beware

SOME "ALTERNATIVE" TREATMENTS seem less than orthodox, like magnet therapy, injections of herbal preparations directly into the cervix, crushed-tomato stomach rubs, enzyme therapy, and dental work. Before you try any unusual treatments, call women your therapist claims to have helped. You may also want to limit your exposure in terms of the amount of time and money you feel comfortable spending, especially as these remedies are not yet proven, and are almost certainly not covered by insurance.

I've also read some success stories in which therapists describe how they've cured fibroids (usually for just one patient) using a laundry list of techniques that may include diet, herbs, homeopathy, acupuncture, visualization, liver cleansing, and natural progesterone.

BONNIE: *In January, I had an ultrasound that revealed a fibroid measuring 6.7 centimeters. I was told that my options were surgery, either myomectomy or hysterectomy, or Lupron therapy. None of these choices was acceptable to me.*

I began to read and research. I started doing castor oil compresses every night. I read Susun Weed's book on menopause and began taking tinctures for fibroids and heavy bleeding, namely Vitex, lady's mantle, shepherd's purse, as well as nettles, dandelion, and burdock, for anemia.

I then remembered the Tibetan physician I had seen for another ailment years ago with great success. He sent me herbs, which I began taking in March. These Tibetan herbs helped more than anything else I tried. Although I was still bleeding daily, the amount was less than before.

In April I went to an acupuncture clinic for an evaluation. I took a comprehensive diagnostic test which determined that my body was loaded with toxins, primarily heavy metals and Candida, and I was put on a strict Candida diet and many supplements to detoxify. I was told, and also read about this, that Candida and metal toxicity, mainly mercury, were thought to be contributing causes of fibroids. I was strongly urged to get my dental amalgams removed and replaced. I had a dental consult for this, but decided against it because of the cost and because I was not convinced that this would solve my problem.

I continued with the strict diet and supplements and also used natural progesterone cream twice daily. Meanwhile I was still bleeding and still desperately seeking an answer to why my body was doing this to me. I thought that my fibroids must be shrinking, with all the herbs, diet, compresses, progesterone cream, etc., that I was doing. So in August, I had another ultrasound. I was devastated to learn that my fibroid had GROWN and was now 8-plus centimeters.

DARBY: *I've tried acupuncture, Chinese herbs, a vegetarian and dairy-free existence, kundalini and hatha yoga, castor oil packs, getting rid of baggage à la Christiane Northrup, etc. I'm still looking for something to make my fibroids go away.*

IMPROVING QI AT HOME

There are some ways you can improve qi on your own, including exercise, massage, sitz baths, and castor oil packs. Some of these may make your fibroids feel better—some may just plain make *you* feel better.

Bodywork

Your car gets it—why not you? Buffing the fenders and polishing the hood—so to speak—can make your whole machine run more smoothly.

Bodywork that can help get your qi moving—and improve your circulation—includes aerobic exercise, massage, walks by the ocean, hikes in the mountains, dancing, Reiki, reflexology, yoga—and let's not forget healthy sex. All of these can help increase energy flow and eliminate energy blocks. Bodywork that helps increase pelvic blood flow and improve lymphatic drainage of the pelvis can remove what TCM calls "stagnation" in the pelvis.

The Touch Research Institute at the University of Miami, Florida, has done studies that suggest massage can relieve chronic pain and fatigue, among other problems. At Weill Medical College of Cornell University, women with early-stage breast cancer received regular massage, which resulted in "higher levels of cancer-fighting natural killer cells, lower levels of stress hormones and . . . increases in their quality of life." Massage can be done by a qualified therapist, as well as by a friend or loved one.

Reflexology is a form of bodywork that just involves your feet. For fibroids, you can try massaging the spots (reflexes) for your uterus and liver. How do you find them? The uterus reflex is in the soft area behind your inner ankle bones. Your liver reflex is on the sole of your right foot, from the middle of the arch to the ball.Press the reflex areas deeply and massage. If nothing else, I can promise you it feels good!

Common Scents

YOU CAN ENHANCE your massage or bath with aromatherapy. Chamomile, lavender, marjoram, and melissa are all scents thought to relieve cramps; rose and jasmine are thought to be good for uterine disorders; rose, jasmine, chamomile, and lavender are also relaxing. Put a few drops of the essential oil of your choice in an ounce of unscented oil, like apricot seed or grapeseed oil, before adding to your bath or using for massage. Remember, essential oils are for external use only.

Sitz Baths

Sitz baths are, yes really, baths you sit in. (The word "sitz" is German and is pronounced "zitz.") The idea is that alternating hot and cold water on your abdomen will stimulate your qi and increase circulation. Rina Nissim, in her book *Natural Healing In Gynecology*, suggests that simply dipping your backside in a pan of cold water every morning for two to three minutes can activate your circulation. This can definitely replace a cup of coffee as a morning wake-me-up.

A more traditional recommendation requires two tubs, each big enough for you to sit in with water up to your abdomen. Personally, I don't know anybody who has an arrangement like this at home, but if you do, you can try this: Fill one tub with hot water and the other with cold, then spend four or five minutes in each tub, switching back and forth four times. (Don't use water that's too hot to sit in comfortably, and don't do this if you have high blood pressure, have a heart condition, or are pregnant.)

Of course, a regular warm bath can also just help you relax. Try adding a few drops of essential oil, plus a cup of coarse salt and a cup of baking soda. This odd recipe is very soothing.

Castor Oil Packs

Castor oil packs are thought to help unblock the energy of the liver and relieve menstrual cramps. Different sources recommend doing it for about half an hour once a day, or at least once a week. Taking the time to lie down and relax will probably feel pretty good, too.

Here's the basic recipe: Spread castor oil, preferably from a health food store, over your whole abdomen. (The oil might be messy, so lie down on something you can clean easily or don't care about.) Put a few layers of warm cloth, like flannel, over the castor oil; top it all off with a hot water bottle or heating pad.

If you want, you can add a quarter teaspoon of scented essential oil to the castor oil before you spread it on; you can also warm the flannel in the dryer before you use it, or gently warm the castor oil in a pot on top of the stove before use—make sure it's warm but not hot, so that you don't burn yourself.

A variation on this theme uses fresh ginger tea. Cut up fresh ginger root, place it in a bowl or pot, and pour boiling water over it; cover and let the mixture steep for about 10 minutes. Once you've made sure the tea is hot but comfortable, soak your flannel cloth in the tea, wring it out, and place it on your abdomen. You can put a hot water bottle over the wet cloth if you like—but not an electric heating pad.

If cramps are troubling you, heat alone may be the operative force here. My own preference is to use a good old hot heating pad.

Homeopathy

In homeopathy, like TCM, the body is said to be integrated by a "vital force" that maintains a state of health. Homeopathy tells us that illness is not unhealthy but a sign of the body restoring itself to balance. As a result, homeopathic therapy pushes the body's defenses to stimulate the self-healing process.

To do this, remedies are chosen according to the law of similars, substances that induce symptoms similar to those of the illness. Doses are diluted to increase their potency. Some remedies might contain no scientifically discernible amounts of the original substance. This

dilution is the reason many Western doctors question whether homeopathy can have any real medical effect.

DR. VICTOR REYNIAK: *I believe in homeopathy because faith heals,
but you can fool a woman only for a little while, a very short while. All
placebos work for everybody, for a little while, until the brain realizes
it's being fooled.*

Who you are is an important part of homeopathy. There are at least
15 different types of personalities that you could fit into, based on looks,
temperament, even body temperature. Different types of people tend
to get different homeopathic remedies. In your first meeting with a
homeopath, you'll probably be asked a range of questions, including
what your relationships are like, what your hobbies are, what kinds of
foods and drinks you prefer, even what you're most afraid of.

According to *The Consumer's Guide to Homeopathy,* "Homeopathic
remedies for fibroids will not always completely get rid of them, but
they do often reduce bleeding or other complications. Homeopathic
treatment of fibroids tends to be more effective when they are not too
extensive."

According to Dr. Judyth Reichenberg-Ullman, there are over 50
homeopathic remedies that may fit an individual with fibroids. *The
Woman's Encyclopedia of Natural Healing* by Gary Null lists two remedies that may help reduce the size of fibroids—*aurum muriaticum*
and *hydrastinum muriaticum*—and another half dozen that may be
able to help reduce different types of bleeding.

While you can use these suggestions as a guide, it's important not to
try homeopathy on your own. In particular, the authors of *Everybody's
Guide to Homeopathic Medicines* caution that women who have fibroids
should find an experienced homeopathic practitioner. If you're taking
any prescription medicines, don't start homeopathy before talking
with your doctor; if you're on the birth control pill, you may not be
able to use homeopathy effectively.

Homeopathy also uses diet to help bring your system back into balance; homeopathic practitioners believe that fibroids, as well as other
growths in the body, correspond to an overly acidic body chemistry.

As it happens, the foods that can make your body too acidic include many of the same foods that, as we'll see in Chapter 8, may be bad for your fibroids: coffee, alcohol, meat, dairy, eggs, and sugar. Staying away from these can also strengthen your immune system.

What are good foods to eat on a homeopathic diet? The basic menu includes complex carbohydrates such as beans, whole grains, and cooked vegetables; some low-fat animal protein may also be good for you, depending on your homeopathic body type. Herbs said to reduce acid and improve immunity include garlic, bladder wrack, and Irish moss.

LAURA: *I went to a homeopath who was also an acupuncturist. I have respect for alternative medicine, but I was not forewarned that they'd need to know everything—I wound up sobbing, I felt so violated. He was asking really personal questions, a little bit singlemindedly: A boyfriend before hit me once and he really wanted that to be the reason I had fibroids. I said, nah, my periods were bad before that. He gave me some pills to put under my tongue and he did acupuncture. For the next two months my periods were better, but then they weren't.*

Naturopathy

Naturopathy, like homeopathy, is based on the principle that our bodies have the power to heal themselves. Naturopaths also believe our bodies have a natural equilibrium, or homeostasis, which can be upset by an unhealthy lifestyle.

Many naturopathic ideas, while around for a long time, are now what we think of as common sense. For instance, naturopaths suggest that an unhealthy diet; lack of sleep, exercise, or fresh air; stress; pollution; and even negative attitudes can allow waste products and toxins to build up in the body, upsetting homeostasis.

For fibroids, a naturopath may suggest a diet low in fat and high in fiber to encourage elimination of excess estrogen. If you're bleeding heavily, you might also be advised to eat iron-rich foods to prevent anemia. You may also be prescribed herbal remedies, yoga, massage, and sitz baths.

Ayurveda

The ancient body of knowledge known as Ayurveda originated in India almost 5,000 years ago; some call it the "mother of all healing" for its influence on Chinese, Greek, Western, and holistic medical theory.

Ayurveda divides us into three primary types based on both physical and emotional characteristics: *pitta, vata,* and *kapha.* Kapha-type women are thought to be more likely to get fibroids—they may be advised to modify their diets by eliminating dairy products and reducing red meat, salt, caffeine, alcohol, and heavy foods.

Kapha, like yin, is cooling, linked to caves, the earth, support. The authors of *A Woman's Best Medicine* say that kapha women are often voluptuous, strong, sweet, loyal, patient, and comforting. Love that part! But don't get too complacent: Kapha women often prefer the living room couch to the treadmill, put on weight easily, tend to be possessive, and are resistant to change.

Regardless of your body type, fibroids are thought to be the result of poor digestion. In Ayurveda, digestion is a complicated process involving the mind as well as the body. A healthy digestion influences *ojas* (also called *prana),* which is the rough equivalent of qi, the life force that keeps our bodies in balance.

How do you improve your digestion? Overall, it's a question of adjusting both mind and body. Depending on an analysis of your condition, an Ayurveda practitioner may recommend a detoxifying program that could include laxatives or enemas, Ayurvedic herbal remedies, and restorative techniques such as therapeutic massage, yoga, meditation, and sunbathing.

In addition to consulting an Ayurvedic practitioner, the authors of *A Woman's Best Medicine* recommend the following simple program to help detoxify your digestive system and bring your ojas back in balance:

○ Sip hot water throughout the day, plain or with lemon.
○ Eat a warm, cooked meal at lunchtime; this should be the largest meal of the day.
○ Take at least 20 minutes to eat each meal; if possible, eat in relaxed,

pleasant surroundings and sit for a few minutes after you've finished eating.

○ Have only liquids after 8 p.m.

Tapping into Your Chakras

The chakras are an energy system that, like Ayurveda, were defined by Hindu philosophers in India thousands of years ago. Seven chakras ascend from your groin to the crown of your head; each one is linked to specific parts of the body and different emotions, colors, and earth elements. Yoga was designed to release and stimulate *kundalini,* the energy that unblocks and balances the chakras.

The second chakra, called the sacral, is the one most related to the uterus. Located in the lower abdomen, the sacral chakra energizes a range of sensual forces—our creativity, our sexuality, our ability to be playful, our capacity for joy. Blocked or imbalanced energy in this chakra is thought to result in fibroids.

Chakra work can be done individually, with a partner, or with a therapist, and can involve both bodywork and meditation. Yoga postures that are associated with the second chakra, such as the Pelvic Lift, Triangle Pose, or Moon Pose, encourage circulation in the pelvic region and may help ease symptoms like bloating or fullness.

The color of the second chakra is orange. A meditation where you imagine breathing in bright orange light can help balance this chakra; orange foods and liquids are also thought to be strengthening.

The sacral chakra is also said to be the home of our inner child. If somehow in the past our inner child has been hurt, part of our creative or sexual growth may have been stifled, or misdirected in the form of other growths, such as fibroids. In working with the sacral chakra, you may be asked to recognize the emotions associated with your wounded child, such as fear, anxiety, anger, and frustration. Understanding the source of the energy block is the key to begin releasing it.

If you resonate with the idea of your wounded child, you may want to meditate on issues from your past that you can then let go of. More positively, you might want to get in touch with the playful side of that cute little girl you used to be, and see if the two of you can't go out and have some fun together.

Bringing Balance to Your Fibroid-Fighting Program

So, can alternative medicine play a part in helping treat our fibroids? As we've seen, the results are hard to calculate. The experience is empowering for many women but provides no satisfaction for others. Since so little is known about most of these therapies, it's wise to find out all you can about the therapy you'd like to pursue and the practitioner you plan to work with—just as you would with any type of medical procedure and doctor.

In *The Fibroid Book,* Dr. Francis L. Hutchins writes that he hasn't found any alternative remedies to be effective in preventing or treating fibroids. But, he says, "if you wish to try one of these alternative remedies, investigate it thoroughly and make sure that there is not a potential for serious side effects. Remember that long-term treatment with something that turns out to be ineffective could prevent you from having the benefit of known and effective treatment."

> **DR. DAVID OLIVE:** *A lot of the women I see are bright, they're accomplished, they read the medical literature, they're on the Internet, they're well versed in the latest randomized trials that we've had and all the different things that we do medically, and then they subject themselves to totally unscrutinized alternatives. And I always ask them, why don't you use the same amount of scrutiny for acupuncture or for vitamins that you do for myomectomy or GnRH agonists? The fact is, sometimes these things work and sometimes they don't—but I think everything has to be held to the same standard.*

Certainly, alternative medicine can make us feel good. It can make us feel like we're taking care of ourselves, and women often report that they feel better after using it whether or not there is an actual change in their condition.

Maybe you'd like to consider taking the best of both worlds. There's no rule that says alternative medicine and Western medicine can't work hand in hand—in fact, many people believe they can do just that. Perhaps we can then think of all types of medicine as "complementary," working together to heal our bodies, our spirits, and our way of life.

~7~

A Question of Estrogen

IN OUR BODIES, OUR MEDICINE CABINETS, OUR KITCHENS

ESTROGEN. IT GOES UP, it goes down. Its impact is biological, emotional, medical, financial, political. You may have heard people talk about estrogen the same way they do about a uterus: It's something you have, and after a certain age, it's something you don't have. But estrogen is far more elegant, more interesting, and more complex than that—just like us.

The word "estrogen" comes from the Latin word *oestrus,* which translates as "gadfly," "frenzy," or "inspiration." High levels of estrogen, especially in the second half of the menstrual cycle, have been shown to stimulate verbal fluency and creativity. The more scientists find out about estrogen, the more we know how truly "inspiring" it is, affecting our bones, brains, and blood vessels. It helps us cope with stress, metabolize food into energy, and maintain our reproductive systems. In fact, estrogen has powerful effects on just about every part of our bodies.

What's more, estrogen is not just one substance but a whole family of hormones, some stronger, some weaker. Our bodies make three major forms of estrogen. *Estradiol* is the most powerful, produced in the menstrual years by the ovaries; *estriol* reaches high levels during pregnancy; *estrone,* made by fat cells, becomes the dominant estrogen after menopause. Beyond these, we make at least 17 other forms of estrogen.

Estrogen doesn't just show up in our bodies. There are also medical compounds that are designed to work like estrogen, plant estrogens (phytoestrogens), animal estrogens, and chemical synthetics that mimic estrogen if we ingest them, which we do, all the time. If you add them all up, scientists have identified more than 200 different kinds of estrogen, all of which can—and do—affect our fibroids.

But estrogen doesn't work in a vacuum. It interacts with the other hormones in our bodies, including progesterone, follicle-stimulating hormone (FSH), and thyroid-stimulating hormone, to name just a few. Some doctors think that the growth of fibroids isn't necessarily the result of too much estrogen alone, but comes from an imbalance of estrogen and progesterone, interaction between estrogen and progesterone, or even how both hormones activate other natural chemicals in our bodies. And those are just some of the possibilities, since scientists are exploring the role of numerous hormones in the growth of fibroids. But for now, estrogen is the one we know most about—and it pays to know as much as possible.

Our Bodies, Our Estrogen

As you know, one of the buzzwords in women's health is *perimenopause,* which describes the time before menopause. For some of us, that time starts in our thirties, for others, in our forties. Perimenopause is not a medical condition; it's a stage in our evolution from birth to older age. But for those of us who have fibroids, the changes occurring in our bodies during perimenopause may be significant.

At some point in our adult lives—usually not a convenient point, in case you were wondering—our estrogen levels start to fluctuate. What happens is this: From the time you began to menstruate, your brain has been sending a messenger called FSH to the ovaries every month when your period ends. The message says, hey there, estrogen's down, time to make more. And thus begins your next menstrual cycle.

As we get older, the ovaries need more of a wake-up call than they used to. The brain figures this out and sends more FSH than it did before. More FSH makes the ovaries produce more estrogen; higher levels of both FSH and estrogen can make your fibroids grow bigger. You also may get more bleeding, since estrogen stimulates blood flow to the uterus, and FSH dilates blood vessels.

Then there's progesterone, the other big part of the hormonal equation. Doctors believe that progesterone may neutralize the effects of estrogen on your fibroids, but progesterone levels start going down right around the same time that your estrogen levels go up. With less progesterone available, your body has more "unopposed" estrogen to fuel those fibroids.

The net result is that fibroids may go through growth spurts, and any symptoms you have may become more noticeable. In some cases, this may concern you enough to consider surgery; the options are discussed in Chapter 5. Other women consider herbal remedies or other alternative therapies; these are reviewed in Chapter 6. You may also want to consider the destressing benefits of meditation, journal writing, or other soothing strategies; we'll talk about these in Chapter 12.

Sooner or later, our hormones stop doing the jitterbug and settle down to a stately stroll. After we stop ovulating, our ovaries still churn out a small amount of estrogen: about 10 percent of premenopause levels. While only the smallest fibroids might disappear after menopause, larger ones don't grow and sometimes shrink.

DR. STANLEY WEST: *In her forties, a woman's estrogen/progesterone hormonal milieu is changing. At age 20, or age 30, your estrogen level rises, you ovulate around mid-cycle, your progesterone rises and depresses the estrogen level. Somewhere in your forties, things begin to change: The estrogen level still rises, but progesterone doesn't rise as much because progesterone is the first to wane. It still depresses the estrogen, but not as much as it used to. And so a woman now has a relative increase in her estrogen production: The absolute amount of estrogen is gradually falling as she approaches menopause, but instead of producing it for two weeks, she produces it for four. And so there can be a "rapid growth" of fibroids.*

Power Surge

THERE ARE CERTAIN benefits to the evolution of our hormones: That energy surge that many of us feel when we turn 40 may be due in part to raised estrogen levels that can be as high as—or higher than—they were when we were twenty. Dr. Susan Love calls this stage of our lives "puberty in reverse." But this time you don't have to ask Mom for the car keys.

Sorting Out the HRT Options

HRT is the term generally used for any form of hormone replacement therapy, but in fact, there are three families of HRT: those made with synthetic estrogen alone *(ERT)*; those that combine synthetic estrogen with progestin, a progesterone-like drug; and those that don't rely on estrogen at all. There's also a group of drugs called *selective estrogen receptor moderators* (SERMs); we'll discuss those in just a moment.

Once we reach menopause, millions of American women take some form of prescription HRT, and many women swear by it. However, the latest available research, from a comprehensive, long-term study by the Women's Health Initiative (WHI), concluded very clearly that women should only use HRT for the shortest possible time; long-term use of any form of HRT is not recommended. (The women in these studies are now participating in a follow-up phase, which will last until 2010.)

All of this will no doubt factor into your decision about whether to start HRT, or continue taking it. HRT remains an option: the decision to take it still depends to a large degree on your own assessment of

Weighing the Risks of ERT/HRT

ESTROGEN REPLACEMENT CAN give you many of the benefits of natural estrogen. But before you get too excited, remember that you have to weigh and balance the not-so-good effects of any type of hormone replacement therapy.

o If you have any of the following conditions, synthetic estrogen may make them worse: liver disease, gallbladder disease, diabetes, migraines, high blood pressure, high blood levels of triglycerides, endometriosis, heart disease, breast nodules, or fibroids.

o Estrogen replacement increases your risk for breast cancer, uterine cancer, ovarian cancer, lupus, and blood clots. It may also increase your risk for asthma, skin cancer, lung cancer, vaginal cancer, and liver cancer.

o The side effects of estrogen replacement can include fluid retention, breast tenderness, cramps, nausea, and dark spots on your skin.

o Progestins in HRT can increase your risk of blood clots and cause fluid retention, breast tenderness, jaundice, nausea, insomnia, and depression. You may also find that menstrual bleeding returns.

the risks, your concerns about aging, and how you feel physically. In addition to risks associated with your fibroids, you may have other conditions, such as a family history of breast cancer, that might make you decide not to take HRT.

As you might expect with something as intimate and individual as estrogen, women with fibroids who decide to take HRT have different experiences. Some have slow increases in the size of their fibroids, or intermittent bleeding, while others see little or no change at all

The scientific findings to date about HRT and fibroids are still a bit murky. One researcher noted recently that "The effect of HRT on fibroids in postmenopausal women is obviously a complicated issue resolvable only by future well-controlled studies." Still, we can start drawing some conclusions from the information that is available.

To begin with, women who have fibroids are generally warned against taking estrogen alone. For instance, the maker of Estrace, a popular drug made from a synthetic form of estradiol, the most potent of our natural estrogens, cautions women who have fibroids (among other conditions) that "You may not be able to take Estrace, or you may require a dosage adjustment or special monitoring during treatment." An identical warning appears in the consumer information for Premarin, another leading estrogen replacement.

A combination of synthetic estrogen with a progesterone-like drug (progestin) is a better bet for women with fibroids. For one thing, this formula imitates our natural mix of hormones better than an estrogen-only drug; some doctors caution that women with fibroids should only take the minimum amount of progestin needed.

There are types of HRT that don't rely on estrogen replacement at all. Tibolone (Livial), for instance, doesn't include estrogen-like drugs; one test of tibolone in postmenopausal women with asymptomatic fibroids showed that it caused less bleeding than an estrogen replacement.

Researchers have also found that how you take HRT might make a difference. Several studies suggest that HRT pills don't make fibroids grow larger (they don't shrink, either), unlike injections, which increased both the size and number of fibroids. Information on how HRT patches (the kind you wear on your skin) affect fibroids is mixed.

Another interesting note: A three-year study of women with fibroids concluded that HRT increased the size of fibroids, but only for two years. In the third year, the fibroids starting shrinking. Go figure.

If you decide to take any type of hormone replacement, talk to your doctor about how often you should get a checkup. At a minimum, doctors suggest one exam per year, including an ultrasound, to measure your fibroids and check for any precancerous changes.

JANIS: *I began estrogen replacement therapy the morning after my hysterectomy—(Estrace, 1 milligram)—so I had no symptoms. I never had any feelings other than euphoria, and I continue to feel that way. I have had no trouble with the Estrace—no mood swings, no hot flashes, nothing unpleasant at all.*

FELICE: *I think it's unfortunate how naive and lazy many women can be about learning about their bodies and their medical options. There was just an ad on TV for estrogen replacement therapy that creates the atmosphere of fear of menopause and that you are doomed to suffer and die a horrible death if you don't get on hormones and that menopause is an unnatural and unnecessary event in a woman s life.*

SERMs

Selective estrogen receptor moderators, or SERMs, are the latest wave of ERT. Also called "designer estrogens," they attempt to send estrogen to the places in your body where it can theoretically do the most good, like your bones, heart, and blood vessels, and keep it from going to your breasts and uterus, where extra estrogen can cause problems. While several types of SERMs are being explored, the two most in use today are raloxifene, prescribed primarily for postmenopausal symptoms, and tamoxifen, which is prescribed primarily to treat beast cancer. Both drugs have shown both a number of benefits, and the potential for serious problems.

As far as fibroids are concerned, raloxifene doesn't appear to increase the size of fibroids, and in some cases, has made fibroids shrink. In laboratory tests, raloxifene shrank fibroids by up to 50 percent. The potential for SERMs as a specific treatment for fibroids, however, is largely unexplored.

> Despite the hip term that is used to describe these drugs, which implies that taking them is no more hazardous than wearing a pair of expensive jeans, much about designer estrogens remains unknown.
> —ROBIN MARANTZ HENIG,
> AUTHOR OF *HOW A WOMAN AGES*

A Cautionary Tale

When Evista, a brand name for raloxifene, was first approved by the FDA in 1997, the product safety information stated that Evista is "not associated with an increased risk for cancer." However, a blistering article in the *Chicago Tribune* alleged that Eli Lilly and Company failed to mention—in both its ads and consumer warning literature—that Evista induced ovarian cancer in animal trials. According to the article, "Lilly's suppression of its own evidence is reckless and threatening to women's health and life. Equally reckless is FDA's December, 1997, marketing clearance. . . ."

As it turns out, the *Trib* was right: the results of the animal studies did show an increased risk of ovarian cancer. Today, that information is included in Evista's patient literature, allowing women—and their doctors—to make an informed decision about the benefits and risks.

In general, manufacturers are (slowly) realizing that consumers want to know all the available information about the drugs we're considering—so that, along with our doctors, we can make intelligent decisions about our health care. For now, to quote Dr. Susan Love, "remember that any time someone tells you they have developed something that sounds too good to be true, it probably is." Read about any new drugs carefully—and don't always believe the very first things you hear.

LEONIE: *My mother had passed away at age 69 with early-onset Alzheimer's, which, as I'm sure you know, is believed to have a genetic basis. Her uncle had also apparently suffered from this. When the new reports regarding HRT having a beneficial effect in slowing the start of Alzheimer's began to come out, I told my gynecologist about my mother's history and that I wanted to go on HRT when I reached menopause. She told me that I should have a hysterectomy if I wanted to use HRT in the future, as the HRT would cause other fibroids to grow.*

ANGELA: *I started taking estrogen a few weeks after my hysterectomy. I'm taking the standard dosage and don't have any problems.*

Plant Estrogens: Do Carrots Have Cravings?

Lest you think, as I did, that only warm-blooded creatures—and our associated pharmaceutical companies—produce estrogen, at least 300 plants produce something called *phytoestrogens* (literally "plant estrogens"). Phytoestrogens are much weaker than our own estrogen or even synthetic estrogens, but they have a similar chemical structure, so they can fool our estrogen receptors into thinking they're the real thing.

Can phytoestrogens help reduce our fibroids? The answer depends on your stage of life.

Before perimenopause, phytoestrogens can help reduce the amount of estrogen in our systems by blocking access to some estrogen receptors; since the "real" estrogen can't get into the blocked receptors, our overall estrogen levels go down. As a result, there may be less estrogen available to feed our fibroids.

During perimenopause, as we saw earlier, estrogen levels fluctuate much more than usual, and declining progesterone levels may make the effect more pronounced. By experimenting with phytoestrogen-rich foods, you may be able to tone down the effects of all those "power surges"—and help reduce or prevent growth spurts in your fibroids.

On the other hand, it is possible to overdo. Even though phytoestrogens are natural, too much can have unintended effects. If you stick to phytoestrogens in food form, such as soy, you'd pretty much have to eat all phyto all the time to hurt your system, but supplements and herbs often marketed as "natural HRT" can be very potent and should only be taken after consulting with a qualified nutritionist, naturopath, homeopath, or doctor of Chinese medicine.

Once you've reached menopause, and the amount of natural estrogen in your system is waning, phytoestrogens can provide a mild form of estrogen. On the other hand, if you're on any form of HRT, too many phytoestrogens can block the effect. The same cautions about working with a qualified health care practitioner apply for any herbs or supplements you'd like to explore at this stage of life.

Food with a 'Tude

COMMON SOURCES OF phytoestrogens include garlic, parsley, soybeans, whole wheat, brown rice and other whole grains, flax-seed, beans, carrots, potatoes, dates, pomegranates, cherries, and apples.

If you'd like to see which foods can affect your estrogen, check out Chapter 8, "Nothing to Eat but Food." For herbs and supplements, see Chapter 6, "But Wait, There's More."

Chemical Warfare

In addition to natural estrogens, which our bodies have spent thousands of years adapting to, there are hundreds—if not thousands—of substances that have been introduced into our environment in the last 75 years or so that have estrogen-like effects on our bodies.

Unlike plant estrogens, which dissolve in water and don't accumulate in our bodies, chemical estrogens dissolve in fat—both animal fat and ours—where they settle in and stay put; the effects of some of these chemicals can last as long as 20 years. These chemicals have come under scrutiny for their effect on wildlife and humans, and if you wonder whether they can be one of the reasons behind your fibroids, the answer is, oh yes.

THE ABCS OF DDT, PCBS, AND APES

The danger of synthetic chemicals certainly isn't news. FDR was president when scientists first found out that some synthetic chemicals could mimic estrogens. Ike and Mamie were in the White House when DDT turned out to be estrogenic. (It would take another 22 years before the use of DDT would be "restricted" as a pesticide.) And JFK was in office when Rachel Carson published *Silent Spring,* describing how synthetic chemicals were contaminating our water and soil. These chemicals, she wrote, were causing severe health problems, especially in species at the top of the food chain—including us.

Despite these early warning signs, the manufacture and use of synthetic chemicals has exploded. Today there are over 100,000 man-made chemicals used in virtually every industry, everywhere in the world. Scientists agree that many of these chemicals are *endocrine disrupters* or *xenoestrogens* (foreign estrogens).

We're exposed to synthetic estrogens in food, water, plastics, and numerous other substances. One of the big problems with these chemicals is that they're sturdy. Even when they're banned, as PCBs (another estrogenic chemical) were in the United States in 1977, they still show up in the food chain almost two decades later.

This is how chemical estrogens can affect our bodies and our fibroids:

○ Since they're stored in our body fat, they can be released at any time, often when we're under stress or when we diet. Tests show that some of these chemicals can spur dramatic uterine growth.
○ Some xenoestrogens mimic estradiol, the strongest type of natural estrogen, raising our estrogen levels.
○ Some may alter our very DNA; this effect may be passed down to our daughters—and granddaughters.
○ Some of these chemicals depress thyroid hormone function. A healthy thyroid is essential to help the liver process estrogen out of our bodies.

> Our bodies reflect or participate in the world's body,
> so that if we harm that outer body, our own bodies
> will feel the effects. Essentially there is no difference
> between the world's body and the human body.
> —THOMAS MOORE, *CARE OF THE SOUL*

Phyto v. Chemical Estrogens at a Glance

Phytoestrogens	Chemical estrogens
Water soluble (disperse in water)	Fat soluble (disperse in fat)
Are eliminated quickly from the body	Stay in the body
May cause reproductive problems if consumed in very large amounts (up to 100% of the diet)	May cause reproductive problems if consumed in even tiny amounts
Found in plants	Found in some pesticides, industrial chemicals, detergents, plastics; also in some meat, poultry, and dairy (see Chapter 8).

Scientists have been raising new warnings about xenoestrogens and their effects on women, including the risk of fibroids, since at least 1993. According to the Tulane/Xavier Center for Bioenvironmental Research, environmental estrogens may cause a wide range of problems, including fibroids, breast cancer, uterine and ovarian cancer, fibrocystic breast disease, polycystic ovarian syndrome, endometriosis, and pelvic inflammatory disease. (Environmental estrogens affect men too, and may be a factor in low sperm counts, testicular cancer, prostate disease, and other abnormal conditions.) In testimony before the Senate Committee on Labor and Human Resources in 1996, government scientists confirmed that these environmental compounds may play a role in a wide range of diseases, including fibroids and cancers of the breast, uterus, and ovaries.

In laboratory studies, certain pesticides seemed to stimulate fibroid growth. Human studies in the 1980s showed that women with fibroids had "significantly higher" levels of DDT in their blood; fibroids also had higher concentrations of DDT than surrounding tissue. A lot more work is being done on how chemicals in the environment affect our fibroids: there's even been a scientific conference devoted to the subject.

Despite the evidence, the U.S. government doesn't require tests to find out if chemicals are xenoestrogens, nor has it banned any but a handful of chemicals, like DDT and PCBs. Unfortunately, even these are still in use elsewhere in the world; the effects reach us through wind and water as well as in some imported products. Although DDT concentrations in people in the United States fell after restrictions were imposed in 1972, the decline has leveled off.

> The American people have a right to know the substances
> to which they and their children are being exposed and to
> know everything that science can tell us about the hazards.
> —AL GORE

LAURA: *I got a book that talks about chemicals and dioxins and all these things, so now when I walk behind a bus I hold my breath. Nobody likes fumes, but I'm thinking, will I be able to have kids? And when I walk into the building and they've just cleaned . . . you know? It's something I'm aware of every day.*

When I started reading about the problems that xenoestrogens can cause—and all the many, many places they lurk in our daily lives—my first reaction was to lower the blinds and hide, or maybe move to Maine and start doing some organic farming. Well, Maine is beautiful, but I don't like farming. The fact is, this is the world we live in.

As with any kind of potential health risk, many factors influence whether we may feel the effects—or if we do, how severely. If you have young children living with you, it may be more important to protect them as best you can, since evidence suggests we're more susceptible to environmental estrogens when we're young. If you're pregnant, environmental estrogens may influence whether a daughter will develop fibroids, among other things.

Minimizing Your Exposure

How can you minimize your—and your family's—exposure to xeno-estrogens? Take a look at the list below for some simple ways to start.

In the kitchen:

o Eat lower on the food chain to limit intake of fatty foods and foods exposed to toxins; meat and dairy may contain high levels of persistent chemicals.

o If you eat fish, choose farm-raised fish, or smaller, younger, wild fish; all of these are typically exposed to fewer toxins. Dr. Andrew Weil recommends limiting consumption of shellfish and avoiding freshwater fish as well as big ocean fish such as swordfish, marlin, and shark.

o Consider buying more pesticide-free, organically produced foods; you can ask your grocer to consider stocking more of these items, or there may be a natural foods store in your area.

o Wash fruits and vegetables carefully.

o Microwave food in glass or ceramic dishes instead of plastic.

o Try to avoid storing food in direct contact with plastic wrap.

o If you can, limit your use of canned foods.

o Consider filtering your water at home.

Around the house:

o Wash your hands frequently, and encourage your children to do the same.

o Try to avoid plastic toys for your children, especially if they're at the age when they chew on them.

o Consider using tempered glass bottles instead of plastic for feeding babies.

o Try using nontoxic cleansers. One key ingredient to watch out for and avoid if possible: alkylphenol ethoxylates (APEs).

Outdoors:

o Use nonchemical pesticides for insect problems around your home, in public areas, on pets.
o Golf courses may use as much as four times more pesticide per acre than farms. If you're a golfer, find out if that's the case on your local course, and try to remember to keep your hands away from your mouth while golfing.

If you're interested in making changes that can help limit your exposure to xenoestrogens, check the Resources section for books and organizations that deal specifically with this issue. This is also an area crying out for consumer activism; if that's something that you're interested in, I've also listed some organizations you can contact.

Learning Our Lessons: DES

DES (short for "diethylstilbestrol," a synthetic estrogen) was a "wonder drug" given to pregnant women to prevent miscarriage; it was prescribed from the late 1940s until it was banned in 1971. If you're a "DES daughter"—someone who was exposed to the chemical in the womb—it may be one of the reasons behind your fibroids.

More than 30 years later, research has shown that DES increased the risk of fibroids (as well as even more serious problems) in the girls—now women—who were exposed. More chilling, DES exposure can alter the very cells and molecules of a developing fetus—allowing the damage to pass down from one generation to another.

Even if you weren't exposed, the DES experience offers some food for thought. As one of the first "designer estrogens," DES was considered safe for over 30 years, yet it was eventually proven to be too dangerous for consumption (though it was still given to animals for a number of years after it was banned for humans). Although DES is now banned in the United States, it raises the question of whether other synthetic estrogens may be affecting us so deeply that they could affect not only ourselves but our children—and our grandchildren.

As a DES daughter myself, I find the thought sobering.

Teach Your Children Well

If you have fibroids, you may pass on the tendency to your daughters. But even without a genetic predisposition, there's evidence that some of the seeds for fibroids and other diseases lie in what we were exposed to as children; like DES, many environmental estrogens can affect young children. So is there anything you can do to minimize the chances that your children will develop fibroids later in life? The answer is yes.

Certainly if you're pregnant, or plan to be, it's important to minimize your exposure to xenoestrogens. In 1995, the National Institute of Environmental Health Sciences said the risk of fibroids—as well as infertility, endometriosis, and other reproductive problems—could be increased by exposure to endocrine-disrupting chemicals "during early development, neonatally, or later in life."

Many diseases—fibroids included—are thought to be a combination of both genetic tendencies and environmental exposure. Consider limiting your children's exposure to plastics, pesticides, and other substances that can have estrogenic effects, and teach them good eating and exercise habits. Your contribution to your children's health from the earliest ages may protect your daughters from getting fibroids as adults—and may keep both your daughters and your sons healthy in all kinds of ways later in life.

～8～

Nothing to Eat but Food

EVALUATING YOUR DIET AND LIFESTYLE CHOICES

CAN THE RIGHT diet help relieve the symptoms of fibroids—or even make them shrink? What about vitamins, exercise—or even enough fresh air and sunshine?

It can be a powerful feeling, a nice feeling, to make choices that are good for you and bad for your fibroids. It can give you a greater sense of control over your body—especially important if having fibroids makes you feel like your body has a mind of its own. And deciding to eat a tomato or go skating is a lot cheaper and easier than relying on medicine or resorting to surgery.

Now, I'm not going to tell you that food can cure your fibroids, or that a run in the park will stop your symptoms. First of all, there's no hard scientific data that shows how food and lifestyle choices affect your fibroids—although that may change after the National Institute of Environmental Health completes its Uterine Fibroid Growth study. (Keep an eye on the Harvard Nurses' Health Study, too; they may look at the link between food and fibroids sometime in the future.)

But there are lots of reasons to believe that some foods are better than others, and some lifestyle choices can make a positive difference in the life of women with fibroids. Making a big difference may require making big changes, but you may find that even smaller changes can leave you feeling better.

Food Fight! Fibroids and Your Diet

For a few years, my mom called me every few days with the latest news about how what I ate could kill me. One day it was toast (the burned parts contain carcinogens), another time it was coffee (I think rats had drowned in a vat of it in some research lab), another time there was some problem reported about the white part of the orange peel. No, I have no idea what that was about. And let's not leave out the national roller-coaster ride about good fats, bad fats, carbs, and how an entire nation of French people can enjoy butter, cheese, and enormous amounts of wine without ever gaining an ounce.

So it was easy to throw up my hands and just eat what seemed healthy. Plus chocolate and ice cream. (Hey, they're brain food!) But if we are what we eat, it turns out that fibroids are even more so. They can grow in response to foods that help create higher estrogen levels in our bodies, and they may shrink in response to a diet that starves them of what they crave.

Now, if you and your fibroids happen to love some of the same foods (which I guarantee you will), you may get frustrated by the idea that you have to completely overhaul your diet. And treating food as medicine, something to be weighed and measured and practically prescribed, can take the joy out of one of our fundamental pleasures in life.

If you want to try changing what you eat based on the information here, try eliminating one food at a time, or changing one habit. On the other hand, if you have the will of a warrior (and I know some of you do), I salute you. You'll see how a focused effort may, over time, make a difference in the size of your fibroids and your symptoms.

FOODS YOUR FIBROIDS FEED ON

Many of the diet issues for fibroids are similar to those you've probably heard from your doctor or in popular diet books. So you probably won't be surprised to learn that dairy products, red meat and poultry, fats, sugar, caffeine, alcohol, and food additives are things to avoid when you're dealing with fibroids. Let's look at how they affect not just our weight and overall health but also our little fibroid friends.

> KIM: *Even though my fibroids were substantial, they weren't interfering in any way, they weren't bothering me. But I went to an acupuncturist and she said you can shrink them, but it's one of the hardest things to do and it requires a major change of diet.*
>
> *I was already a vegetarian so I always ate pretty well, but I always ate a lot of sugar. Not a lot of dairy, but I did eat some. I use soy milk. I don't drink caffeine. She thought I should go on a macrobiotic diet, combined with herbs and progesterone cream. But I think I want instant results and of course fibroids don't shrink right away, it takes a very long time and I wasn't committed to the change, going macrobiotic. She said it could take two years, at least. And now that it's four years later, I should have done it! But there were no guarantees.*

> ANITA: *I asked if diet affects fibroids and I was told no.*

Dairy Products

Through no fault of Flossie, Bossie, or Elsie, milk and many milk products seem to be on the minus side of the fibroid and food equation. (I say this despite my deep and powerful affection for Ben & Jerry's Vanilla Heath Bar Crunch.)

Both Dr. Christiane Northrup and Dr. Susan Lark advise women with fibroids to avoid dairy products made from cow's milk, since they can lead to higher levels of both estrogen and prostaglandins, the hormone that helps cause cramps.

In Eastern cultures, milk products are considered very "yin," as are sugar and alcohol. Since fibroids are considered partly the result of having too much "yin," Eastern tradition suggests that dairy foods can overload your system.

Do you have to give up every kind of dairy food? Not necessarily. Ann Chopelas, a chemist at the University of Washington, says that nonfat yogurt, cheese, and milk products are safe bets because they don't contain *arachidonic acid,* the type of fat that produces prostaglandins. She also suggests that small quantities of Parmesan, mozzarella, and shelf milk are fine, as are sheep's cheese (such as feta or Romano), goat cheese, and yogurt.

Now, apart from the natural properties of cow's milk, there may be another problem. In the United States, about one-third of our nine million dairy cows are given something called *bovine growth hormone* (BGH) to promote milk production. The problem? BGH produces a hormone called *insulin-like growth factor-1*, which may have a role in fibroid growth, as well as in prostate cancer and breast cancer.

According to the FDA, milk from treated cows is "safe for human consumption," so much so that products made from BGH-treated cow's milk aren't labeled as such. But there's a wrinkle: The FDA's approval relied largely on information from the Monsanto Corporation, the company that sells BGH.

Canada, a country that clearly cares about its milk, investigated unpublished documents and found that BGH was absorbed into the bloodstream of almost a third of the animals that Monsanto studied in lab tests. In January 1999 the Canadian government decided not to approve the use of BGH. The FDA takes strong issue with the Canadian findings. But until dairy food producers start including BGH on their labels, you might want to try calling your dairy company to find out if they are selling BGH-treated products, or consider buying organic dairy products.

KATI: *I eat a good diet. Lots of chicken, fish, and veggies, and not much red meat. Ice cream is my weakness, but I know it's not good for my hormonal levels so I'll have it maybe once a month. I don't really miss it like I thought I would: I've integrated the changes over a three-year period.*

DONNA: *I went to someone who was an MD and also holistic—he talked about a variety of things you could do for your fibroids, including diet modification that might reduce them, especially eliminating dairy products. Probably if I were a better person I would have done that, because it was a nonsurgical alternative, but he couldn't tell me how much the fibroids would shrink or if they would shrink, and it would take a year before seeing any results.*

Meat and Poultry

Many animals raised for food in the United States are treated with drugs called *anabolic steroids* to make them bigger. The FDA, as well as two separate groups of international scientists, report that the level of drugs used is no threat to humans—even children. So why do we need to question whether eating treated meat or chicken is safe?

While the FDA maintains that any extra hormones are excreted before the animals are slaughtered, scientists tell us that when animals ingest any kind of substance like antibiotics, pesticides, and growth hormones, these substances accumulate in the fat. Some of these chemicals may have estrogen-like effects, as we saw in Chapter 7. If we eat treated animals, the fat in our own bodies accumulates these substances.

A study in Italy found that women with fibroids tend to eat more meat, including beef, other red meat, and ham; these women also ate fewer green vegetables, fruit, and fish than women without fibroids. The researchers weren't sure if the women with fibroids were getting too much estrogen and fat from meat, or too few phytoestrogens from vegetables.

We do need protein, and not all of us are cut out to be vegetarians. If you don't want to or can't cut out meat and meat products, consider cutting down. These three tips may also help when you choose to eat meat:

o Select lean meat or skinless poultry.
o Broil or grill meat until well done to help cook out any remaining fat, and don't use the drippings.
o Look for organically raised meat to avoid the steroids that may be present in commercially raised meat.

The Facts on Fats

Fat is one complicated subject, so sit tight.

It starts off simply enough: There are only two basic kinds of dietary fat, saturated and unsaturated. Saturated fats tend to be in animal foods, while unsaturated fats tend to show up in plants and seafood. Unsaturated fat is divided into two types: monounsaturated (also called omega-9) and polyunsaturated. And then, just to make life interesting, polyunsaturated fat is divided into three groups: omega-6, omega-3, and trans fats.

Still with me? Good. Millions (maybe billions) of words have been written about fat—but how does fat relate to fibroids?

o Fat from animal products is where any toxins or extra hormones may be stored for convenient transfer to your body.
o Fat can raise cholesterol levels; cholesterol can convert into estrogen, raising your overall estrogen levels.
o Saturated and polyunsaturated fats are easily oxidized into "free radicals," which may weaken your immune system.
o Omega-6 and trans fats produce prostaglandins, which can cause cramps.

But on the plus side . . .

o Omega-3 fats produce antiprostaglandins, which can help control pain.
o In animal studies, olive and canola (monounsaturated) oils didn't promote tumor growth the way polyunsaturated fats did.

DR. STANLEY WEST: *Cholesterol is a fat. Estrogen is made from cholesterol. So if you decrease fat and cholesterol and so forth in your diet, you will at least slow the growth of the fibroids.*

But fat is everywhere, so let's be realistic. Most sources suggest keeping fats of all kinds down to 30 percent or less of your total calories. Dr. Andrew Weil recommends focusing on the healthier omega-3 fats and keeping your fat consumption between 44 and 67 grams a day (as part of a 2,000-calorie diet). Of all the fats we eat, saturated and trans fats are the ones to consider minimizing. Of course, those are the ones that are hardest for most of us to give up, showing up as they do in fries, pizza, tacos, ice cream, cheese, and every kind of meat and poultry. But if you want to reduce your intake of these fats, check labels, avoid fried foods, choose skim or fat-free dairy products, and in general try to keep these foods to a minimum.

The following chart shows the different types of fats and common food sources. As you'll see, the fats are divided into three categories: The Good, The Not-So-Bad, and The Ugly. You'll also notice that some foods fall into more than one category. Use your judgment, and if you want to cut down fats in your diet, err toward the middle and left side of the chart.

Fats

The Good	The Not-So-Bad	The Ugly
Omega-3 fatty acids, found in salmon, tuna, rainbow trout, mackerel, herring, sable, whitefish, eel, sardines, bluefish, swordfish, haddock, rabbit, wild game, flaxseeds and flaxseed oil, walnuts and walnut oil, leafy greens, fish oil supplements, canola oil	**Monounsaturated fats,** found in olive, canola, sesame, and peanut oils, high-oleic sunflower seed oil, high-oleic safflower seed oil, almonds, olives, avocado, hazelnuts and macadamia nuts, chicken, beef, pork

Omega-6 fatty acids, found in corn, safflower, sunflower, cottonseed, soybean, and sesame oils, blue-green algae, evening primrose oil, blackcurrant oil | **Saturated fats,** found in animal products such as meat, chicken with the skin, regular milk, cheese, ice cream, eggs, butter, and coconut, palm, and cottonseed oils

Trans fats, found in partially hydrogenated oil, margarine, vegetable shortening, commercial baked goods, fried foods, many fast foods, and most prepared snacks, mixes, and convenience foods |

Sugar and Spice and Everything Nice

If sugar were only in lollipops and birthday cake, it would be so easy to smile sweetly, say no thanks, and move on. But there it is, in so much of what we eat, either as processed sugar or, more subtly, as carbohydrates in bread, pasta, potatoes, rice, and fruit. Too much sugar may take its toll on us and our fibroids in four ways:

○ Too much sugar raises insulin levels. Extra insulin decreases something called *sex hormone–binding globulin,* which binds free estrogen. Less of this hormone means more estrogen circulating in your bloodstream.
○ Extra insulin has been traditionally associated with weight gain, and extra body fat may increase your circulating estrogen.
○ Sugar reduces levels of vitamin B, which can make it harder for your liver to process estrogen out of your body.
○ Sugar depletes our bodies of the nutrients needed to keep our immune systems intact.

But the idea is not to eliminate sugar. First of all, most of us probably can't. Second of all, feeling deprived is not part of the recipe for feeling good. And unless you're diabetic or at risk, the benefits of eating moderate amounts of foods like fruit or even pasta outweigh the effects of the sugars they contain.

But if we're anything like the "average American," whoever she is, we consume something like our body weight (120–160 pounds) of sugar every year. And how sobering is that? If you want to consider reducing the amount of sugar in your diet, here are a few suggestions:

○ Think about reducing your intake of refined sugar, the kind in candy, cookies—you know, the good stuff.
○ Remember that there's a lot of sugar in regular soda, regular fruit juice, juice drinks, and sweetened tea and coffee.
○ Consider cutting back on white-flour products in favor of whole-grain foods.
○ When you eat complex carbohydrates, try eating them along with some protein and vegetables; eating carbohydrates as part of a balanced meal can slow down insulin production.
○ Think about it: Are sugary foods your "comfort food" when you're stressed or sad? It so, maybe you can pick a healthier alternative—and have it in the kitchen for when those cravings hit.

o If by any chance you need another incentive to exercise, know that
  it can help keep your insulin levels in check.

Coffee, Booze, and Red Dye #3

I happen to love the taste of coffee. And have I mentioned chocolate?
Caffeine—whether in coffee, tea, sodas, or chocolate—is a controversial substance, but even heavy caffeine use doesn't seem to have more
than a slight impact on fibroids. Still, there are a few indirect ways that
caffeine may affect fibroid-related symptoms. Though the information
that's available isn't definitive, you may want to consider this:

o Drinking a lot of caffeine can interfere with how well your liver
  functions; it can also aggravate fibroid-related cramps.
o Drinking coffee or tea after eating can reduce the amount of non-
  heme iron your body can absorb; this is important to know if you're
  anemic.
o Drinking four to five cups of coffee a day can increase your stress
  levels; we'll talk about how stress can affect your fibroids later in
  the chapter.

Green tea contains some caffeine, but there's more and more evidence piling up that it has a number of general health benefits. Herbal
teas don't contain caffeine.

Are you a fan of an after-work margarita now and then? You
should know that consuming alcohol increases the risk of fibroids,
especially—I kid you not—drinking beer.

In a four-year study of 22,000 women, those who drank one beer
a week had an 11 percent higher chance of developing fibroids; seven
beers a week increased a woman's risk for fibroids 57 percent over her
teetotaling peers.

So if you don't drink, you're ahead of the game. Most of us know
that alcohol is bad for the liver, and as we've seen, being kind to your
liver is a key component in keeping your estrogen levels down. If
your fibroids are causing cramps, fatigue, or bleeding, alcohol can
make them worse. But if your fibroids aren't bothering you, enjoying

an occasional drink shouldn't hurt, as long as it's part of a generally healthful diet—see the chart on page 198 for a tip sheet to see
how you can balance what you eat and drink to work against your
fibroids.

Additives, preservatives, artificial coloring, artificial flavoring, and
artificial sweeteners are tough to avoid. They're in just about everything you don't cook yourself from scratch. At least one may have a
direct impact on fibroids: Dr. Chopelas reports that aspartame, the
ingredient in popular sugar substitutes, has been linked to increased
incidence of tumors in the uterus as well as the brain and pancreas.
It's pretty doubtful that any of these products will kill us, but if you
eat a lot of prepared or processed foods, you might want to consider
putting them on your "buy less often" list.

And Now for Something Completely Different

So what changes can you think about making in your diet that don't
involve cutting foods out? You can include lots of things. Delicious
stuff, fun stuff. Oh, and lots of water. Let's eat.

Soy Ahoy

In the *Fibroid Tumors & Endometriosis Self Help Book,* Dr. Susan
Lark tells us that soy foods "have been found to help reduce bleeding
problems" in women with fibroids. Why? According to Jane Brody,
author of *The New York Times Book of Health,* soy foods include
something called *genistein* that, at least in tests, blocked the growth
of new blood vessels.

Soy may have an even more protective effect. As we saw in Chapter
7, some plants—soy in particular—contain phytoestrogens (plant
estrogens). Phytoestrogens are much weaker than our estrogen or
even synthetic estrogens, but they have a similar chemical structure,
so they can block the absorption of "real" estrogen into our systems,
even though plant estrogens themselves don't have a strong estrogenic
effect on our bodies.

The benefits of eating soy got yet another a boost from a 1997 study

Getting Started on Your Fibroid-Fighting Diet

HERE'S A LITTLE GUIDE to the foods and drinks that you might want to consider cutting down or avoiding, and those that you might want to include more of, in a fibroid-fighting diet.

Keep an eye on...	Think about including...
Dairy products, especially cow's milk	Soy foods, including tofu, tempeh, soy milk, soy ice cream, and soy yogurts
Meat and chicken	Fish, especially salmon and tuna
High-fat foods, including pizza, fries, burgers, tacos	Olive oil, canola oil
Carbohydrates, especially food made with white flour, like white bread, pasta, cookies, and cakes	Complex carbohydrates, found in whole grains, beans, vegetables, and fruit
Sugar	Fiber, found in beans, pears, dried figs, oat bran, flaxseed, apples, and cooked whole grains, among other foods
Alcohol	Water—lots of it
Food additives	Vitamins A, B, C, E
Caffeine	Potassium, found in fruits, dark-green vegetables, dandelion, celery, parsley, and seaweed, among other foods

by the Cancer Research Center of Hawaii, which found that women who ate the most phytoestrogen-rich foods had a 54 percent reduction in their risk of getting endometrial cancer. A later study in San Francisco had similar results.

If you decide to eat soy for its protective benefits, it's important to be consistent, making soy products a part of your daily diet. How can you do that? Jane Brody suggests that you aim for 25 to 50 grams per day. Four glasses of soy milk would give you about 30 grams; a drink made from soy-protein powder offers about 20 grams per cup (check the label). Other sources include tofu, tempeh, and miso, or you could try soy burgers (veggie burgers) or even soy hot-dogs, soy-based cheese, soy ice cream, and soy yogurt.

It you're in menopause and still have your fibroids, you may need to consider soy and other phytoestrogens in a slightly different light. No one knows the effect of eating large amounts of phytoestrogens while on HRT therapy, but if phytoestrogens block absorption of HRT, it may affect your results. If you're not taking HRT, eating soy and other phytoestrogens can act as a mild form of estrogen replacement. In either case, talk to your doctor about whether you should monitor your fibroids on a regular basis.

> **ROBIN:** *I started doing the soy protein drink every morning, but even though I didn't see any chance that my fibroids would get smaller, I've stayed with it because of the benefits of soy.*

Mmm, Pass the Fiber

I still have a childhood idea of fiber that makes me think it means eating cloth. Fortunately, the reality is a lot more tasty. (OK, it's still not chocolate.) Apples have lots of fiber, as do just about every other fruit, most veggies, whole grains like brown rice, whole-wheat products, old-fashioned oatmeal, nuts, and seeds. Increasing dietary fiber from 15 to 30 grams per day reduces blood estrogen levels, one of the things that may help fibroids grow.

How does it work? Dietary fiber is the express bus that moves waste products through our bodies: If that waste sits in our intestines, the accumulated toxins sit there too, and some of them get reabsorbed through our intestinal walls. Fiber picks up all those toxic little passengers, including fats, and gives them a quicker ride out of your body. (As a result, fiber can also help relieve constipation, a problem that affects up to half of all women with fibroids.)

And how to flush all this good stuff out of your system (if you'll pardon the expression)? Drink plenty of fluids: At least eight glasses (64 ounces) of clear, uncarbonated water a day will help your body detoxify. And water, by the way, means water—nothing else works as well, not soda, juice, coffee, tea, or the best French champagne drunk out of your lover's shoe.

Max the Flax

SPRINKLE UP TO two tablespoons of ground flaxseed (available at health food stores) on food every day: perhaps on top of cereal, or in a salad. It's a healthy and simple remedy that seems to relieve bloating, aid digestion, and help reduce fibroid growth.

ROBIN: *I believe part of the problem with constipation is physical pressure on the colon from the fibroids. Always drink lots of water. A high-fiber diet is key to continued normalizing of the colon. Try eating more raw food, and oatmeal—I mean real oatmeal!*

Eat Your Veggies

Vegetables are a major source of almost all the vitamins, minerals, and natural chemicals that may play a role in helping control fibroid growth and symptoms. The vitamin and mineral chart on pages 202 and 203 gives lots of examples of vegetables that provide a host of different nutrients, but an easy way to remember what you need is to think in color: yellow, red, and green.

Yellow and gold vegetables like carrots, butternut squash, and yams, just to name a few, contain the powerful *beta-carotenes,* defenders against the rebel molecules called the free radicals. *Free radicals* are molecules that trigger cell abnormalities, possibly including fibroids. Dark-green leafy veggies like spinach and kale are also good sources of beta-carotenes.

Broccoli, arugula, cabbage, kale, and other green vegetables also include something called *indole-3-carbinol,* a chemical that does two things: It prevents the development of cells that respond to estrogen, and it converts estradiol, a powerful form of estrogen, into the milder form called estrone.

Do you like tomatoes? Eat up—the same substance that turns tomatoes red can help reduce the free radicals in your system, even more powerfully than the beta-carotenes.

Fruits are also nutritional treasure troves. The only thing to remember as you work out a balanced diet is that fruits contain more sugar than vegetables.

V is for Vitamins

While vitamins and minerals won't reduce your fibroids, they may help relieve some of the symptoms, including heavy bleeding and cramps. Some of them may prevent future fibroid growth by helping your body manage estrogen more efficiently.

The following chart shows a list of vitamins, minerals, and a couple of other important elements, how they may help your fibroids or fibroid-related symptoms, and which foods you can find them in. Though this list doesn't necessarily include every food in each category, it should give you a good idea of where to start. You'll also notice that many foods contain a lot more than one vitamin.

In general, if you can get your vitamins and minerals from food, they'll be more effective. But since eating a balanced diet is more a goal than a reality for many of us, you may choose to take some supplements. (For a doctor's-eye view of how vitamins affect your body, take a look at Dr. Allan Warshowsky's *Healing Fibroids*.)

Remember, popping vitamins won't make up for a gooey, fatty, sugary diet (if only!). Also bear in mind that excess amounts of some vitamins or minerals can be counterproductive or even toxic, depending on your diet, any allergies, and other medical conditions, so please, consult your doctor or a trained nutritionist about the right amounts to include in your diet. Also ask if he or she can recommend a brand or brands of supplements. Since these so-called nutraceuticals aren't regulated, quality control varies widely.

Vitamins and Minerals

WHAT THEY DO AND WHERE TO FIND THEM

Vitamin or Mineral	May Help to ...	Some Common Food Sources
Beta-carotenes	Reduce heavy menstrual bleeding	Carrots, squash, yams, cantaloupe, bok choy, sweet potatoes, apricots, spinach, corn, kale, turnip greens, citrus fruits
Bioflavonoids	Replace some of your natural estrogen with milder phyto-estrogens	Most fruits and vegetables, including citrus fruits, grapes, carrots, broccoli, cabbage, cucumbers, squash, yams, soy products, tomatoes, eggplant, peppers, cherries, berries
Calcium	Relieve cramps	Dairy products, collard greens, canned salmon and sardines (with the bones)
Fiber	Eliminate excess estrogen	Whole grains, most vegetables, fresh fruit, beans, lentils, split peas, seeds, nuts
Gammalinolenic acid (GLA]	Decrease estrogen by controlling insulin levels	Black currant oil, evening primrose oil
Indole-3-carbinol	Reduce estradiol	Broccoli, arugula, cabbage, cauliflower, kale
Iron	Reduce anemia	Beef, lamb, pork, turkey, chicken, beans, soy, whole grains, dried fruit, dark-green leafy vegetables, black cherries
Linolenic acid	Regulate prostaglandins	Many fruits and vegetables, flaxseeds
Lycopene	Reduce free radicals	Tomatoes, paprika, red peppers, watermelon

Vitamin or Mineral	May Help to . . .	Some Common Food Sources
Magnesium	Relieve cramps	Kale, collard, Swiss chard, watercress, whole grains, beans, nuts, seeds, fruit, chicken, seafood, potatoes
Potassium	Prevent fibroid growth, reduce cramps	Bananas, oranges, cantaloupes, spinach, potatoes, bran flakes, prune juice, tomato juice
Selenium	Strengthen immune system	Garlic, scallops, barley, whole wheat, lobster, Swiss chard, brown rice, mushrooms, radishes, carrots
Vitamin B complex	Reduce estrogen in your system	Whole grains, beans, peas
Vitamin B_1 (Thiamine)	Relieve cramps	Whole-grain cereals, especially wheat, rice, and oats, lean meats (especially pork), fish, dried beans, peas, and soybeans.
Vitamin B_6	Relieve cramps	Meat, grains, beans, bananas, leafy green vegetables, corn, peas, nuts, fish, garlic
Vitamin C	Reduce bleeding, menstrual cramps, and pain	Citrus fruits, broccoli, leafy green vegetables, tomatoes, peppers, strawberries, cantaloupe, potatoes
Vitamin E	Reduce heavy bleeding, menstrual cramps, and pain	Wheat germ, oatmeal, nuts, brown rice, soy, asparagus, cabbage, leafy green vegetables
Zinc	Strengthen immune system	Meat, chicken, shellfish, dairy products, beans, fortified cereals

NANCY: *The fibroids were causing me so much pain that I was taking narcotics, something I was very reluctant to do, but I needed to do something. And the bleeding was intense. I'd start hemorrhaging.*

I realized I could change my diet. I never ate much meat, but about a year ago I cut it out entirely. And the other big thing, which was much harder, was cutting out dairy—believe me, giving up ice cream was one of the hardest things in my life! Well, at least in my dietary life. I also added whole grains to my diet. Apparently, whole grains absorb excess estrogen in your system and help your body flush it out. I think flaxseed can also do that.

I noticed that the first month after I changed my diet, the bleeding was a little less, and the pain was a little less. After six months, the doctor told me that the fibroids had shrunk by a third. I think if I'd kept going another six months, they would have been reduced even more, but at that point I agreed to have a myomectomy. Since the fibroids were smaller, my doctor was able to operate through my vagina, so I had no incisions or scars. I've kept up the diet, and so far I haven't had any more symptoms.

Now that you know which foods might have an effect on your fibroids, what other things can you examine in your life that may make a difference? Will you be surprised if the answers are weight management, exercise, and stress relief? I didn't think so. Funny how all roads lead to Rome. Let's look at how these well-worn topics relate to fibroids, and how we may be able to use that information to make some new decisions.

LEAN AND MEAN: FIBROIDS AND BODY WEIGHT

We're obsessed with weight in this country. Now *there's* a news flash. When it comes to fibroids, though, weight counts.

Enlightened doctors will tell you that there's a big grey area between "just right" and "way too much," but studies around the world show that the more fat you carry, the more likely you are to have fibroids. (Some women tip the scales because they have a lot of lean muscle mass; that doesn't count.)

What it boils down to is that your risk increases up to 20 percent

Can Fibroids Actually Make You Gain Weight?

IN ANN CHOPELAS'S SURVEY of women with fibroids, weight gain was one of the biggest commonalities, occurring in 40 percent of the participants.

for every "extra" twenty pounds, and 6 percent for every increase on the Body Mass Indicator (BMI) scale. (Let the good folks at the National Institutes of Health calculate your BMI in a jiffy at http://nhlbi support.com/bmi/bmicalc.htm.)

Where you carry extra weight can also make a difference: fat concentrated around the middle rather than thighs and hips increases your risk for fibroids, especially if your waist-to-hip ratio is over 0.80. You can find out your waist-to-hip ratio by dividing your waist measurement by your hip size: a 30-inch waist and 40-inch hips have a ratio of 0.75.

Last but not least, because I know you want to know, researchers at the Harvard School of Public Health found that the risk of fibroids was somewhat higher for women who'd gained weight since age 18. (If you do not fit into this category, please raise your hand.)

Why is extra weight an issue? Because body fat is not simply a passive, cuddly substance that helps us support the clothing industry (at least those of us who routinely have a range of four sizes in our closets). Body fat actually converts *androgens,* a male hormone we have in small amounts, into estrogen. The more body fat we have, the more of this conversion takes place and the more our risk for fibroids increases.

KACI: *I read that if you carry more weight in your stomach, you're more prone to problems. Fibroids are linked to fat, so it makes sense to me.*

But why should things be simple? Not every study confirms that heavier women are at greater risk for fibroids. And not all women with fibroids are heavy—far from it. The only thing that the information about weight suggests is this: If you're carrying extra weight—and I mean 20 pounds or more, not just the results of last night's slice of mud cake—and that weight is concentrated around your middle, you might want to consider some weight reduction.

Some women do report that after losing 20 pounds or more, their fibroids shrank. But guess what? Other women found that losing weight aggravated their fibroid-related symptoms.

But even if you're not going to make huge changes, should you do nothing? Of course not! (You knew that.) Even women who make modest changes in their diets find that they feel less tired and more upbeat. Focusing on improving your diet may also help reduce the time and energy you spend thinking about your fibroids.

If you don't want to make big changes, consider choosing one or two foods that you want to cut out or cut down on (like soda or chips, for example) or add in (broccoli). If you're not overweight, but don't think you eat as healthfully as possible, this could be a good experiment for you to consider too.

But always, be gentle with yourself. In a 1998 paper, the American Diet Association and the Canadian Diet Association put the whole issue of women and weight in perspective:

> Under the influence of [a] strong cultural bias for thin-ness . . . large numbers of women diet almost continuously. Instead of dieting, [focus] on normalizing eating behaviors, eating more healthfully, becoming more physically active and building positive self-esteem.

This advice is not only good for our fibroids, but for our whole way of life.

SHAKE IT UP, BABY: FIBROIDS AND EXERCISE

Fibroids hate exercise. That's one good reason you can like it more—or learn to! According to the National Institutes of Health, athletic women seem to have fewer fibroids than women who aren't as active. (You may be familiar with this latter group by its technical name: "couch potatoes.")

You don't need me to tell you that exercise helps reduce fat and cholesterol; it also lowers insulin levels. As we've seen by now, all of these changes can help lower the amount of estrogen available to feed your fibroids. Asian medical traditions associate fibroids with stagnant blood; exercise is a great way to get your blood and oxygen to circulate more freely.

If your fibroids are causing cramps or pain, exercise can help there too. Taking a brisk walk or getting on your bike may not be the first thing on your mind if you've got cramps, but you'll be doing yourself a favor by increasing your circulation, relaxing your muscles, and releasing pain-killing beta-endorphins. You can choose any aerobic activity that's fun and relaxing for you and that you can manage to fit into your schedule, whether it's roller skating, dancing to oldies on the radio, swimming, even pushing a vacuum around with a little extra oomph.

Whatever you choose, remember that the objective is to feel better, not worse. If you push your body too hard—a level that will be different depending on whether you're an experienced athlete or a beginner—it can make your pain worse. If your fibroids are large, running, step-aerobics classes, or similar exercises might feel jarring. Use your judgment, and slow down or stop if you're in any pain. If you're anemic, bleeding heavily, or have other medical conditions, check with your doctor before starting any exercise program.

Gentle exercise is a perfectly good option. Dr. Susan Lark recommends flexibility and stretching exercises for fibroid-related cramps and lower back pain; yoga can be a good way to introduce yourself to or practice these kinds of moves.

If you're concerned about the time it takes to exercise or are worried about your fitness level, it's just as helpful if you start small, maybe with a 15-minute walk every day or a few minutes of stretching before bedtime. If you have children of grade-school age or older, you may want to enlist them to join you on a daily walk or bike ride, which will not only give you company and time with your children, but can help start their good exercise habits.

Last but not least, exercise is a great stress reliever; we'll talk more about stress and fibroids next.

CAROLYN: *Walking is the big difference for me 'cause I get really constipated in the two weeks between ovulation and the start of my period. If I can walk enough, along with eating lots of fruits and veggies and other fiber, I'm okay. If I miss one or more of the elements—ouch.*

TAKE A CHILL PILL, LIL: FIBROIDS AND STRESS

I think stress may be the number one complaint in America. We all have it—and not many of us know what to do about it. But can stress also affect your fibroids? You bet.

Ann Chopelas found that 44 percent of the women she surveyed could identify periods of significant stress in which their fibroids seemed to grow or actually did. More than half of the women reported that they were under continuous stress; 27 percent said that simply having fibroids increased their stress levels.

Stress isn't just "in your mind." It sets off a complicated chain reaction in your body that can make your fibroids grow and any symptoms get worse. I've noticed that my own symptoms are considerably worse when I'm under extra stress; figuring this out has helped me postpone surgery more than once, as I waited for life to even out and my symptoms to bother me less.

Stress does three other things that work against us if we're trying to control our fibroids. First, it depresses the immune system, which reduces our ability to fight off infection and increases the severity of fibroid-related symptoms. Second, lots of us manage stress with the kinds of habits our fibroids just eat up. You know what I mean—things like eating too much; eating fatty, sugary foods; drinking more alcohol; and not exercising. Third, there's evidence that stress may release some of the stored toxins we carry in our bodies, potentially raising estrogen levels.

And as many of us know, just having fibroids can add stress to a life that's already complicated by working a job, having a family, having a relationship (or not), dealing with car trouble, saving the rain forest, taking the dog to the vet, and chipping a manicure. And that's the short list.

NANCY: *I spent a lot of time thinking about my life. To me, there was something seriously wrong with what I was doing—or there was a cumulative effect of years of doing something wrong.*

I really do think lifestyle is a big factor in having fibroids. I mean, think about it: We don't know how stress affects the body, but it makes sense to me that it can affect us systemically.

Now, I know this is extreme, but I actually decided to leave my job to reduce some of the negative energy in my life. It's not that I'm working less—since I'm going to graduate school and working part-time, I'm probably putting in more hours than ever—but I'm doing something that makes me feel better about myself and about how I'm spending my time.

Just smiling more can strengthen your immune system. So can a hug. Studies prove that a loving touch boosts the immune system as well as your mood. Amazingly, something as simple as a friendly handshake can make you feel better all day. Regardless of whether you have a partner, kids, or live alone, see if you can introduce a Minimum Daily Touch Requirement into your life.

The Impact of Violence

THE HARVARD NURSES' Health Study is currently reviewing data from over 65,000 women to see how—or whether—a history of emotional, physical, or sexual abuse affects their risk for asthma, high blood pressure, and fibroids.

Get Your ZZZs, Louise: Fibroids and Sleep

Are you a night owl or a lark? Would you ever dream that what time you tuck yourself in at night could make a difference to your fibroids? Well, stop dreaming. *Melatonin,* a hormone your body only produces in noticeable amounts in darkness, may tone down some of the effects of estrogen.

According to the *Women's Health Advocate* newsletter, night-time light exposure can interrupt your body's natural production of melatonin—and melatonin may slow tumor growth. The secret seems to be a question of lighting conditions. Lab experiments showed that animals who were allowed periods of complete darkness had slower tumor growth than animals exposed to stray light during sleep periods.

So how can you get the most melatonin moments? Dr. Russel Reiter, author of *Melatonin: Your Body's Natural Wonder Drug,* suggests getting regular amounts of sleep, light-proofing your bedroom or using eyeshades, keeping alcohol to a minimum, and taking a few moments every day to relax or meditate.

Let the Sun Shine In: Fibroids and the Great Outdoors

Now that you've gotten a good night's sleep, don't forget to enjoy some daylight. An hour of natural sunlight a day can increase serotonin levels in the brain, which in turn can lead to better emotional and physical well-being.

Native Americans believe that the rays of the sun help balance us spiritually and emotionally, as well as physically. There's a Cherokee belief that when the sun is highest in the sky, we have the opportunity to be most in harmony with nature.

Can you spend an hour outside taking a walk with your children, riding a bike, tending a garden? I know, you don't have time. Can you park the car a few blocks from work and walk the rest of the way? Eat lunch outside? Whatever you decide, remember that a little fresh air and sunlight can restore your energy, optimism, and peace of mind.

You Make the Call

As we've seen, a healthier lifestyle involves choices, and you're in charge. (Personally, I've always thought that one of the major benefits of being a grown-up is that I get to decide what to eat for dinner.) You can look at it this way: Would you rather make your fibroids happier—or yourself?

Making changes and making choices is not always easy. It feels like you need time, money, and energy to do the right thing sometimes. And I can't tell you that's not true. What I can do, though, is ask you to ask yourself one question: Are you worth it?

The answer is Yes, you are.

~9~

Sex and the Single Fibroid

CAN FIBROIDS AFFECT YOUR SEX LIFE?

WHY IS IT, do you think, that your doctor is more likely to ask whether your grandmother had breast cancer than if your fibroids are affecting your sex life? It can't be because they're embarrassed—could it? Gina Kolata, writing in the *New York Times,* reports that doctors have "a huge resistance to understanding women's sexual responses" and "it's easier and more socially acceptable to study psychological problems than the physiology of sexual responses in women."

Women don't seem to be much more eager to bring up issues or questions about how their fibroids might affect their sex lives—or how surgery for fibroids might change their sexual response. Most of the doctors I spoke with said that women rarely brought up questions about sex, even in discussions about surgery. In a discussion about fibroids and sex in an Internet chat room, women who logged on to participate were surprisingly reticent about the subject at hand. Are we that shy? Or have we bought into some of the myths about the uterus and the role it plays in our sex lives?

And yet the uterus is a major part of our sexual system, and for many of us, a major part of our sexuality as well. Clearly, if you have fibroids, there's a chance that they'll disrupt your sex life. If you're facing the possibility of losing your uterus, you need to think long and hard about how that kind of change will make you feel during sex—and how it may make you feel *about* sex.

DR. SCOTT GOODWIN: *When you learn about human sexuality in medical school, most of the emphasis is on clitoral orgasm. You do hear something about uterine contractions, but this idea that some women have a large amount of their sexual experience dependent on uterine contractions is something I wasn't really aware of until my patients started talking to me about it.*

Fibroids Interruptus

If you're worried about your fibroids, or think that having them somehow makes you less feminine, sex can remind you that you're a whole, functioning woman. Sex can help you relax, enjoy your body, get closer to your partner. If you're feeling some pain, vaginal and cervical stimulation can block it (thank you, beta-endorphins).

As an added benefit, orgasms can relieve cramps by releasing muscle spasms. Unfortunately, sex can also sometimes cause muscle spasms, giving you cramps that can be, if anything, worse than before.

For some women, fibroids can make sex—or even the prospect of sex—less pleasant. Fibroids can interrupt the way the uterus is supposed to work, giving it less room to elevate or expand. They can also prevent the normal contractions of your uterus during orgasm. Women have told me about a variety of problems that affect sex, including bloating, pressure, pain during penetration, a feeling that the uterus is shifting around, and uterine, ovarian, and back pain.

If your fibroids are too large, sex can be painful, or just, well, weird. During intercourse your fibroids can press up against adjacent organs, like the bladder or rectum. They won't cause any damage, but the feeling may be distracting. Your male partner may feel a difference too, though you'd have to talk to him to find out if they affect his pleasure.

Fibroids can also make the choice of birth control a significant problem. Since birth control pills may cause fibroids to grow, they may not be an option. If your fibroids have distorted the shape of your uterus by tipping it back or changing the shape of the cervix, a diaphragm isn't an option either, since it can't be fitted properly and can cause pain or pressure. So if condoms and foam remind you of that messy sex in high school, you're not alone, but you may not have much choice.

Then, of course, your fibroids may mean you'll choose not to have sex at all, because of bleeding, pain, fatigue, or plain old lack of interest. Bleeding is a serious damper. Even being worried about whether sex will trigger bleeding can tamp down the ol' libido.

Of course, anything that affects your sex life can affect your self-esteem, your feelings of femininity, and your relationship, if you're in one. Worst of all, you can start feeling like there's something wrong with you as a person.

CAROLYN: *I am in so much pain that I have little interest in sex at all.*

LAURA: *I had to give up sex, because it would just make me bleed. And I was losing weight, I was very thin, I was anemic. I wasn't sure if I looked pale, but I felt like I looked pale. I felt very dried up, like being a woman is sort of round and I felt dried up and skinny and brittle and I think at some level I also felt that this was what I got for ever being sexual in the first place.*

ROBIN: *I was having more and more pain with intercourse. My diaphragm didn't fit because my cervix had tipped so much it was going in the opposite direction. It created more tension in my relationship—the physical pain associated with sex turned me off, and there was the fear that my birth control wasn't working. We'd had a frequent, active, relaxed, and happy sex life, so that put a big strain on us.*

KATE: *My cervix was in a different position, so I couldn't use a diaphragm. During sex, certain positions were painful and I felt like there was something in the way. The partner I was with told me they bothered him, it didn't feel natural. His saying that bothered me, it made me feel out of control.*

Ladies, Start Your Engines

Now we all know that good sex is a whole-body experience. It's about touching and being touched, the triggering of hundreds of different physical sensations, deepening the emotional bonds with your partner. Orgasms can be stimulated in your vagina, your clitoris, your nipples, your skin. And we all know how important the brain is. Even paralyzed women, who have no feeling below the rib cage, are capable of having an orgasm. So why should you worry about treatment for your fibroids? What's the role of the uterus in your sex life, anyway? Sit back, relax, and get ready for a little sex ed.

You know the feeling. Your body starts reacting as soon as you start to get excited. Your heart beats faster, your adrenaline starts flowing; your arteries dilate, filling your uterus, vagina, and the rest of your pelvic muscles with blood. This extra blood flow is the beginning of that tingling feeling you get when you're excited. The top third of your vagina swells, while the uterus grows almost twice as big as it was before.

And then your uterus actually starts to elevate, pulling up and back toward your spine; in the process, your vagina lengthens about an inch. In some women, this creates a distinct physical sensation. (Does any of this sound familiar? Two hundred years ago, the uterus was actually thought of as an "inverted penis.")

Researchers are beginning to gather evidence that the uterus is a player in its own right when it comes to sex, with its own set of nerves and reflexes that can work together with other responses, or separately.

DR. GARY BERGER: *I can tell you that in relation to orgasm, the uterus is the female analog to the prostate, which is extremely important in orgasm for the male. And the uterus obviously contracts, and it would be ridiculous to imply or suggest that women don't feel the activity of the uterus during contractions, during orgasm; I think it's probably an essential part of orgasm.*

Now, when you have an orgasm, the muscles of your uterus contract, clenching and unclenching in quick waves from the top of the uterus down to the cervix. Some women feel these contractions very strongly, defining the intensity of their orgasms by the strength of the contractions. (By the way, stimulating your nipples can also cause uterine contractions, another source of touch and pleasure.) The contractions, in turn, increase the pressure inside your uterus. Dr. Sylvia Helena Cardoso of the Center for Biomedical Informatics at the State University of Campinas in Brazil writes that "a specific deeply satisfying female orgasm is associated with intrauterine pressure change."

Dr. Cardoso defines orgasm in general as "a state of heightened sexual excitement and gratification, followed by relaxation of sexual tensions and the body's muscles . . . marked by a feeling of sudden and intense pleasure." Since the uterus is largely muscle, it makes sense that it would contribute to these feelings.

Uterine orgasms seem to be particularly strong when your G-spot, that coin-sized nerve center on the front wall of your vagina, is stimulated. In what doctors call a "traditional" orgasm, brought on by clitoral stimulation, the uterus is apparently pretty quiet. But when your G-spot is stimulated, the uterus gets more involved, with deeper contractions and increased internal pressure. If you have multiple orgasms, one reason is that the blood flowing to your pelvis while you're still excited keeps your uterus enlarged and extended, which in turn keeps you primed for additional orgasms.

So listen: If you're considering treatment for your fibroids, keep in mind the possibility that your sex life may be affected. And if your doctor—or anyone—says there's no such thing as a uterine orgasm, or that the uterus plays no role in sexual satisfaction, here's my suggestion. After you finish laughing, look them straight in the eye and tell them that they're sadly limited by a failure of imagination—or experience.

DR. STANLEY WEST: *If you go back and look at Masters and Johnson, in the '50s, you know they did some scandalous, at the time, research in which they had a bunch of co-eds from the University of St. Louis come to their lab and masturbate. Terrible, absolutely shocking. And they hooked up all kinds of wires and cameras and they found out how a woman works. For the first time. No one had ever looked before. And they found that when a woman has an orgasm, the uterus rises away from her vagina, undergoes a series of contractions and then relaxes again. You ain't got it, you ain't going to get it. And it's as simple as that.*

LINDA: *The thing I thought was really ridiculous—that's the kindest word I can say—is that when doctors talk about the uterus, the function is for kids, a home for the baby, and it MAY have something to do with sex and sexual pleasure. And I thought, what, are you kidding? That women can't feel it contracting? After my first kid, that was the only thing I was dismayed about—it took a long time for my uterus to get back in shape—I really enjoyed those hard contractions!*

Isn't It Hysterical?

THE UTERUS HAS strong connections with the erotic. The annual festival of Aphrodite, the Goddess of Love, was called Hysteria, which also means womb. Hysteria got its present meaning from Hippocrates, who believed that the womb wandered about the body, causing uncontrollable reactions. And what's more "uncontrolled" than sex?

The Role of the Cervix

Did you know you have a Frankenhauser uterovaginal plexus? Does it make you happy now that you do? It should. When it's stimulated it contributes to sexual arousal and orgasm.

And that's just one of the ways your cervix contributes to your sexual happiness. The cervix, that little ring of muscle, is a little like the O-ring on the space shuttle: It may not look like much, but boy, is it important.

The cervix is the circular end of the uterus that connects with the vagina; it's also a source of pleasure for many women. Some of this is from the physical sensation that can occur during penetration; beyond that, this surprising little ring of tissue also releases beta-endorphins during intercourse, heightening your feelings of pleasure.

The cervix also produces a thin mucus that provides about half the lubrication you feel during sex; fluid from your vaginal walls provides the rest. And if that weren't enough, scientists have identified a nerve, called the *vagus nerve,* which goes directly from the cervix to the brain stem. (How's that for a mind-body connection?!) The vagus nerve is thought to be an independent pathway for the sensations of orgasm.

Removing the cervix in a hysterectomy deprives you of all these happy things. In addition, if your cervix is removed, it's replaced by scar tissue, which is just not as elastic. So losing your cervix may also prevent full expansion of your vagina—another sensation of arousal. Removing the cervix can also shorten the vagina; even a decrease of as little as 1 centimeter (about half an inch) can make sex difficult or painful.

Will Treating My Fibroids Do Anything for My Sex Life?

If you decide to treat your fibroids, what can you expect to happen to your sex life? In general, if you've been plagued by fibroid-related problems, your sex life should get better—simply because the pain or discomfort that prevented good sex has been relieved.

But how about your ability to achieve really great sex? Sad to say, in this sex-obsessed world of ours, women's sexual pleasure after fibroid treatment has only been studied in a limited way. We know the most about sex after hysterectomy, but not how it compares to other, less invasive procedures.

One antidote to the lack of available information about sex after surgery may be more and better communication. Doctors and women both report that there isn't enough conversation about sex either before or after fibroid treatment. Many doctors don't discuss it unless asked, and many women just don't ask. So unless your doctor is Dr. Ruth, you may have to bring up the subject of sex yourself. But be forewarned: Your doctor may minimize any potential problems after treatment—either to "sell" you on the procedure or because he really doesn't know the aftereffects.

While information is still emerging about how the different treatments for fibroids may affect you sexually, let's look at what we do know.

DARBY: *Well it's a Hobson's choice, isn't it? I keep hearing that treatment might affect my sex life, but now the darn fibroid is beginning to interfere with sex, so I'm damned if I do and I'm damned if I don't.*

SEX AFTER UAE

A number of recent studies have shown that the majority of women are happy with their sex lives after UAE (uterine artery embolization). Is this just because their symptoms are better? Does UAE affect your ability to have orgasms that are as good or better than before? Now that UAE has been practiced in the United States for about 15 years, doctors are starting to answer those questions

Data from the Georgetown University Medical Center suggests that sexual function after UAE most often stays the same—with about equal numbers of improvements and disappointments. Sixty women responded to a questionnaire from Georgetown researchers six months after they'd had UAE: 64 percent reported that their orgasms felt the same as ever; 6 percent said their orgasms were more powerful; 8 percent had weaker orgasms; and 6 percent had none at all. Desire certainly was healthy: 92 percent of the women responding were interested in having sex at least once a week. Interestingly, self-image also seems to improve after UAE, which may also have a positive effect on sex.

The fact that UAE is minimally invasive is also thought to affect women's feelings. When the procedure is complete, all you have to show for it is a small incision—and maybe some temporary black and blue marks at the same spot. In addition, a relatively fast recovery period means that most women are ready to get back to business—and I'm not talking about the office—within a couple of weeks, if not sooner.

One concern some women have consistently expressed—and experienced—is a change in uterine orgasms. A small number of women seem to lose the ability to achieve either uterine or clitoral orgasm at all.

Dr. Scott Goodwin thinks that if a woman has problems achieving orgasm after UAE, one possible reason could be damage to the nerves going into the uterus. Dr. Goodwin explains, "A nerve is a living tissue and it needs blood supply like any other living tissue. So if you embolize and block the blood supply to the nerves going into the uterus, those nerves may very well be damaged. And if you were feeling something in your uterus that was pleasurable, you may no longer feel that after the embolization."

Not all women experience uterine orgasms; some sources suggest that the sensation is only felt, or noticed, by about a third of all women. But if you're in that third, be sure to have a strong heart-to-heart with your doctor before the procedure.

The FIBROID Registry is currently examining issues related to sex and sexuality after UAE on a broad scale.

ROBIN: *I was so turned off because of my association with pain. I had zero libido. I didn't care if I ever did it again. But after my UAE, when I resumed sexual relations, I enjoyed it for the first time in years. I said, "I forgot! This feels good!" And my partner said, "Oh yeah? Oh really?!"*

SEX AFTER MYOMECTOMY

A confession: When I think about sex, I can pretty much guarantee that I don't think about Bialystock, Poland. But researchers there found that after myomectomy, both the pressure inside the uterus and the intensity of contractions increased when the women they studied were sexually excited. So in this case, getting rid of your fibroids can bring your sex life back to life.

Dr. Victor Reyniak concurs: "You can't have the famous uterine contractions that accompany orgasm with fibroids, because the uterus cannot contract even if it tried. Once a woman has a myomectomy, the contractions resume." If you've been bleeding heavily, myomectomy, like the other procedures available, can also improve life dramatically.

If you have an abdominal myomectomy, you will probably have to avoid sex for 4 to 6 weeks, while your wound heals. Vaginal and laparoscopic myomectomies will probably not put you out of commission for more than a week or two. After surgery, when you're healed, you're healed. You might feel anxious the first time you have intercourse after your operation, but after that, it should be just like riding a bicycle. Trust me.

SEX AFTER HYSTERECTOMY

Sometime around 1950, a Dr. M. E. Davis wrote, "The complete removal of the uterus does not interfere with a normal sex life." The quality of sex after hysterectomy is a strangely polarizing issue. For decades, if not longer, doctors and researchers have seemed determined to convince you that hysterectomy has nothing to do with your sex life—or can even improve it. On the other hand, there are a number of individual women, women's activists, and yes, some doctors, who insist that hysterectomy will spell the end of whatever sex life you enjoyed before. The truth, not surprisingly, lies somewhere in the middle.

DR. SCOTT GOODWIN: *It does seem to me if you are a woman whose orgasm depends on uterine contractions and you have a hysterectomy, then that's going to be gone.*

DR. JOSEPH FESTE: *There's no evidence in the literature that hysterectomy affects sexual response, but it's unclear. We certainly can't disregard it as a possibility, and women who have a fear of sexual disruption shouldn't ignore it.*

Your Male Partner

MEN MAY NOTICE the effects of hysterectomy as well. Michael Castleman, author of *Sexual Solutions: A Guide for Men and the Women Who Love Them,* writes that men may be affected by both the physical and emotional changes in their partners. Intercourse can be more difficult because of reduced lubrication, which can be easily addressed, or a shorter vagina, which may require more surgery. Emotional changes, including loss of libido, can affect either male or female partners.

NORA COFFEY: *The uterus is a hormone-producing sex organ that supports the bladder and bowel, so at a very basic level, it has these very important functions all of a woman's life. And women are not educated about the impact of losing it. Like when a woman tells me that a doctor recommends a hysterectomy and she asks specifically, will I be changed in any way, will it affect my sex life? And she's told, absolutely not, you'll be exactly the same, you just won't be able to have children. That's so interesting that we could accept that idea. Tell a man that you're going to cut off his sex organ, and that he will be unchanged, he'd just find the idea ludicrous. But a woman somehow is expected to believe that you could remove her sex organs and she would still be unchanged.*

LEONIE: *I felt that my gynecologist didn't even consider the possible effect of surgery on my level of sexual satisfaction. This was a negative message regarding women and sex which fit right in with my upbringing that never spoke of women enjoying sex or having a right to sexual satisfaction. Can you imagine any doctor suggesting to a man that he give up a good part of his sexual organs because it's a "convenient" way to treat a benign condition?*

HILLARY: *Christiane Northrup says that in a study in England 30 percent of women lost their sex drive after hysterectomy. I mean, why screw around with this? You can't get it back if you give it up. Sometimes it takes the threat of surgery to make us appreciate these things.*

The fact is, in many cases you can plan on having a satisfying sex life after a hysterectomy. Surveys do show that 50 to 60 percent of women report better sex lives after hysterectomy, though we don't know how these women would have felt after a less invasive procedure. And a certain number of women experience no change.

But that leaves a fairly large percentage of women whose sex lives go downhill. According to the *American Journal of Obstetrics & Gynecology*, 33 to 46 percent of hysterectomized women have partial or total loss of sexual function due to losing their uterus. A review sponsored by the Bill and Melinda Gates Foundation found that anywhere from 10 to 46 percent of women have reported a decreased sexual response following hysterectomy or oophorectomy (removal of the ovaries). As many as 15 percent of women may not start having sex again for months or years—if ever. Online postings from women in various Internet forums often include reports about sexual problems after hysterectomy, with stories about everything from lower libido to loss of physical sensation. Believe it or not, even kissing might be affected. One study showed that all types of sexual behavior decreased after hysterectomy, including kissing, touching, hugging—even daydreams. Dr. Judith Reichman, author of *I'm Too Young to Get Old* and *I'm Not in the Mood: What Every Woman Should Know about Improving Her Libido*, says, "I think women know how they feel sexually . . . About two-thirds of the women who have had hysterectomies say it made no difference, but one-third say it does."

DR. MITCH LEVINE: *After hysterectomy, there are many reports of sexual dysfunction. Despite what some doctors may say, many women will tell you their sex life really became dramatically worse after hysterectomy.*

Does the type of hysterectomy you have make a difference? Most studies suggest that all of the different types of surgery—vaginal, laparoscopic, abdominal—generally improve your sex life (though none of these, as far as I know, has been compared to myomectomy or other techniques). Unfortunately, as Dr. Anne D. Walling reports in an article in *American Family Physician*, all three techniques also leave women with "bothersome sexual problems"— loss of lubrication, arousal, and/or sensation—about 40 percent of the time.

A French survey of 170 women did indicate that a laparoscopic hysterectomy was least likely to affect a woman's sex life. While only about 8 percent of the women studied had sexual difficulties after laparoscopic hysterectomy, the number rose to 13.5 percent after vaginal surgery—and to a whopping 24 percent after abdominal hysterectomy.

If you're able to have laparoscopic or vaginal surgery, however, the shorter recovery period means you'll feel better—and more sexual— sooner, and the smaller scar—or complete lack of one—is likely to make you feel more feminine. Supracervical hysterectomy probably has the least impact on your sexual feelings and response, since the cervix and vagina are left alone.

Surgical errors can occur during any type of hysterectomy, of course, and these can also create sexual problems. Perforated vaginas, bowels, and bladders are the most common. Accidental perforation of the vaginal walls can result in a significant shortening of the vagina, leading to painful and difficult penetration, a real problem that can't be solved by K-Y Jelly, sex therapy sessions, or visits to a psychiatrist.

JANIS: *My sex life since the hysterectomy has been great . . . the best ever since the kids have been out of the house in college. I have been married for 30 years and my hubby is wonderful. He mirrored my reactions . . . had NO thoughts whatsoever of me being less feminine or less sexual. He thinks I am one amazing old broad!*

ANGELA: *Truthfully, after the hysterectomy, sex is different. And we are struggling a little with it. It's not horrible, it's just different, and different in probably not as good a way.*

The Role of the Ovaries

Once you agree to have a hysterectomy, you need to have a frank discussion with your doctor about whether or not your ovaries need to come out; the outcome of this discussion can have a big impact on your sex life too. As we discussed in Chapter 5, about 50 percent of hysterectomies include a double oopherectomy, the removal of both ovaries. But your ovaries aren't part of the flotsam and jetsam of surgery; they also make an important contribution to your sex life.

Why do you want to consider keeping your ovaries? First of all, they preserve the hormonal levels you had before surgery. In addition to estrogen, the ovaries produce androgens, a hormone that plays a part in your sexual arousal. Your ovaries also help keep your vaginal walls strong and your lubrication level normal. Unfortunately, even if you keep your ovaries, there's some evidence that they need the uterus to survive. About a third of the time, ovaries left in place after hysterectomy stop functioning.

Still, in a study of almost 700 women, those who kept their ovaries had a much better attitude about having had a hysterectomy than those who didn't. How much you want sex, how often you have it, and how easily you achieve orgasm all seem to be easier when you have your ovaries.

That Big Sex Organ Called Your Brain

Now, I wouldn't want to suggest that feelings play no part in how your sex life recovers after surgery. As you've seen, though, that shouldn't be the easy answer for any problems you may experience.

Here's something from a medical journal that sounds on the surface like a self-fulfilling prophecy: Women who are most concerned about their sex lives changing after hysterectomy seem to get more depressed than others afterward. Left out of the article were these questions: How active were their sex lives before? How much of a change did they experience? We don't know, but one possibility is that good sex lives became colder, hence the depression.

Another study found that how much you enjoy sex after surgery depends on how much you enjoyed it before. But is that the whole story? Fibroids can, as we discussed, make such a dent in your sex life that it's possible to have forgotten how good sex used to be, or could be.

The good news about these types of issues is that a caring partner, friend, or even therapist can help you sort out your fears and feelings. Don't overlook the nurse, either in your doctor's office or in the hospital. Many women feel that nurses are the most valuable source of information about sex after surgery. And most important, consider this part of your life just as carefully as you would any other aspect, and make sure your doctor understands and shares your concern—and interest—in your having a happy, fulfilling sex life.

∽ 10 ∾

And Baby Makes Three

FIBROIDS AND PREGNANCY

Fibroids . . . are significant causes of infertility in women.
—*DISEASES OF REPRODUCTION IN WOMEN,*
NATIONAL INSTITUTES OF HEALTH

PREGNANCY AND FIBROIDS are linked in any number of subtle, complicated ways. Having fibroids can be the reason for getting pregnant before you're emotionally or financially ready, or they can be one reason you might not be able to conceive or carry to term.

The fact is, fibroids are one of the most common conditions among women of childbearing age. Dr. Marjorie Greenfield, writing on the Internet site DrSpock.com, says, "Most [pregnant] women with fibroids deliver normally." And even the cautious American College of Obstetricians and Gynecologists notes that "If you are pregnant and have fibroids, they likely won't cause problems for you or your baby." And here's a fun fact: the more often you're pregnant, the less likely you are to get fibroids—talk about incentives!

It's reassuring to know that most women with fibroids are able to deliver healthy babies. But it's important to know when, and how, fibroids can affect your pregnancy, from conception to delivery, and even after. Let's take a look.

How Can Fibroids Complicate Pregnancy?

BEFORE:
- o Infertility
- o Miscarriage
- o Ectopic pregnancy

DURING:
- o Uterine inversion
- o Red degeneration
- o Abdominal pressure
- o Sciatic pressure
- o May require you to rest in bed
- o Restricted exercise
- o Restricted sexual intercourse

IN DELIVERY:
- o Prolonged labor
- o Obstruction of labor
- o Need for cesarean section
- o Premature rupture of membranes (water breaking)
- o Premature labor
- o Placenta may separate prematurely from the uterine wall
- o Breech or another difficult-to-deliver position

AFTER:
- o Postpartum bleeding and infection
- o Low-birth-weight baby

JENEANE: *They told me if I had any more fibroids, they'd be coming out of my mouth. I felt horrible. My ultrasound technologist admitted later that she didn't expect a positive outcome. She had rarely seen so many fibroids and a full-term pregnancy. After the pregnancy, she told me,*

"You're an enigma. It's a miracle you made it." I just figured our baby was as stubborn as we were.

BEFORE PREGNANCY

One day, during an otherwise normal checkup, my ob-gyn told me that if I ever wanted to try to get pregnant, I should have a myomectomy before my fibroids got too large. Unfortunately, she also said she couldn't guarantee that I wouldn't wind up with a hysterectomy. She was quite firm about it and wanted to schedule the surgery as soon as possible. In fairness, she was trying to preserve my ability to have a child, but at the time I was too upset about the idea of "needing" surgery to have a thoughtful conversation. (And no, I didn't follow my own advice—I was there at the appointment by myself.)

Even though I wasn't trying to get pregnant at the time, I decided I'd better get some other opinions. I saw three other doctors: They all said, in effect, don't worry about your fibroids, go ahead with your life.

They didn't all get points for courtesy, consideration, and kindness: One doctor said some pregnant women carry fibroids as big as watermelons and don't worry about it. I wanted to know: Had this guy ever seen a watermelon? Another (female) doctor told me not to worry about my fibroids, but at my age, I'd better "hurry up."

Finally, I met Dr. Richard Levine, a leading ob-gyn at NewYork-Presbyterian Hospital, who gave me what seemed like a balanced point of view: That is, that fibroids can sometimes cause problems, but the prudent course would be to try to get pregnant—when and if I was ready—and only consider having surgery if the fibroids actually proved to cause problems.

Not all the women I spoke with were able to get a similarly reasoned answer, even after consulting several specialists.

JENEANE: *A fertility specialist said, "DO NOT GET PREGNANT with a uterus the size of yours. It won't work. It's too risky, you need to get a myomectomy."*

Then I went to a doctor who said, "We can do more testing. Here are the risks if you get pregnant: pain, bleeding, miscarriage."

I went to a third doctor and asked, "What's the worst thing that could happen if I got pregnant?" She said, "Well, mortality is the only absolute—I like to start from there and work backwards." I was like, okay. I didn't go back to work that day.

Can Fibroids Cause Infertility?

Certainly infertility is an issue for many people. Twenty percent of couples—one in five—have trouble conceiving a child even after a year of trying consistently.

Many sources say fibroids aren't a factor in infertility, but others differ. Dr. Joseph Feste, for example, told me that in his experience, "Ten to twenty percent, on average, of all infertility is caused by fibroids. More common reasons for infertility are endometriosis, which accounts for about 70 percent, or adhesions, but fibroids can definitely play a part."

In studies of women who have fibroids, there's a high rate of infertility and spontaneous abortion. A study of 60 pregnant women with fibroids revealed that 43 percent had a history of infertility and another 25 percent had a history of miscarriage. In her book *Having Your Baby: A Guide for African-American Women,* Dr. Hilda Hutcherson says, "The presence of fibroids can make it very difficult or even impossible to get pregnant."

Some doctors think fibroids don't prevent pregnancy simply because they believe that pregnancy isn't an issue for women "old enough" to have fibroids. Dr. William H. Parker, author of A *Gynecologist's Second Opinion,* writes, "Fibroids most often occur in women in their late thirties and forties, at a time when many women have already completed their families."

The reality is, women aged 35 to 39 are the fastest-growing group of pregnant women in the United States, followed closely by women aged 40 to 44, and women aged 30 to 34 (yes, in that order).

Scars and Infertility

IF YOU'VE HAD abdominal surgery, such as a myomectomy, the internal scars (adhesions) can sometimes cause infertility. If this is a significant problem for you, a skilled doctor can clean up some of the adhesions laparoscopically.

And while fibroids can affect women of any age, they are most often an issue for women in their thirties and forties.

There are four major ways in which fibroids might interfere with your ability to get pregnant:

Blocking the tubes: One or more fibroids—usually inside your uterine cavity—could be blocking or compressing your fallopian tubes, making it impossible for an egg to be released into your uterus. (One uncommon but possible result of this is *ectopic pregnancy*, a dangerous situation in which a fertilized egg begins developing in a fallopian tube.)

Changing the physical landscape: Some types of fibroids can change the lining of your uterus so that there is no place for a fertilized egg—a tiny zygote—to make a home for itself. Result? The lining of your uterus—the endometrium—changes from a warm, inviting surface to a cold, smooth, hard wall. The zygote needs a place to attach and burrow into your uterus so that it can start growing and developing. The more fibroids, the less chance that the zygote will land in, well, fertile ground, for lack of a better term. And unfortunately, zygotes don't have fallback navigational systems. If the zygote does find a comfortable place that's close to a fibroid, this can also cause problems as the fetus and fibroid compete for the same blood supply.

Changing the chemical environment: Fibroids can release chemicals called prostaglandins, the hormone that triggers pain. (Some analgesics, like Advil, are "antiprostaglandins," because they work on this pain mechanism.) Prostaglandins can also induce contractions of smooth-muscle tissue—which includes your fibroid—making it about as easy for your zygote to settle into your uterus as it would be for you to stay on a surfboard in a thunderstorm.

Sending in the troops: Although fibroids are almost never cancerous, like cancer cells, the cells of a fibroid divide faster than the "normal" cells in your body—hence the growth you can often see in a fibroid from one ultrasound to the next. This rapid cell division can trigger a response from your immune system, sending the body's natural defenses to try to deal with the perceived invader. This reaction is bad news for another "alien" in your body—your fertilized egg.

FERTILITY TESTING

The tests that you can take to rule out—or determine—whether fibroids are the cause of your infertility are ultrasound, magnetic resonance imaging (MRI), hysterosalpingography (HSG), and hysteroscopy (see Chapter 4 for a full description of these tests).

- Ultrasound can usually tell you whether your fibroids are inside the cavity or changing the wall of the uterus; MRI can provide a more precise view.
- HSG can help determine if fibroids are blocking your fallopian tubes, preventing eggs from being released into your uterus. If you have both ovaries, you only need one tube to be open to release an egg. However, a spasm may give the appearance of a blockage, causing a false-positive test result. Since HSGs can have false-positive results 10 to 20 percent of the time, you may have to confirm the diagnosis with another test.
- Hysteroscopy lets your doctor see whether a fibroid is affecting the uterine lining.

If your doctor tells you not to worry about your fibroids, that they shouldn't affect your ability to conceive—or haven't been proven to be a problem—that may be good news and good advice. But it's in your best interests to stay aware of your symptoms, if any, and chart your progress on conception.

If you've been "watching" your fibroids and trying unsuccessfully to conceive for more than 12 months, it may be time to explore stronger options, possibly including drug therapy with GnRH agonists or myomectomy. But—and this is a very important "but"—even if they're present, even if they're big, fibroids may not be the cause of infertility.

FELICE: *By September, we started trying to get pregnant. I bought a basal thermometer and started charting my temperature religiously, reading every book I could find on getting pregnant, reading the pregnancy newsgroup online, and getting disappointed month after month.*

It's now the eleventh month of trying, and I can tell that my period is just about to start. The cramps are intense, and I've started taking my double dose of Aleve and a light spotting has begun. So I called my gynecologist and we will do an HSG—the "X-ray dye test"—in 10 days from the start of this period and a progesterone test this month and start figuring out if it is the fibroid/adenomyosis that is stopping me from getting pregnant or something else. Then we'll see if I should have surgery or an embolization. Maybe we'll get the problems cleared up ahead of time and have a safer pregnancy.

Other problems that can affect fertility include endometriosis, salpingitis (an infection of the fallopian tubes), and a host of other factors, including, by the way, your partner's fertility.

In their book, *It's Your Body: A Woman's Guide to Gynecology*, Dr. Niels Lauersen and Steven Whitney stress that if you're experiencing infertility, your husband/partner/donor needs to take a sperm test. In a sad but telling aside, Dr. Lauersen and Mr. Whitney say that "countless women" have undergone surgery rather than ask their men to go through a painless fertility test. You're not planning to get pregnant all by yourself (even if you're planning to become a single parent). Don't assume you're the infertile partner.

Fibroids and IVF

In-vitro fertilization, or IVF, has gone from being a wonder of modern medicine to an almost commonplace occurrence. In my neighborhood, it's not unusual to see parents pushing twins in strollers, a reminder of the everyday miracle of assisted reproductive technology.

But does it work if you have fibroids? Studies show that having fibroids reduces your chance of success anywhere from 30 to 50 percent; if your fibroids are changing the shape of your uterus, your chances of becoming pregnant drop as low as 9 percent.

Other factors that can affect your ability to become pregnant include—surprise!—the size and location of your fibroids. A recent study in Brazil concluded that fibroids larger than 4 centimeters may affect the embryo's ability to implant. An Australian study showed that women with fibroids inside the uterine cavity or the lining had a much lower rate of success with IVF, even when the shape of the uterus was not changed. Subserosal fibroids—the ones on or near the outer wall of the uterus—are least likely to affect IVF.

The problem is that in addition to the emotional trials and physical stress, IVF can be shockingly expensive, so you don't want to go in under anything less than optimal conditions. If your fibroids appear to be the type that could cause a problem, your doctor may recommend a myomectomy or a course of GnRH agonists before trying—or proceeding with—IVF. We'll talk about both of those possibilities shortly.

Tick-Tock: Time to Get Pregnant?

Ironically, fibroids are often the reason women try to get pregnant, sometimes sooner than planned. When fibroids are discovered, some doctors suggest that their patients try to get pregnant as soon as possible—ready or not. The emotional, physical, and financial toll can be enormous, putting a huge strain on relationships and career plans. Some women have been told that their choice is a stark one: Have a baby or have a hysterectomy.

Only you and your partner can judge your situation and decide if you are ready to start a family. As we've seen, fibroids can prevent pregnancy, but they don't have to. At the end of the chapter, you'll read about options that can prolong your fertility by removing or

> ## *Maintain Your Own Health File*
>
> **A GOOD IDEA** in general, maintaining a health file can save time, money, and confusion during a pregnancy, especially if you go for second opinions or if for some reason you have to change doctors midway through your pregnancy. Each time you have an appointment, ask your doctor's office to send you copies of every report. If you're keeping a pregnancy log, jot down each appointment, test, and result there.

shrinking your fibroids—letting you and your partner prepare to have the family you want.

FELICE: *In January, during a regular annual exam, I found out that I had fibroids. The ultrasound showed my uterus to be enlarged to about a 12-week size. My gynecologist told me to come back in three months and we'd check it again. In the meantime, she suggested that if I was thinking I might want to have children, I should start trying as soon as possible because this thing could grow and get worse and cause more problems.*

Well, that was a mind-blower for my husband and me. We had started thinking more seriously about having children in the future, but the future still seemed far away. My husband sank into a depression later that summer as the overwhelming reality of life and age catching up with us set in, and we tried hard to face all sorts of issues in our relationship in preparation for feeling ready to start trying to make a baby.

JENNIFER: *My symptoms were minor. My doctor suggested trying a pregnancy ASAP if we were financially and emotionally ready. I had an HSG that showed that the largest tumor was not blocking my right tube, and the lining was only minorly distorted. I went off the Pill two weeks after that, and four weeks later, I learned I was pregnant.*

MARY: *My husband and I married relatively late, after doing all the things we wanted to do without the constraints of marriage. Within 12* *months we decided to try to have children. Boom! Surprise!! I had no problem getting pregnant.*

What about Miscarriage?

Location, location, location. Fibroids take up valuable real estate inside your body, space that nature allocated for a developing baby. The size, number, and placement of fibroids determine how much they might affect a pregnancy.

Just because you have fibroids, you're not automatically at risk for having a miscarriage, but they don't help. New research from the University of North Carolina at Chapel Hill estimates that fibroids increase the

The Emotional Toll of Infertility and Miscarriage

The failure to conceive at the desired time
(or early loss of a pregnancy) puts women at risk
for anguish and a variety of social pressures.
—NATIONAL INSTITUTES OF HEALTH

EVER SINCE THE time of Sarah and Abraham, infertility has put an emotional strain on women and their partners. Now that medical technology has advanced beyond stone knives and prayers, we have even higher expectations that we can conceive and carry children. If we have trouble, it can be not only a personal tragedy but a social failure.

The experience of losing a much-wanted pregnancy affects each woman—and man—differently, as does the strain of not being able to conceive. Some people will need time to themselves, others may find support groups—either formal or informal—helpful and comforting. Some resources for support are listed in Resources, but no matter what you decide to do, it's usually important to acknowledge your grief and disappointment—at least to yourself.

risk of miscarriage 55 percent. (Fibroids are not the only reason women miscarry, of course: 15 to 30 percent of pregnant women in the United States have miscarriages every year.) While earlier research showed that large or multiple fibroids increased the risk of miscarriage, the North Carolina study points to small fibroids as the primary culprit. (Thanks to a grant from the NIH, the study is being expanded to track thousands of women over a five-year period—although that does mean we'll have to wait until about 2010 to find out the results.)

MARY: *My doctor followed me very closely, with numerous ultrasounds to check the growth of the fibroids, until the thirteenth week when I started spotting. She admitted me to the hospital, where after three days I lost my first baby on Mother's Day. The doctor explained that both the baby and the fibroids needed blood to survive and the fibroids had been more aggressive in their need.*

If a fibroid causes a miscarriage, it's more likely to happen in the first or second trimester; in fact, fibroids can cause miscarriage so early on, you might not even realize you'd been pregnant. Later in pregnancy, fibroids tend to cause pain or preterm contractions rather than miscarriage.

LINDA: *I was late, miscarried, but I didn't realize it for a few weeks or a month, when my body flushed out what had been the developing embryo. That's when I realized I had been pregnant. I called my physician, and he said that I needed an ultrasound: The upshot was that I had a very large fibroid.*

Oh, You've Got That Glow: Fibroids and Pregnancy

Many women have uneventful pregnancies, fibroids and all; some women don't even know they have fibroids until they start getting fetal ultrasounds to check on the progress of their pregnancy.

Fibroids are reported to cause physical problems during pregnancy anywhere from 10 to 30 percent of the time; they can cause psychological problems a bit more frequently. (To put that in some perspective, the CDC says that "at least 30 percent" of all the women who get pregnant in the United States each year have a "pregnancy-related complication.") Some women are able to stay calm and collected when they hear they've got fibroids; some spend nine months fearing the worst. "It really wasn't bad, except for the worrying, and the perinatologist shaking his head in disbelief," one woman said of her pregnancy.

Of course, some women do have experiences none of us would wish for. Some of the most moving stories I've heard in my research about fibroids are those that involve the struggle to be or stay pregnant, and to manage some of the complications that fibroids can cause, before, during, and after.

The good news is how many of the stories have happy endings, with full-term, healthy babies.

LINDA: *During my pregnancy with my last child, now 12, I found that I had a fibroid. I had three kids, she was my fourth pregnancy. The fibroid was on the outside wall, high up, difficult to palpate manually but still small. We had to watch it, but it didn't interfere with the pregnancy. The baby was fine. In fact, she was the healthiest baby and the best delivery of all four kids.*

JENEANE: *I worried about everything during my pregnancy—would I lose the baby? Would the baby be healthy? Would I have her early? Everything. I coped by taking lots of warm baths, though not too hot, as that could be bad for the baby. Sometimes I took four baths a day! That and reading. I never had time to read before and never since, but I didn't sleep much during my pregnancy, so I read novels—*The Firm, The Client, *every Grisham book and then some. It kept my mind occupied while the baths soothed my sore back. I had appointments at the perinatologist every four weeks, and of course the usual checkups at the OBs every month—more frequently at the end. Seemed like I was always going to an appointment.*

JENNIFER: *The pregnancy was tough. I started bleeding and having pain in my second month. As my uterus grew, the largest tumor was pushed up further and further and ended up living in my rib cage, on my ribs, wherever. It had nowhere else to go as it took up sooo much of my uterus and body at that point! I had a prescription for Tylenol with codeine and cyclobenzaprine to relieve the pain, but it was hard to take the meds as they made me tired and I had to teach 100 students a day.*

I was placed on many restrictions and was finally pulled out of work at 30 weeks because of how low the baby was. I was worried about my students, my career, and that being home was taking time away from my maternity leave. And, of course, the financial worries. I got my last paycheck in December. I am not the type to sit around and watch TV all day, but that is exactly what I was supposed to be doing to protect the baby.

I had a few close calls, when I thought I'd deliver, at the end of the second trimester. Then I developed a bad case of gestational diabetes, made worse by the steroid shots I was getting in case I went into labor preterm.

Is Your Pregnancy High Risk?

AMAZINGLY, IN THE United States, 20 to 25 percent of all pregnancies are high risk—up to a million every year. If you have fibroids, does that automatically place you in a high-risk category for pregnancy? The answer is probably, certainly to the extent of being monitored by your doctor on a regular basis.

Among other things, being at high risk means you can expect some high stress, high anxiety, and a high chance of some pretty dramatic disruptions in your life. Work, home, and relationships can suddenly take second place—even though all of those parts of your life still need as much attention as ever. It can mean going to the doctor every week instead of every month—and coming up with new ways to cope with pain, stress, and fatigue.

DONNA: *The advice you get and the decisions you have to make because you have fibroids can affect a pregnancy. I've talked to other women who've had fibroids during pregnancy, and everyone's kind of on alert, everyone's kind of on a watch. It's never easy. You worry about it, and it's not uncommon among people I know that they've needed to spend a couple of days in the hospital at one time or another directly related to their fibroids. You really need to get information and talk to different people.*

What Are the Risks of Fibroids When You're Pregnant?

As we've said, fibroids can cause many side effects during your pregnancy, some more serious than others, most of them manageable with the right care.

If you're pregnant now and experiencing problems from your fibroids, this information may be able to help shed some light on what's happening, why, and what you can expect. If you're not having a problem pregnancy or are not yet pregnant, it's important to know that these side effects are possible but not inevitable. Read this section the way you might read the warning label on a prescription: to be informed, not frightened.

Bleeding during Pregnancy

Bleeding is one of the more common effects fibroids can cause during pregnancy. Depending on how far along your pregnancy is, bleeding can signal different problems; the American Nurses Association recommends that you call your doctor for any vaginal bleeding during pregnancy. Bear in mind that slight bleeding, or spotting, can be normal, especially in the first trimester.

JENEANE: *I started bleeding when I was six weeks pregnant and had bleeding episodes for about two weeks. They wrote "threatened mis-*

carriage" on all my forms you get at the visit. I had to go to the doctor each time for an ultrasound, and that was very scary. My doctor told me, well, either the baby will keep growing or it won't. It's really that straightforward. I cried and cried about it that day. But from about nine weeks on, I didn't bleed again.

Carneous (Red) Degeneration

This colorful term is simply what doctors call fibroids that degenerate during pregnancy, meaning those fibroids that outgrow their blood supply and begin to die.

While the pain of red degeneration is one of the most common complications fibroids cause during pregnancy, that doesn't mean you'll definitely get it. One study following pregnant women with fibroids showed that it affected one woman in ten.

How will you know if you're experiencing red degeneration? Pain is a good indicator (sorry!), usually beginning around 20 weeks. While it can be severe, it may not be distinctive: The pain is usually centered over the fibroid and may also radiate into your lower back. You may notice some light bleeding—always a sign to talk to your doctor during pregnancy—as well as nausea, vomiting, and low-grade fever. At worst, the degeneration could set off preterm labor, hemorrhage, and shock, but these are not considered everyday side effects.

DR. VICTOR REYNIAK: *Red degeneration doesn't affect the baby—the baby does well. It's the woman that suffers—sometimes you even have to hospitalize her.*

Regardless of the pain you may feel, you can take comfort that red degeneration doesn't hurt your baby. The pain may last from a few days to over a week, and many doctors simply suggest bed rest and acetaminophen or ibuprofen, though these don't always conquer the pain. A word of caution: Dr. Hilda Hutcherson points out, "You should not take ibuprofen without speaking to your practitioner first, and never take it after thirty-four weeks of pregnancy."

If you are simply in agony, call your doctor fast. She may be able to give you a prescription to provide some relief. Make sure you ask about any possible side effects, as certain drugs may carry some risk of miscarriage. The other option for pain relief is hospitalization, where you can get pain medications and fluids through an IV line. You may also need antibiotics if you have a fever or other signs of infection.

Uterine Crowding

Fibroids that take up space inside your uterus can cause uterine crowding; in pregnancy, preexisting fibroids can increase three to five times in size.

What can happen to your baby? The most severe possibility is that the baby's lungs may not develop fully. Other severe effects could include a misshapen skull or face, a dislocated hip, bowed legs, a club foot. Fortunately, the effects are usually mild. Delivery and the passage of time will reshape the baby's head and other parts that seemed abnormal at birth.

Having a large fibroid pregnancy can feel like you're carrying twins. You'll get bigger sooner and will often get bigger than you would normally. This means that symptoms that are more common in late pregnancy can happen to you sooner, like back pain, hemorrhoids, varicose veins, difficulty breathing, and heartburn.

Placenta Previa

Normally, the placenta forms at the top of the uterus, the part farthest from the cervix. But if you have fibroids where the placenta is supposed to be, it may form in the "wrong" place, lower in your uterus and closer to the cervix, where it can block the entrance to your vagina. When this happens, it's called placenta previa. It's not too uncommon, happening to 1 in every 200 pregnant women.

How can you know if you have placenta previa? There are a few warning signs. The first possibility is bleeding, often bright red, although not necessarily heavy, usually starting around the sixth month. Why does this happen? Because as you get into the third trimester, your cervix begins to expand: If the placenta is near the cervix, it can tear loose, creating a raw spot that bleeds. The other things to watch out for are:

○ pain that comes on suddenly and doesn't go away, in the area of your uterus and lower back;
○ a feeling of tenderness in your uterus; and
○ early contractions.

Your doctor can tell where your placenta is by doing an ultrasound. A word of caution: If you or your doctor think you have placenta previa, you should not have a pelvic exam, as this can make any bleeding worse. Keep this in mind if you are examined by any unfamiliar doctors. You'll also need to avoid intercourse for the rest of your pregnancy.

The effects of placenta previa can range from mild to severe. You may have to be confined to bed for the rest of your pregnancy, possibly even in a hospital. You might need drugs to prevent premature labor; you might need an emergency C-section. The worst-case scenario includes severe bleeding. While painless, it can put you at greater risk for infection and deprive your baby of adequate oxygen, affecting his or her growth and development. If your blood loss is severe, you might need a transfusion.

Sometimes the placenta can move again, basically solving the problem on its own. Even so, the majority of women whose placenta shifts in this way will still have to deliver early.

If placenta previa occurs after the 37th week, your doctor will probably try to induce labor, though you still have a good chance of delivering normally.

Premature Rupture of the Membranes and Uterine Rupture

The extra size of fibroids can put pressure on the flexible but delicate container surrounding your unborn baby. In extreme cases, fibroids can cause the membrane surrounding the fetus to break open, or rupture.

If your doctor is concerned about this possibility, you may find yourself having the longest bed rest of your life, to avoid putting the extra pressure of gravity on your uterus. This, plus close observation by your doctor, will normally protect both you and your baby. Most women find bed rest frustrating and boring, as well as a big disruption at work and around the house. If you have other children, you'll have to line up someone else to help care for them.

If your membrane does get damaged, some of the amniotic fluid will begin to leak. Your first sensation could be a gush of fluid, followed by continuous dripping, like a leaky faucet. The two big problems this can cause are premature delivery and infection, so a prompt call to your doctor is critical.

Less common is the risk of uterine rupture during labor or early contractions. You're generally only at risk if you've had surgery on your uterus. The scars from a cesarean section, myomectomy, myolysis, or cryomyolysis can weaken your uterus so that it can't withstand the pressure of labor.

Your risk after myomectomy is in direct proportion to how many incisions your doctor had to make in your uterus to remove your fibroids; if you had an extensive myomectomy, your doctor may recommend delivery by C-section to avoid the possibility of uterine rupture. The danger of rupture is great enough from myolysis that it's not recommended as a procedure for women who still want to get pregnant; pregnancy is also not recommended after cryomyolysis, since the dangers are currently unknown.

What are the warning signs of uterine rupture? Severe pain in your abdomen is the first. You may even feel a sensation of something tearing inside you. You may faint, and your heartbeat and breathing may become rapid. Once again, call your doctor immediately.

Fibroids and Delivery

You're almost there. It's been quite a trip, but your destination is in sight. But just as a ship has to navigate shallow water before it can land safely, you and your baby have to make your way through delivery.

If your fibroids haven't caused a problem so far, you may be able to deliver normally, though this is a subject you'll discuss with your doctor. There's also a possibility that your delivery will be a little different than you'd planned, either because of premature labor, the possibility of needing a C-section, or the danger of bleeding after delivery.

> FELICE: *I had always thought that when I had a baby it would be with a midwife at home, but now I was having second thoughts. My doctor is the head of gynecology at the Medical University Hospital in Portland—he's on the certification board for midwives and is open to home births, so I asked him his opinion on that. He felt that it was not a good idea, that this falls into a high-risk pregnancy category and would need to be closely monitored. Also, there is a potential for severe hemorrhaging during and after a fibroid pregnancy, which must be taken into account. So I gave up on the home-birth fantasy.*

PRETERM LABOR

"Preterm" deliveries are those that begin any time between 20 and 36 weeks, as opposed to the "normal" full-term pregnancy, which lasts from 37 to 40 weeks. Women with fibroids have a higher risk of preterm labor; your risk is also higher if you're over 40 or have had abdominal surgery.

But being at risk doesn't mean it will definitely happen to you. About 12 percent of pregnant women are likely to go into labor early.

To the Batmobile!

ONCE YOU REACH your third trimester, you might want to have a plan in place in case you have to make a quick trip to the hospital. This includes having someone you can call to take care of your other children, if you have them; knowing the fastest route to the hospital if your partner or a friend plans to drive you; and keeping the number of your doctor and a local ambulance service on a pad next to the phone or some other handy place.

According to the authors of *Intensive Caring: New Hope for High-Risk Pregnancy,* fibroids pose only a "mild" risk to pregnant women.

How will you know if you're going into preterm labor? It may be difficult to tell, but here are some of the warning signs:

o Uterine contractions every 15 minutes or faster
o Menstrual-like cramps
o A dull ache in the lower back
o Pressure or a feeling of fullness in your lower abdomen
o Increase or change in vaginal discharge

If you do go into labor early, bed rest and extra liquids may help stop the contractions. If not, your doctor may suggest a drug called a *tocolytic.* While this is often helpful, the side effects can be unnerving, including headaches, rapid pulse rate, nervousness, dizziness, and shortness of breath.

As for any preemie, the earlier the birth, the more the potential complications, and the more care your child will need. But with the right medical attention and care from you, most children born after 24 weeks should be fine.

JENNIFER: *My daughter was born about five weeks early. She was sent to NICU with blood in her lungs and a heart condition. She stayed there for 16 days. She was still battling a heart condition at four months and was REALLY hard to take care of. Preemies need so much more than full-term babies! We did have a throwing away of the heart medication and syringes ceremony when her EKG came back normal. We just chucked all the stuff into the garbage . . . like kids on the last day of school throwing away their notebooks! She's doing great now—I think her one-year birthday party will be a celebration for us as well.*

CESAREAN SECTION

If you have fibroids, do you automatically need a C-section? Not necessarily. Dr. Hilda Hutcherson writes, "Women with fibroids are usually able to go into labor spontaneously and deliver vaginally."

What if you've had a myomectomy? Is that an automatic ticket to a cesarean? Again, not necessarily. So how can having fibroids increase your risk of a C-section?

○ Fibroids in the lower part of your uterus can block the baby's descent.
○ Many fibroids can keep your uterus from contracting properly, preventing progress in labor.
○ If fibroids change the shape of your uterus, they can influence the position of your baby, so that instead of being positioned normally (head down), he or she could be positioned feet first, in the breech position, or sideways, in the transverse position.
○ If you've already had a cesarean delivery or myomectomy, especially if your myomectomy was for intramural fibroids, the scars might make your uterus too weak for a normal delivery.

C-sections are the number one operation women get (hysterectomies are second). So obviously, C-sections are fairly common, but there are some risks. Complications from C-sections can include infection, excessive bleeding, reaction to a possible transfusion, and reaction to anesthesia. There are fewer dangers to the baby. The general anesthesia that you get could affect your baby by reducing her oxygen supply or depressing her breathing; fortunately, this is rare, and if it does happen, it can generally be managed successfully.

Interestingly, women seem to recover much faster from C-sections than from other types of abdominal surgery, possibly because they know their new baby is depending on them, or even because the surgery was for a happy reason rather than to fix a problem. In any case, you will need at least a week of complete recovery time, and experts suggest that you'll recover faster if you don't rush it.

JENNIFER: *My amnio fluid level dropped steadily from weeks 33 to 35. I was in for my weekly biophysical profile and the perinatologist told me that the fluid was down to 3.0—how did I feel about having a baby tonight? Two hours later, I was in labor and delivery, being prepped for a C-section.*

The fibroids caused a lot of bleeding and pain. I measured 51 weeks at 35 weeks when I delivered. It was like having twins! The tumors prevented the baby from turning, so she was breech. Plus, the tumors tricked my body into thinking that I was WAY too pregnant, so all systems began to shut down. I'm lucky I lasted so long!

JENEANE: *The docs decided to do a C-section in my 38th week since the baby was breech. They don't do versions with fibroid women—too risky. A version is when they try to turn the baby around manually from the outside. With fibroids, it's too risky to do because the baby is usually turned breech for a specific reason—like there isn't room for him or her to turn around due to the fibroids.*

It was hard getting her out—they had to pull her out by her feet, but she made it. She's a tough little baby. She was 6 pounds 13 ounces and 18.5 inches.

Thank God we had a healthy baby. I was in the hospital for four days after my C-section. Unfortunately, my incision got infected and I had to go back to the doctor several times so they could clean it out. They put me on antibiotics—after a while, it healed up, though it looked horrible.

ANITA: *I learned that I had fibroids when I went for my first ultrasound scan when my fetus was nine weeks. I was told I had a 5-centimeter posterior fibroid. About six weeks later I had another scan and learned that I had two fibroids—each about 7 centimeters.*

I haven't had any obvious complications. Last week I had an examination and the OB said that the fibroid was not in the cervix. Therefore, I can proceed with a normal vaginal delivery.

POSTPARTUM HEMORRHAGE

Bleeding is a common complication after delivery, but if you have fibroids, you might have a greater risk. Why? When the placenta separates from the wall of the uterus, the exposed blood vessels bleed freely. Normally, your uterus should contract and shut the vessels off; fibroids can keep that from happening. If you've suffered from placental previa, premature labor, or uterine rupture as a result of your fibroids, you may also be at risk for postpartum hemorrhage.

What happens if you're bleeding too much after delivery? The first thing your doctor may do is give you a rubdown. A vigorous massage may help your uterus contract, shutting off open blood vessels. Your doctor may also inject a drug to slow down the bleeding, pack your uterus with gauze, or tie off the uterine arteries. In extreme cases, your doctor may have to perform a hysterectomy.

If your doctor thinks you may be at risk for excessive bleeding when you deliver, discuss the pros and cons of donating your own blood for a possible transfusion.

JENNIFER: *The tumors bled a lot and I lost lots of blood quickly, about a liter. Much more than average. I needed saline to bring up the blood volume.*

Pregnancy after Fibroid Treatment

Maybe you've already taken steps to treat your fibroids; maybe your doctor is advising treatment before you try to get pregnant. What are your treatment options—and what do you need to know about each of them?

AFTER MYOMECTOMY

If you've been trying to get pregnant without success, you may be a candidate for surgery. Conservative doctors will want to know if you've tried to get pregnant for a year before suggesting any radical treatments, including those for fibroids.

The tricky part about surgery is that the cure can be worse than the disease. Cutting into your uterus for a myomectomy—surgery that is like a "lumpectomy" for fibroids—for example, can be more dangerous than doing nothing. On the other hand, it may be the best route to keeping your reproductive options open.

If the fibroids aren't giving you any trouble, you may not need to do anything. But if they're large enough to distort your uterus, creating problems like heavy bleeding, or are actually inside the uterine cavity, taking up potential baby-space, you may need to explore having them removed surgically. A skilled doctor can remove them, repair your uterus, and help create a much friendlier environment for a fertilized egg to implant. See Chapter 5 for more about myomectomies.

While myomectomy offers no guarantees, about two-thirds of the women who want to conceive after myomectomy are able to. But once you've conceived, miscarriage is still a possibility. Estimates of delivery rates—successful pregnancies—after myomectomy range anywhere from over 50 percent to almost 90 percent. The results of one recent study suggest that the results are best for women who've had large intramural fibroids removed; results were also better for women who had laparoscopic myomectomies. It's even possible to give birth vaginally after a myomectomy, although it's important to be in a hospital delivery room, in case of complications.

If your doctor wants to rush you into a hysterectomy, remember that it's not your only option. Many women went to doctors who recommended an immediate hysterectomy, only to have a second opinion that allowed them to preserve their fertility—and they have the happy, healthy children to show for it.

DONNA: *By the time I really wanted to have a child, I had quite a number of fibroids, all external to the womb. The largest one was the size of a plum, which I later discovered was not that large.*

In talking to different doctors in a group practice, they were very mixed about whether I would need surgery or not. One said I should absolutely without question have the fibroid surgery, because given the hormone changes when you get pregnant, they would only get larger. I also had two fibroids around my cervix and that was a concern as well, because they didn't know if my cervix would open early or not.

Another physician pretty much said that I was on the borderline and that I could or couldn't have the surgery; a third physician advised me against it because the elasticity of the uterus could be affected by the fibroid surgery, so that I could be trading one set of problems for another.

So in asking different questions, I came to the following conclusion. If I had the surgery, I'd probably be incapacitated for three to five weeks. And my perspective was, why go through all this pain and suffering and time in the hospital and maybe still never have a child? I asked the doctors what was the worst thing that could happen if I were lucky enough to get pregnant without the surgery, and they said I might have to spend two to three months of bed rest at the end of the pregnancy.

The pregnancy proceeded very well. The last two and a half months, the doctors advised me to be within an hour of the hospital, so I pretty much limited my traveling. When we got past 28 weeks, we all kind of celebrated, my doctors and I, and when we got past 32 weeks we celebrated even more. I wound up going 39 weeks and having a 6-pound, 6-ounce baby.

FELICE: *I started meeting women who'd had nightmare pregnancies because of fibroids and who told me that if they could have known they would have had them out before going through a pregnancy.*

DR. MITCH LEVINE: *We have a lot of pregnancies: We've had hundreds of women get pregnant after myomectomies.*

But Don't Fibroids Come Back after Myomectomy?

This is a frequent question. One of the reasons doctors often discourage myomectomy is that fibroids can grow back after surgery. More likely is that microscopic fibroids, impossible to detect during surgery, continue to grow.

But not everyone gets new fibroids after a myomectomy. As we have seen, the general consensus is that fibroids grow back in about 20 percent, or one woman in five. Even if you do get new fibroids, they may not interfere with your chances of conceiving. There's often a window of opportunity after you recover from surgery and before any new fibroids have a chance to grow large enough to affect you. (Interestingly, an Italian study found that women who had a child after myomectomy had half the recurrence rate of those who did not.)

All that being said, it is probably helpful to time a pregnancy as soon after surgery as you're ready. If you wait too long, and if your fibroids do come back, larger ones may interfere with your ability to carry your baby to term without complications.

MARY: *I had a myomectomy in November. The fibroids were successfully removed, one 12 centimeters, the other 8 centimeters; my uterus was "rebuilt," and one year later, in December, my son was born. Two and a half years later, my daughter was born. Both of my kids were delivered by C-section because of the myo. I had a tubal ligation during the second C-section, since my ob-gyn didn't think my uterus could support another pregnancy.*

CAROLYN: *I was 39 when I had a myomectomy. My time was really running out, age-wise! I got pregnant about six months later. Now I have a beautiful five-year-old daughter. So yes, pregnancy is possible after myomectomy.*

KATE: *I always thought I'd have kids and I wanted to preserve my fertility, but every year my fibroids were getting bigger and my gynecologist said I should consider taking them out. That was weighing on me.*

My gynecologist said I should have the myo—but it was incredibly scary because he said there was a 5 percent chance I'd have serious blood loss and need a hysterectomy. The doctor I went to for a second opinion said he could do a myo and that he'd never had to do a hysterectomy on a woman who needs a myomectomy. So that was like bells in my ears. He said the bigger the fibroids are, the more difficult and the more scarring, but you won't need a hysterectomy.

AFTER TREATMENT WITH GnRH AGONISTS

Gonadotropin-releasing hormone (GnRH) agonists, drugs that temporarily shut down your natural production of estrogen, can give you a brief window to try to get pregnant. If your doctor thinks that one or more fibroids is the reason for suspected infertility—for instance, by blocking one or both fallopian tubes—three months of taking GnRH agonists may shrink the offending fibroids enough to allow for conception.

The timing of this strategy is tricky. Obviously you can't get pregnant while you're in "menopause," so the idea is to start trying as soon as you finish the GnRH agonist treatment. If you haven't conceived within three to six months or so, your fibroids are likely to come back (though not necessarily in exactly the same position).

Asherman's Syndrome

ANOTHER POSSIBLE CONSEQUENCE of surgical procedures is called Asherman's syndrome. This is a scarring of the uterine lining; it can be caused by an infection following a birth or miscarriage, a D&C, or potentially any invasive procedure that involves the lining of your uterus. While this syndrome is considered rare, moderate scarring can lead to miscarriage; severe scarring can cause infertility. Check with your doctor if you have reason to believe you could be affected by Asherman's syndrome, including either the absence of your period or a much lighter period than usual. Asherman's syndrome can be diagnosed and, if not too severe, corrected through hysteroscopy.

While there aren't any guarantees, there's some evidence that GnRH agonists, either alone or as a treatment before myomectomy, can restore fertility in some women. Small studies are not the best barometer, perhaps, but the ones available show a 50 percent success rate in getting pregnant after myomectomy (where fibroids were the sole cause of infertility), as well as some cases where GnRH agonist treatment alone did the trick.

It's important to know that the side effects of using GnRH agonists can be severe, and that there are doctors who can perform myomectomies without using GnRH agonists first. You can read more about this topic in Chapter 5.

CAROLYN: *After losing one pregnancy because the fetus could not attach—due to a huge, cone-shaped fibroid inside my uterus—I was on Lupron*

for three months and then had a myomectomy. One of the male, older
doctors in the practice wanted to do a myomectomy immediately, but my
doctor convinced me to do the Lupron first. She took out a softball-sized
glob of stuff: small, medium, and large shrunken fibroids from all over my
uterus, abdomen, cervix, vaginal canal, everywhere. I had a noticeably
flatter tummy for a while—loved that! I turned 39 that summer. Seven
months after the surgery, I got pregnant with my daughter.

AFTER UAE

As we saw in Chapter 5, UAE [uterine artery embolization] is not currently recommended if you want to preserve your fertility—but at the
moment, that's only because we don't have enough information on how
UAE affects your ability to conceive and deliver a healthy child.

According to Dr. Robert Worthington-Kirsch, "There are women
who have become pregnant after UAE, and their outcomes have been
no different than would be expected in the general population. The
fertility rate after myomectomy is better documented, but may not be
any higher than the fertility rate after UAE." In fact, women do report
healthy pregnancies after UAE; the results of the FIBROID Registry
study will shed some much-needed light on the subject.

AFTER FUS, MYOLYSIS, OR CRYOMYOLYSIS

There's no apparent reason that FUS (Focused Ultrasound Surgery)
would affect your ability to get pregnant, but until it has been in wider
use for a longer period of time, doctors suggest that you avoid it if you
still want to have children.

Myolysis and cryomyolysis are alternatives to myomectomy or
hysterectomy for women who aren't planning to have children. Some
women have conceived after these procedures against their doctors'
advice, running the risk of uterine rupture. Until the risks have been
fully explored, you might also want to pass on both myolysis and
cryomyolysis if you want to conceive in the future.

Reach Out and . . .

HOW TO TALK ABOUT HAVING FIBROIDS

> Life . . . is a community, a struggle to
> preserve intimacy and avoid isolation.
> —DEBORAH TANNEN, PH.D.,
> *YOU JUST DON'T UNDERSTAND*

In the last couple of decades, we've been able to start having open discussions about topics like breast cancer, condoms, and oral sex, subjects that were unthinkable to talk about in public in the Puritan days of, oh, 1985 for instance. But talking about the uterus still feels a bit taboo. I think it's partly because it's not a visible organ, partly because it's part of our reproductive and sexual lives, partly because it can simply feel reductive—after all, women have spent a lot of time and energy to avoid being identified as just a "walking womb."

Fibroids in particular are an awkward topic. In an article in *BWH*, a publication of Brigham and Women's Hospital in Boston, Dr. Cynthia Morton notes, "Women don't like to complain about fibroids. They don't make for good cocktail party conversation."

ROBIN: *I've made such a point during this, I tell everyone. I find there are so many women who've had fibroids or the symptoms; the statistics of how many women have them is unbelievable. I tell women all the time about my fibroids and no one knows about them, they don't have any information. It's so bizarre in this open society how taboo it is to talk about it.*

But not talking about your fears and feelings can heighten stress and anxiety, which, apart from the physical symptoms, may be among the chief side effects of having fibroids. And if that's true for you, it's not something to ignore. As you may know all too well, these feelings can affect almost every aspect of your life.

You may feel your fibroids are your business and no one else's. It may be embarrassing to talk about something so personal, so private. You may have been disappointed in the past when you asked for help and didn't get it. If your fibroids aren't interfering with your day-to-day life and aren't fatal, you might feel like they're not a real problem—not as serious as, say, your father-in-law's heart condition or your best friend's broken leg. You may be on the receiving end of some well-meant but misplaced attention. Or you may simply feel your fibroids are no big deal.

The last thing I want to do is suggest you have to feel weak and unempowered. I do believe, though, that there's strength in numbers. So how do you explain you have fibroids—and how do you get the kind of support you need from the people in your life?

Write It Out

IN *THE ARTIST'S WAY,* Julia Cameron recommends keeping a notebook and pen next to your bed. As soon as you open your eyes in the morning, before you stretch, yawn, brush your teeth, or make coffee, grab the notebook and pen and just write. Write anything that comes to mind. Write at least three pages, more if you feel like it. If you try this even once, you'll probably get some surprising clarity; try doing it every day for a week to explore the complex layers of feelings that you have about having fibroids.

MARY: *I urge all women—and men—to do a lot of asking and talking. Talk to anyone and everyone who has gone through this, or who is going through this, and with this open exchange of thoughts and ideas, it all seems a little easier to bear.*

FELICE: *I would say that the best advice is just to keep talking a lot and not hold anything back. My husband is very supportive and listens all the time, but it was also good to have other friends to talk to about what was going on separate from my husband.*

Lucy, You Have Some 'Splainin' to Do

If you were to get really sick, God forbid, you could turn to your best friend and say, "I have cancer." You know you would fall into each other's arms and cry, and talk for hours. If you turn to someone and say, "I have fibroids," they may look at you innocently and say, "Excuse me?" (Or as one smart aleck said to me, *"Gesundheit!"*)

This can be frustrating, to say the least. While many people seem to have heard of fibroids, most don't know exactly what they are. Beyond that, if someone hasn't dealt with fibroids themselves, they may not have the faintest idea of what you're going through. Don't expect your friends to be mind readers: If you want them to help, you're probably going to have to step up to the plate.

Sometimes, even with the best intentions, the people who want to help the most need you to explain what fibroids are and why they can be a problem. You may get frustrated by feeling that you have to give so much information before you can get the support you want. And sometimes it's simply hard to ask the ones you love to focus on you and what you need.

Are you sad, worried, confused? Perhaps you're weighing a decision about surgery, pregnancy, or drug therapy. You may want to take some time for yourself to explore how you feel so that you can explain it to the people who are close to you.

Be prepared: It's possible that your news about fibroids may worry the people you confide in; it may mystify them, make them feel helpless. Fibroids can be surprisingly stressful on relationships, partly because they're so poorly understood. The more your friends and family can understand what fibroids are, what they're doing to you, and how you're feeling about it, the more likely they are to respond in the right ways.

LINDA: *For my husband, everything I was going through to avoid a hysterectomy was mystifying and frustrating. There wasn't really much he could do—he could see it was very emotional for me and that was hard for him to deal with. He's good in terms of info and straight talk. So in terms of making decisions, he was supportive and helpful. In terms of emotions, it was anxiety provoking for him.*

FELICE: *My husband has been great through all this, but he has his moments of fear and stress and anxiety like any normal person.*

KACI: *Let me tell you my personal feelings about discussing this with friends . . . I have a few women friends with whom I felt close enough to talk about this. They'd sympathize, but sympathy was not what I was looking for. Their gynecological dealings consist of a yearly Pap smear, like most women. They really didn't know what I was going through. So I'd ease away from the conversation or minimize the issue so they'd be more comfortable. This didn't make me feel any better, so after a while, I just stopped sharing. It became like, "Well, I'm going into the hospital on the 5th. Could you stop by the house and water my plants?"*

SHARON: *It's hard, because it seems like there's nothing anyone can say to make you feel better. If they say, "Oh, I'm sure you'll be fine," you think, "Easy for you to say!" Or if they say, "Oh, you poor thing, that must be absolutely HORRIBLE!" you think, "Hey lighten up, I don't plan on dying!"*

Rabbi Harold Kushner, author of *When Bad Things Happen to Good People*, says that our own sense of helplessness and inadequacy may keep us away from the people who can help us feel better. After being disappointed by people you've confided in, it can feel easier to shut down and just handle everything on your own.

The fact is, talking about your fears, your rage, your anxiety, is good for you. Beyond the commonsense aspect, studies show that feelings of stress and isolation actually depress your immune system, and let's face it, fibroids can definitely stress you out. On the positive side, caring conversation can change the physical circuitry of your brain, literally creating connections for more positive thoughts and feelings. You don't even have to say a word. Hospital studies show that just having a friend close by doubled a patient's ability to tolerate pain.

As sociologists know, telling stories is part of who we are. Sometimes our stories include pain, fear, shame, anger, loneliness; not every tale is a Hollywood romance. Not telling your story means that part of you remains invisible, kind of like being in the closet. And closets are dark, small, lonely places. Rabbi Kushner recommends opening the door and letting the world in "so you can tell and retell and retell again, and by the 30th or 40th time it doesn't hurt as much."

So let your friends in on the secret. Sure, tell them "everybody" has fibroids, but they're bothering you. Tell them they're benign 99 percent of the time, but you can't help thinking about cancer anyway. Tell them you have a certain number of treatment options to decide among, including doing nothing. Tell them if you're in pain, or bleeding, or scared. Tell them if you're worried about not being able to have children. Tell them if you feel like less of a woman. Tell them if you want a hug, a neck rub, or a glass of really decent wine. Tell them if you want them to cheer you up, stay upbeat, or to keep the conversation focused on safe subjects, like politics.

ELLEN: *When I decided to get a hysterectomy, my family and friends supported me by staying light. My sister came over with a funny little flower thing made up as an ice cream soda with a tampon topping.*

CAROLYN: *I just asked friends to take me to the grocery store and made darn sure I got several days' worth of stuff each time, because I hated riding in a car for several weeks after the surgery. . . . I found it very uncomfortable.*

JENEANE: *During my pregnancy, my family was a source of strength. My mother and sister live in the same town as us. They helped me clean the house when I was on bed rest, from 36 weeks on. They shopped for me. Helped in lots of ways.*

Paging Dr. Freud...

Sometimes, it helps to talk to a pro. And not just for the facts, ma'am. There's a difference between information and understanding. Take this little quiz:

Who had the best recovery from hysterectomy?
a) Women who got a factual rundown of the surgery and what to expect afterward
b) Women who got counseling about the feelings they had and could expect

If you guessed (b), give yourself two points. Make it three.

But do you need a therapist when you're thinking about surgery? Can't your doctor help you sort out your questions? Dr. Leon Hoffman of the New York Psychoanalytic Society explains that gynecologists are actually trained to depersonalize you in order to treat you objectively, that is, without developing sexual feelings toward you.

"Doctors have to learn how to objectify the human body," Dr. Hoffman says. "The patient has to uncover her body, the doctor has to look at her in a nonsexual way. That creates an attitude in the doctor where the psychological aspects of the patient can be minimized."

In therapy, there's talk but no touching. As a result, Dr. Hoffman says, "A woman can reveal her deepest secrets."

Therapy isn't for everybody, but a compassionate social worker, psychologist, or psychiatrist can help you articulate fears and concerns, even anger, that you didn't know you had, whether or not your fibroids are causing physical symptoms, whether or not you're scheduled for surgery.

So You're Not the Touchy-Feely Type

IF SOUL BARING isn't your style, you can still ask people to give you a hand.

Experiment with asking for something specific: a ride to a doctor's appointment, getting some extra groceries, picking up the kids from school, even keeping you company for something relaxing and fun, like a manicure or a movie.

You might be surprised how good it feels when a friend shows up at your front door with a bag full of stuff you need from the supermarket.

JENEANE: *I was so depressed after the fifth or sixth day in the hospital that I wanted to die. I cried. I told my husband to take me home. I even thought of suicide. Isn't that bizarre—here I had narrowly escaped bleeding to death and I was so depressed I thought about dying. I did confide in my doctor, who asked if I wanted to talk to a psychologist on my insurance plan. I said yes. One came to visit me and talked with me and my husband a couple times. It helped me get through the rest of the time there.*

ROBIN: *I was seeing a therapist twice a month just for general reasons, but the common thread he always came back to was that everything rests on your health. Until you can get your health stabilized, you can't make other decisions, you've got to focus on getting this health thing fixed.*

LAURA: *I was in therapy while I was trying to get my problem diagnosed, so I just talked to her a lot—I was still pretty hysterical about how much I was bleeding, but if I hadn't talked that much I probably would have killed myself. I mean, I was really worked up, suicidal. I talked to my friends, and then I started telling people I knew peripherally. That's when I started finding out how many women have fibroids and I started getting enraged—why was this so hard to figure out?*

But Dahling, I VANT to Be Alone!

When there's something wrong, whether it's physical or emotional, we often need some time to ourselves, to think things through, allow our feelings to surface, whatever they may be, to baby ourselves a little. Lots of us like to curl up at home and mend when we're in pain. And it's okay. You don't have to give up all your obligations. Just try not to neglect your most important one: yourself.

Do you feel like you're "not allowed" to have some down time? How many of these things sound like something you would say?

○ If I take off just one day from work, things are a disaster.
○ I can't ask anyone to look after my kids while I take a couple of hours off just for myself.
○ My family expects me to have dinner ready in the evening.
○ If I don't clean the house, no one will.
○ I said I would volunteer, and there's no one else to fill in.
○ If I don't get to the gym, I feel really guilty.

Though it may rarely feel like it, you are the goddess who organizes and manages your life. And you can take a look at your schedule, your obligations, and make some decisions. Really, you can. Really!

It's mostly a question of expectations, our own and those of the people around us. We can't be Superwomen (as super as we all may be). I know it's hard to accept, but the world won't stop spinning on its axis, if, for instance, you play hooky from work for a day. Or even if you take an hour off for lunch—something that most of us have the right to do, but many of us don't take advantage of. (After all, there are all those extra memos you can write at lunchtime.)

So instead, get in your car and take a drive. Take a walk around the block. Whether you bring your lunch or buy it, eat something healthy. Eat something naughty. Do the thing that will make you feel good.

Take a look around your home. Do you feel better when the house is beautiful? For some of us, cleaning is very calming—and the results are aesthetically satisfying. If you don't love to clean, can you survive a messy house? Yes, you can (I'm living proof). Can your kids pick up after themselves? Can your partner? Is there anybody else in the house who knows how to work a washing machine? A vacuum? (I mean, they can drive a car, can't they?)

Whatever you choose to do, the idea is simple: Take a look at how you spend the day, and figure out where you can grab five minutes for yourself—or half an hour—or an hour. As they say, every little bit helps.

CAROLYN: *I have no family nearby at all, and none of my good friends were around when I was scheduled to have my surgery, so I was pretty much on my own. I arranged for a few casual friends to check on me for a few evenings after I was home to be sure I was okay, and my boyfriend at the time came over a couple of times, too. But I am one of those people who just wants to be left alone when I don't feel well.*

IRIS: *I didn't look for stress reducers as I was so busy trying to work full-time, take care of three elementary school–aged daughters, be a home-maker, and so on. I did use humor a lot, that's my coping mechanism. If you can laugh or see the humorous side of things, it seems to make them easier to bear. I've since discovered that's also my way of denying what's going on. I eventually slowed down at home, rested a lot more, and let my house turn into a pigsty! My girls were really too young to understand what was going on, they just knew their mother was bleeding a lot and was tired and sick. I tried to make light of it, since I did not want to scare them. My husband was his usual aloof self. To his credit, he didn't complain about the messy house or my weakness; to the best of his ability, he was supportive.*

That Old-Time Religion

If you belong to a church, synagogue, mosque, ashram, or any other type of religious or spiritual community, you can often find comfort and support there. Many congregations have a weekly prayer list, where the names of people needing prayers for healing are read out loud during services. There may be a weekly healing service that takes place outside of regular hours of worship. If not, consider organizing one yourself; there will be other people who'll appreciate it. Fibroids may not be the worst problem in the group, but that's fine—you deserve healing and attention too. As my father likes to say, my headache hurts just as much as your toothache.

A word of advice: If you're considering doing anything like this for a friend, talk it over with her first! Not everybody appreciates the attention. You can also create a service for yourself; ask a friend to help you organize the group at your home or hers.

JENNIFER: *I didn't rely on my church, but family members, on both sides, were praying for the baby and my health. It was great to know people were rooting for us! Dan's great-aunt even lit a candle at church, if I remember correctly.*

ANGELA: *This is pretty funny—I had my surgery on a Monday and on Saturday I got a call from someone who said, I heard your name read at the synagogue this morning; are you okay? And I, of course, didn't call to give my name, a friend of mine did without asking me. I'm sure he thought it was a very nice thing to do, but I was mortified. And I thought to myself, the rabbis just announced in front of 2,000 people that I had a hysterectomy, thank you so much! I didn't think of myself as sick, and I really wasn't inclined to share.*

Organized religion offers one place to find community, but it's not the only one. Dr. Dean Ornish tells us, "Anything that promotes a sense of love and intimacy, connection and community, is healing." Belonging to any kind of group where you feel free to express yourself can ease anxiety and possibly reduce stress hormones, whether it's a sewing circle that you've been in for 10 years or a fibroid support group that you organize next week.

E-Support

In this electronic age, you knew I couldn't leave out the Internet as a source of support. Weird as it is, the virtual relationships that develop online can often feel just as strong as, or stronger than, some of our "real-life" encounters. Maybe it's not so weird: After all, there's another human being out there, typing away on her keyboard, thinking about you.

There are a few resources on the Web for women with fibroids; by the time you read this, there may well be more. You can even start your own group, and you don't have to be a computer genius to do it.

KIM: *One thing that was really interesting was that Internet site I found. It's not really a Web site, it's a chat room that AOL designed. One woman I met online had a myomectomy and she sent me a list of all the vitamins and herbs and natural supplements she took prior to the operation—she healed immediately, right after her myomectomy. Of course, she may be in better shape than I am to begin with!*

JENEANE: *Man, the Internet is a lifesaver for anyone with anything. I remember the first forum I joined—it was for women who were pregnant, or trying to get pregnant, with fibroids. I joined as soon as I got the news about my fibroids being 16 weeks' size. The group of us e-mailed each other and the hosts of the forum kept a digest that they e-mailed out once a week with everyone's questions. It was amazing. SO many stories. It was like being adopted into a family of women who were just like you. I felt hopeful from all the successes I watched happen before my eyes. I became anxious when I lost touch with women who dropped out in the middle of their pregnancies. Mostly, I would come home from work with pages I had printed out that my husband and I would study and learn from.*

One caution: It's great to listen and be open to what other women have to say, but consider whether their situation is the same as yours. The Internet can be a great source of information, but it can also attract people who need to discuss their problems. Their issues and yours may not be the same, and you may get a distorted sense of whether a treatment works, since success stories don't always find their way into the electronic world.

Fibroids and the 9-to-5

Bleeding episodes. Problem pregnancies. Cramps. If only you could schedule them in your day planner. Even more than an irate client or a moody boss, fibroid symptoms can really mess up your work day, and can sometimes make you miss work for weeks.

If you do wind up being out for any significant period of time, it's important to know your rights. Check with your personnel department about how many sick days you're entitled to, whether vacation days can be rolled over into sick days, when you're entitled to short-term disability. You may need to know the laws about employment in your city: You can call the local Bureau of Labor or attorney general's office. Since finding the information may be time-consuming, it could be useful to do your homework before any possible problems occur.

If you're self-employed, you might want to consider having a contingency plan in place. This could include a list of important clients or contacts that a friend can call for you if you're out of commission for a couple of days.

IRIS: *Luckily, the general manager of the company I worked for was a woman and she was very understanding and supportive. When I was just too exhausted and weak to come in to work and would call in sick, she would always say, listen to your body, stay home and rest.*

Staying home was hard for me to do. I had always been fairly healthy, energetic, and had a strong work ethic. I believed I was strong and could overcome anything.

JENEANE: *Four weeks after I got back to work, I was laid off. I had been there four years and had gotten 5 out of 5 on my last review. I sued; we settled. I know what it was really about—everyone did—and any work-*

ing woman who has ever had a baby knows what it was about. I felt betrayed for having four years of stellar performance—managing the "star" group in the company—wiped away because I decided to create another human being and didn't have as easy a time of it as a 20-year-old would have. You'd think a woman-owned company would have behaved differently, but I'm here to tell you, watch out. While you're out of sight—especially if you have to be on bed rest early—you're soon out of mind. So make your plans accordingly.

When All Else Fails, Have a Party

I know you think I'm kidding. Not long ago, I would've thought I was kidding. On a recent vacation, I started chatting with two women from San Francisco while we were all waiting for a table at a restaurant. We wound up having lunch together; when I told them I was working on this book they looked at each other and burst out laughing,

"You have to talk to our friend Ellen," they said. "You'll never believe what she did!"

They were right: It was the first time I'd ever heard of anyone throwing a bon voyage party for her reproductive organs.

ELLEN: *After 10 years of problems, I finally found a doctor who took me seriously: He found a fibroid the size of a fist pressing against my bowel. Since I was 48, I decided to have a hysterectomy. I was relieved to be free of my bowel problems, and I felt extreme joy about never getting my period again! I decided I wanted to celebrate, so I had a bon voyage party. Friends got me a cake with a little uterus and ovaries on it that said "Bye-bye Junior"; we had a Tampon Toss, played "pin the tampon on the uterus" and did a tampon hunt. We gave out little erasers as prizes. I had a really good time, and as a parting gift, my guests re-hid all the tampons around the house . . . I'm still finding them!*

~ 12 ~

Know Thyself

THE MIND-BODY CONNECTION

Everything psychological is ultimately biological.
—DR. DAVID G. MYERS, AUTHOR OF
THE PURSUIT OF HAPPINESS

ANYBODY WITH A brain knows there's a mind-body connection. When we're happy, most of us feel pretty good—or great; when we're down, every little ache and pain can get thrown into sharp relief.

Anxiety, anger, fear, worry, resentment, hurt—all emotions that, for the sake of simplicity, I'm labeling "stress"—have an impact on our bodies. Most of us are at least familiar with coping strategies like meditation, prayer, and yoga—even working out. The question is, how do these traditional balms for the mind fit in with the healing of our bodies? Do our minds have any influence over our fibroids? Can mind-body medicine—whatever that is—help us, heal us, cure us?

I imagine you've come across individuals or books that insist we each possess miraculous healing powers—and if we don't know how to put them to use, it's our own fault. We're made to feel guilty of being hopeless, unspiritual, limited. Mind-body medicine, as it's evolved within the medical community and as it's described in this chapter, is not a substitute for treatment or a declaration of our invincible powers of self-healing. Rather, it's an area where medical science, philosophy, psychology, and spirituality merge.

Alice Domar, Ph.D., and Henry Dreher, authors of *Healing Mind, Healthy Woman*, define mind-body medicine as "any method in which we use our minds to change our behavior or physiology in order to promote health and recovery from illness." The mind can influence the way we choose to live, the therapies we choose to pursue—or not—and who we choose to listen to for guidance, including our own intuition.

Doctors exploring the use of mind-body medicine make a distinction between "curing" and "healing." While mind-body medicine may not make your fibroids go away—that is, cure you—it may help restore you to a more generally healthy condition. Dr. Bernie Siegel, comparing two common choices, says that people "who want to get well through the doctor alone or God alone are minimizing their chances." This simple reminder allows us to explore how our emotions, beliefs, and attitudes can have a role in healing ourselves, while not rejecting the many other tools at our disposal.

The organized study of the mind-body connection is growing fast, although as you might imagine, the mind-body connection for healing women with fibroids is not exactly at the top of the research agenda. But looking at the evidence and research that exists, we can draw some conclusions that apply to us—and perhaps gain some surprising insights as well.

None of the mind-body techniques we'll discuss are presented as a substitute for medical treatment or a healthy lifestyle. At the same time—since your mind is a part of your body, after all—you may find that one or more of these techniques can make everything else work even better.

Some people use the power of faith, a power outside themselves, to cope with physical problems. Others join a support group that provides the strength of community. Others use their own imaginations to redirect their lives and their thinking, so that either living with fibroids or making treatment decisions becomes an active choice, a choice that feels good instead of bad. You can choose one of these directions, or all of them; unlike drugs, there aren't any dangerous interactions.

East and West, We've All Got Stress

You may already know that more than two-thirds of visits to the doctor are directly related to stress. It's not that we want to get sick, or that our problems are psychosomatic, but that our emotions trigger complex chemical reactions that have far-reaching effects in our bodies.

Our bodies release hormones under stress that can suppress the immune system, impair memory, trigger skin problems, and heighten muscle tension. When people are under stress, cuts and bruises tend to heal more slowly and latent viruses like herpes can become active again.

The Pleasure Principle

THOMAS MOORE ASKS, "Are you fighting pleasure somewhere or in some part of your body that is seeking pleasure? . . . We could imagine disease . . . as the failure of the body to find its pleasure." Studies show that the effects of stress can be offset by laughing—so if you can't find something to tickle your funny bone, get someone to tickle you.

Stress is also a key factor in infertility. How many people do you know who struggled to get pregnant, only to have a biological baby after adopting? Or who conceived while they were on vacation? In fact, women dealing with infertility can have as much anxiety and depression as women dealing with heart disease, cancer, and HIV.

So here's the zillion-dollar question: Can stress cause fibroids? Based on cancer research, it's possible that stress can be a factor in triggering disease in people who are already susceptible. So although it's probably not accurate to say that stress causes fibroids, if you're already predisposed because of your genes, body type, or other factors, stress might be the match that lights the fuse.

Can stress make fibroids grow? Once again, studies give us a quali-fied maybe. As we discussed in Chapter 7, there is evidence that stress can release toxins stored in our body fat. Estrogen imitators in these chemicals can spur the growth of fibroids. When animals were put in stressful situations—those in which they had no control or were helpless against repeated injuries—their tumors grew, an indication that feelings of having some control over our situations and having options are important for our health.

And finally, since stress can make you tired, cranky, and depressed, you may stop taking care of yourself and not do things like eat right, exercise, and have a few good giggles—all of which, as we've seen, might make a difference to your fibroids, and do make a difference to your quality of life.

BONNIE: *In June I separated from my husband after 13 years of a very difficult, stressful marriage. In August I began to gush blood toward the tail end of my period. By October, I was dropping clots of fresh blood the size of a baseball during my period; my next period was extremely heavy with some flooding. My hemoglobin was very low and I was tired a lot.*

The next January I had an ultrasound that revealed a large fibroid measuring 6.7 centimeters. Now I knew what I was dealing with.

Be Here Now: Living in the Present

If you wait for tomorrow, tomorrow comes.
If you don't wait for tomorrow, tomorrow comes.
—WEST AFRICAN SAYING

Two-thirds of the sources of all your stress are 100 percent under your control. How can I be sure? Because while our bodies exist solely in the present, our minds allow us to live simultaneously in the past, present, and future.

Deepak Chopra writes, "Both past and future are born in the imagination; only the present, which is awareness, is real." There's more to this than philosophy: The events that we remember or anticipate can affect our bodies just as surely as events in the present.

Think about the power of memory: It makes us laugh about things that happened to us as kids or cry over an old heartbreak. When we develop a picture in our minds, even if it's just an image of something we remember, our bodies react: Blood flows to the visual centers of the brain, the nervous system gets moving, and there go our emotions—just as if we were seeing something happening right in front of us.

Our brains are also able to visualize the future—something we normally call anticipation. If you've ever felt your heart beat faster while you were waiting for someone special to show up for a date, or felt your palms sweat while waiting for a job interview to begin, you know that anticipation can cause a physical reaction.

When you start thinking about stress in the three dimensions of past, present, and future, you can start to see how much time and energy we spend on events that are taking place only in our minds.

So how can we apply this to fibroids? For starters, if I'd known how to distinguish my fears from reality, I would have spent a lot less time getting upset in doctors' offices. (At one point, a rather famous doctor told me that my fibroids were like a big block of concrete dangling over my head—and the rope was fraying. Instead of crumpling up in his guest chair and anticipating being crushed to a powder, I looked at him and laughed. "Don't you be talking like that to me," I said. "Don't go trying to scare me." After that we had a grown-up conversation. And I was able to think about my options calmly.)

The first time most of us learned we had fibroids, we didn't have a clear idea what they were and, without that education, developed a perfectly normal fear of the unknown. For many of us, our fibroids became our monsters in the closet. Hopefully, that's behind us, and armed with an education about what fibroids are, we may be able to help the next person we know who's diagnosed with them.

Another way we can start using mind-body techniques is to sort out the kinds of stress we're reacting to and how we want to deal with each one. Some of us may decide that we're carrying around old emotional wounds that we're tired of packing in our daily luggage. Some of us may have the constant tension of bleeding, pain, or other symptoms. Many of us may be caught up in our fears of the future—whether we'll need surgery, start having symptoms one day, or not be able to get pregnant.

Once you discover the source—or sources—of your stress, it may become easier to come up with ways to deal with them. Less stress can mean fewer symptoms; you may also be able to manage your decisions about treatment with a clearer mind. Once you're off the high-stress track, you may find you have more free space emotionally to make positive changes in your life. This too may not heal your fibroids, but it could be the single most productive, creative side effect of having them.

Say Amen, Sister: Faith in a Higher Power

Faith has many shapes and forms. One of them is belief in a higher power outside ourselves, often expressed, though not always, by being a member of an organized religion. A 1998 survey found that 86 percent of us believe that prayer, meditation, or other spiritual practices can improve the results of medical treatment (though we may think it can work for other people better than ourselves, since only 58 percent of us say we're strongly committed to religion). A 2004 survey showed that almost half of us have prayed for someone's health—including our own—in the last 12 months.

Dr. David B. Larson, president of the National Institute for Healthcare Research, suggests that religious belief can play a role in coping with illness, recovering from surgery, handling stress, and managing depression. At Duke University, doctors found that patients with some religious link had hospital stays that were only half as long as patients who didn't.

Incorporating religious tools directly into the healing process may also be effective. A study of Muslim patients showed that those who prayed and read from the Koran as part of their treatment program improved more quickly than those who received medical treatment alone. Even remote prayer may improve the results of medical treatment. Researchers in Durham, Virginia, found that cardiac patients receiving prayers from sites as far-flung as the Western Wall in Jerusalem, a Buddhist monastery in Nepal, and a Carmelite convent in Baltimore recovered better after surgery than patients who didn't receive such prayers.

You can even create your own prayer team. In Kansas City, researchers recruited a group of 75 local people (mostly women who went to church at least once a week) to pray for patients in the cardiac care unit. The "intercessors" only knew the first name of the patients, which they included in a daily prayer for four weeks. All together, the group prayed on behalf of almost five hundred patients, asking for a "speedy recovery with no complications." So what happened? The patients didn't leave the hospital any sooner than a control group—but their symptoms were somewhat less severe.

Can faith alone help you leave your fibroids behind? Mary Baker Eddy, founder of the Church of Christ, Scientist, once said, "Health is not a condition of matter, but of mind." Christian Scientists believe that God provides the "mental medicine" which leads to a healing change in the body. Other religious traditions, such as Pentecostalism, also rely on the power of God, and faith in God, as their primary "physician."

Other faith traditions don't promise physical healing, but do offer a spiritual and emotional connection with both the divine and human forces around us. People with a strong faith in God may have more hope, better coping skills, less depression—even enhanced immune function. If you're part of a faith community, you can choose to ask members of your congregation to pray for you, cry with you, laugh with you—or just talk with you.

I'm not suggesting you run off and join the religion of your choice to help you feel better about your fibroids. The baseball legend Satchel Paige once said that you can't pray when it rains if you don't pray when the sun shines, and studies bear out that religious or spiritual faith seems to work in healing only if it's already a part of your life.

KIM: *Every now and then I'll go to a healing session and I'll do a misha berach—a healing prayer—for my fibroids, but it's not something I do regularly. And I don't know why, because it's sort of up my alley to do that.*

Thinking about my fibroids is sort of included in my general spiritual practices, but I haven't focused specifically on them, maybe because I don't really believe that prayer alone would make them shrink. I think I have to do more than that.

JENNIFER: *I always prayed that the baby would make it and be okay, which, thank God, happened, even though it was a rough start. Both my husband and I think that she was an act of God, or a miracle, at least to us. I always knew I was tough, but this was by far the most physically and emotionally draining thing that has ever happened to me or my husband. I cried a lot and asked God why A LOT. My hubby is a lot more religious than I, but we both believe that this baby was meant to be. I've resigned myself that if I'm not able to have another child, that is what is meant to be and we'll be happy with the way things are. This baby was a gift and we really treasure every moment we have with her.*

KACI: *I broke up with my significant other a few months before my second surgery, and it was a very stressful time for me. So, yes, I did pray—and take long walks. I concentrated on keeping a positive frame of mind and not giving in to self-pity, because it accomplishes nothing.*

HILLARY: *I started paying attention to what I was eating, I focused on meditation, on prayer, and on having faith that I would be safe. Part of what I'm trying to learn about my faith in God is that I'll be safe. Even if I have to have surgery and have the fibroid out, I'll be safe.*

Believe You Me: Positive Expectations

Sometimes I've believed as many as six
impossible things before breakfast.
—THE WHITE QUEEN, IN
THROUGH THE LOOKING-GLASS

Another way to talk about faith is to look at belief. Medical technology, whether drugs or surgery, obviously has a physical effect, but belief in whether a treatment will work has a dimension all its own. Even when a treatment has no known medical value, it can work from 30 to more than 50 percent of the time: This is the famous "placebo effect," which depends purely on belief.

Belief—or if you prefer, expectations—does have a physical effect. It turns out that placebos can trigger the release of dopamine in your brain. And what is dopamine? It's a natural chemical that—among other things—makes us feel happy. Other experiences that release dopamine into our systems include—you'll love this—food and sex.

So perhaps that helps explain why belief can affect how well you weather a procedure. For instance, a study of women having laparoscopy showed that the amount of pain they had after the procedure could be predicted by each woman's beliefs about pain and how serious she considered her condition.

Positive expectations can also affect how well a treatment will work for you—even if it doesn't work for everyone. One study found that patients with AIDS who had faith that their treatments would work stayed well longer than the patients who stopped believing that the treatments were effective. Perhaps one of the lessons for us is that treatments for fibroids—none of which is 100 percent satisfactory for everybody—may be affected by each woman's belief in whether it can work for her.

Dr. Dan Molerman of the University of Michigan, quoted in the *New York Times,* says, "The physician is an agent for optimism and hope and a great inducer of beliefs." In tests, people told by their doctors that a medicine would definitely work had much better results than patients with identical symptoms whose doctors told them they weren't sure if the treatment would be effective. If your doctor says you "only" have an 80 percent chance of having a successful myomectomy, that may send a different message than saying, for instance, four out of five women have successful long-term outcomes.

So what does that say about how we approach our decisions to treat fibroids? Since so many doctors are most comfortable prescribing hysterectomy—or their own preferred method of surgery—it's critical that we form our beliefs about treatment separate and apart from our doctors' recommendations. Of course, your doctor can be a valuable source of information. But be aware of how his or her own beliefs can influence your feelings and subsequent decisions.

Decisions, Decisions

Don Koberg and Jim Bagnell, authors of *The Universal Traveler,* say there are only two real choices in life: "To accept things as they exist or to accept the responsibility for changing them."

Well, maybe it sounds easier than it is. But making the effort is the first step. Accepting the way things are means giving up blame, regrets, and fears—the negative memories and visualizations of past and future. I'm not talking about a victimy kind of acceptance, the feeling that you just have to take whatever gets dumped on you. Think of it as an active acceptance: living in the present, evaluating things as they are, and accepting the fact that you have the ability to make changes.

"Ability" may sound like you need some kind of special skill. But Deepak Chopra offers us a fresh perspective, telling us that "we have the *ability* to have a creative *response* to the situation *as it is now.* . . . [this] awareness allows you to take the moment and transform it to a better situation or thing."

And how cool is that?

KACI: *I do believe there's a mental connection to illness and health. The friends I have stuck with me "through sickness and health." I have a full-time job, am involved in real estate, and write in my spare time—though I haven't been published yet! These activities give me a sense of gratification. Right now there's still no "significant other," but getting married and having babies is not an all-consuming passion like it was even a couple of years ago. I don't know when exactly I made my peace with that, but it just happened, just as the prospect of having a hysterectomy used to scare me to death, and I can now accept it if it's inevitable. I realize I have a pretty good life. It hasn't always been a bowl of cherries, but whose is?*

Making choices often means making trade-offs. More time with the kids or more time working out? A week of caffeine withdrawal or the comfort of a coffee jolt? Accepting that you can live with your fibroids—and the symptoms—or going through surgery? Accepting that surgery is the right option for you—or living with symptoms that wear you down?

As we've seen, there are a lot of creative choices you can make about your fibroids, including accepting them as part of who you are right

Design the Future You Want

GET A REALLY big piece of paper. Starting at the top right-hand corner, draw an "S"; make sure it fills up most of the page. Now, starting from the top right-hand corner again, write in everything you do on a typical day, following the shape of the S, from the moment you wake up until you go to sleep at night. This is your daily road map. You can use this to look at habits that might affect your fibroids, from how often you're able to exercise to how often you prepare a healthy dinner. When you're done, sit with a cup of tea and take a look at the way you're spending your time. Is this ideal? Are there things you'd prefer to change? If you want to do things a little differently, here are five steps to help you change course:

o Accept the situation. This is where you are today, and there is no blame or guilt attached to that. It simply is.
o Clarify your goals. Do you want to lose weight, get more sleep, even change jobs? Choose one or two things to focus on at first; you can always go back and do more.
o Plan your action. Using a different color pen, edit your road map to show the changes you'll make. Simple changes are good, like taking a 10-minute walk in the evening or writing one job application letter every day.
o Put your map somewhere where you'll see it, or write your plan in your date book for the next few weeks.
o Think of your "dates" as being with a friend. You wouldn't stand up a friend, would you?

now. But whatever your decision is, once you've made it, accept that it's a good one. My aunt Rita once gave me a Zen-like piece of advice. She said, "Whatever decision you make, at the time you make it, is the only decision you could have made at the time." Deepak Chopra puts it like this: "There is only one choice, out of the infinity of choices available in every second, that will create happiness for you as well as for those around you."

So trust yourself that once you've done your homework, talked to the people you care about, to your doctor, herbalist, homeopath, or other professionals, that the combination of your research and your instincts will lead you in the direction that's right for you.

And if that doesn't work, you can almost always change your mind later.

The Power of Positive Thinking

If we only have one choice left in life, it's how we'll react to the situation we're in. I'm not talking about being a Pollyanna Purebred, unless you look especially good in braids and an apron. You can acknowledge that something stinks while deciding to make the best of a bad situation.

A lot has been written about "the power of positive thinking," but it's a term that's often misinterpreted. We can't change what's happening around us because we have sunny attitudes: Feeling positive won't stop bleeding or relieve cramps. But positive thoughts help put us in control of our actions. Do we give up or look for options?

A positive attitude is associated with a stronger immune system—and how well we take care of ourselves overall. Actors know that pretending to be happy can wind up feeling like the real thing. Try this: Walk down a busy street or through the mall with a glum look on your face. Check out how people react. Then think of something that makes you smile and see what happens. Creating a positive attitude in the people around you can reflect right back at you, like a smile in the mirror.

Laurie A. Baum, M.S.W., author of *Astrological Secrets for the New Millennium*, says, "Our thoughts can make us feel better. I walk around feeling the way I want to feel: it starts to happen and the world reacts."

HILLARY: *I'm very aware that my emotions can make my fibroids more of a problem: I'm more attuned to what causes stress. I became aware of how I could change my attitude with positive thinking, basic stuff. And affirmations: I am safe. I will be taken care of. I will be all right. I will find a doctor I can trust.*

BETH: *I had to climb out of a H-O-L-E to get W-H-O-L-E.*

There's always one good thing to think about.

DO YOU SEE the glass as half-empty or half-full? Or are you one of those people who see the glass cracked, with the water running all over the mahogany table and making a stain that will never come out? A negative attitude, a prolonged bad mood, even long periods of stress are bad for your health. Wounds heal more slowly, your resistance to colds and infections is poor, and when you do come down with something, it's worse. Doctors say that even if you're depressed, even if you have true, justifiable, irrefutable reasons to feel negative (and don't we all, from time to time), *you can change your mind* . . . and start to heal physically, as well as mentally.

The Relaxation Response

Man is a thinking reed, but his great works are
done when he is not calculating and thinking.
—DAISETZ T. SUZUKI, FROM THE
INTRODUCTION TO EUGEN HERRIGEL'S
ZEN AND THE ART OF ARCHERY

Meditation, visualization, conscious breathing, chanting a mantra, or the rhythmic footfall of a steady run can all help stop the noise in your mind, toning down the drumbeat of your fears, so that you can get perspective on your situation. And as Jimmy Buffett might say, changes in attitude can lead to changes in latitude.

"The relaxation response" is a term coined by Dr. Herbert Benson, president of Harvard's Mind-Body Institute and author of *The Relaxation Response*. According to Dr. Benson, "When a person engages in a repetitive prayer, word, sound or phrase, and when intrusive thoughts are passively disregarded . . . there is a decreased metabolism, heart rate, breathing rate and slower brain waves." The relaxation response has been shown to help relieve the effects of, among other things, chronic pain, PMS, infertility, anxiety, and depression. Students of Eastern religions will recognize the basic technique as being a secular application of Buddhist religious practice, where meditation, breathing, and mindfulness are central tenets.

Robert S. Ellwood refers to this process as finding the "Quiet Mind." He writes, "Giving time to the Quiet Mind will bring the stress level of the whole of your day down a few notches . . . What it can do is affect the way the mind works so that it responds differently . . . with more calmness, with greater access to reservoirs of inner joy and strength."

Researchers at the University of Wisconsin at Madison put meditation to the test. They recruited 25 volunteers to take part in an eight-week program, which included weekly meditation training classes and a one-day retreat. The participants were also asked to meditate on their own for an hour a day, six days a week. When researchers measured the electrical activity in the participants' brains, they saw increased energy in the left, frontal region—the spot associated with reduced anxiety and positive feelings.

Can meditation actually improve your health? Taking things one step further, the Wisconsin volunteers all got flu shots at the end of the training. Blood tests taken a month later showed that they had produced more anti-flu antibodies—showing a higher level of immunity—than a group who also got the flu shot, but did not meditate.

Ellwood cautions, "Meditation is not magic, and will not magically remove the causes of anxiety, depression or lethargy." But meditation in all its forms—including prayer, mindful breathing, and other

Trying the Relaxation Response

DR. BENSON DESCRIBES the relaxation response in two basic steps:

○ Repeat a word, sound, prayer, thought, phrase, or muscular activity.
○ Simply return to the repetition when other thoughts intrude.

relaxation or focusing techniques—can help us break the train of negative thinking by giving us room to focus and listen to ourselves. A daily meditation may be just as good for our minds as good food and exercise are for our bodies.

KIM: *A friend sent me a book on fibroids. It's a little "if you relax and meditate they'll go away" and I don't believe that happens. Because I do relax and I do meditate and they don't go away.*

You're Getting Sleeeeepy, Verrry . . .

Feeling drowsy? Hypnosis has been the subject of a lot of jokes, but it's a technique that shows how the power of suggestion can help us meet specific goals. Stephen M. Kosslyn, associate psychologist in neurology at Massachusetts General Hospital, explains, "The world is not just what's there, it's how we interpret it. Your mental imagery can set your physical systems in motion."

Before anesthesia was invented, people sometimes used hypnotherapy to minimize pain during surgery. Even now, people use hypnotism instead of anesthesia for procedures from dental work to C-sections. People who get hypnotherapy before cardiac surgery often leave the hospital sooner, needing less pain medication than other patients. Under hypnosis, some cancer patients even experience reductions in tumor size.

What can hypnosis do for fibroids? Some hypnotists believe that it's possible to control both bleeding and pain. One practitioner suggests that you can visualize your blood vessels squeezing shut, stopping the blood flow from your fibroids. You can also imagine the fibroids being reabsorbed into your body, molecule by molecule. You'd need to try this over a period of several weeks before expecting any results. If you're going to an acupuncturist to relieve bleeding, you could try this type of visualization during your treatments.

You can use hypnosis as a relaxation technique, a way to clear out everyday distractions and get in touch with your goals. You might want to start having a more positive attitude, put aside a past hurt, or envision a future success. It starts by getting into a receptive state. Then when you're ready, you tell yourself what to do; over time, you should see your suggestions taking hold. You can go to a qualified hypnotherapist, but you can also try some self-hypnosis. Here's one very basic recipe from *The Universal Traveler* that you can try at home (approximate time, 20 minutes):

○ State your goal clearly (perhaps in writing).
○ Make sure you won't have any interruptions: unplug the phone, shut the door.
○ Relax, lie down, close your eyes, let your breathing get deep and even. Let go.
○ Say your suggestions out loud. Talk to yourself in a soft but firm tone.
○ When you're ready, open your eyes and acknowledge your new plan.

How you react to a suggestion also depends on who's doing the talking. As we saw earlier, doctors usually have a lot of influence over us, partly because we grant our doctors a lot of authority and power due to their expertise. Deborah Tannen, Ph.D., points out that in situations "when an expert man talked to an uninformed woman, he took a controlling role in structuring the conversation." Being informed and asking questions will not only help you react to your doctor's suggestions objectively, but help your doctor become a better partner in your health care will also.

Picture Your Pain

IF YOU TRY picturing your pain, you might be able to change how it feels. Imagine what color it is . . . what shape it has . . . whether it's rough or smooth, hot or cold. Now imagine how can you change it. If it's hot and fiery, try making it a cold ocean breeze; if it's small and hard like a stone, try making it softer, lighter, bigger . . . until it's so big and light it floats away like a big balloon.

Creative Visualization

Shakti Gawain, in her book *Creative Visualization,* explains that this technique is nothing new, exotic, or even difficult. In fact, she says, we use it every day. She defines creative visualization as "using your imagination to create what you want in your life." Why can this work? Because every action is preceded by a thought. You think about reaching for a pen, and your arm moves. You think about going to the movies, and off you go.

Do you want to see yourself eating more healthfully, exercising more, taking time out to relax? Visualization can help you "see" yourself there, creating a blueprint for the future. Visualization, like hypnosis, can help put our minds on the positive track we'd like to be on—sooner or later, our actions follow. Visualization can also help relieve anxiety and reduce pain. Dr. Allan Warshowsky suggests that focused visualization can also help control bleeding, even when you're under sedation during surgery.

You can also use visualization to get in touch with any emotional issues your fibroids raise. In a world full of diseases, Ann Chopelas, Ph.D., asks us to consider why we get fibroids and not something else. This, she says, "is the emotional aspect attached to the uterus." If you'd like to try bringing creative visualization to work on this question, here are a few suggestions to get you started. The only trick to preparing for creative visualization is to relax and get comfortable. Make sure you won't be interrupted. Let your imagination be creative, free, and uninhibited.

○ Picture a time in your life when you didn't have fibroids. What was your life like then? Is there anything about that time that you'd like to recapture in your current life?

○ What do you want your life to be like in six months? a year? What would you have to change to get you there?

○ Imagine that you have a twin who doesn't have fibroids. Were her choices in life different from yours? How does she compare to you when it comes to eating well, exercising, getting enough sleep, dealing with stress? Is there anything you could learn from her?

○ Imagine that your uterus is a garden. What kinds of plants are your fibroids? Are you helping to fertilize them in any way? Do they fit into your landscape, or are they overrunning the other plants? Talk to the gardener. Do you want to tear them out by the roots, bulldoze the entire garden—or just leave everything alone?

○ Imagine that you're in a comfortable beach chair, sitting by the ocean. The sun is warm but not hot. There's a second chair next to you; another woman is sitting in it. She starts talking to you. She tells you how she feels about having fibroids, why she thinks they grew, and what would make her feel best going forward. If you have questions, you can ask her. When you're done, lean back in your beach chair. Feel the sun warming your skin. When you're ready, open your eyes and remember the insights and advice you got from the wise woman by the ocean.

When you're done, don't talk or move for a little while—stay with the feelings and the thoughts that came up. It might be helpful to write your experience down in a diary; you might want to talk about it with a good friend. Don't worry if you don't draw any conclusions right away. In a few days or weeks, you'll experience an "aha!" moment and have one more clue about your life and, perhaps, your fibroids.

Home Sweet Home

IN ANCIENT CULTURES, homes were often equated with the womb. You can think of your home as the womb that nurtures you, the environment that refreshes and restores your senses. Pick a project that you've been planning to do around the house—painting a room, buying some plants, making some new pillows—and start making your home even more beautiful. If you like yellow, go for it; it has a positive effect on the mind and an energizing effect on the body.

Journaling

We might place more importance on the stories
we tell about our illnesses and the history of our
bodies. We might notice dreams that occur at
the time of an illness. We could tone down the
masculine heroics in the modern practice of
medicine and allow some freedom of imagination.
—THOMAS MOORE, *CARE OF THE SOUL*

When I was a kid, I had one of those red fake leather diaries, with a little lock and key. There was a tiny little pocket for a miniature yellow pencil; the pages had light blue lines to write on. Every entry started like this: *"Dear Diary . . ."*

Well, we've grown up since then. You may keep a journal already, either regularly or when you feel like it, or you may hate writing—in which case, if you like, you can try talking your thoughts into a little tape recorder.

There are a million things you can accomplish by keeping a journal, but here are a few ways that may help you shed some light on the parts of your life that are affected by—or that affect—your fibroids. (You may even improve your physical health. Studies show that writing for twenty minutes a day, for just three days, promotes faster healing and relieves certain symptoms.) Choose one or all of them, or maybe you'll have your own approach. If you want to try more than one of these suggestions, I would space them out, maybe doing one a day or one a week. Two reasons why: First, your insights from one set of entries will make the next entry deeper and more interesting. Second, if you do all this self-examination at once, it may trigger more stress. I would be compelled to eat at least a pint of ice cream. So here goes.

LOOK ON THE SUNNY SIDE

Oprah Winfrey suggests keeping a gratitude journal to have a record of the things that make life better for you. This kind of writing can help retrain your mind to emphasize the good things about your life and put any negative areas into better perspective. If your fibroids aren't troubling you, or you've decided you don't need surgery, you might feel grateful for that. If you've had a successful surgery, or have realized the strength of an important relationship, those would qualify too.

HOW DO YOU COPE?

Get comfortable. Flex your writing hand—shake it out. Now take a deep, slow breath, and start thinking about everything that stresses you out. I know, how much time do you have? Here's one way to get started: Write down five life changes or events that have caused the most stress in your life—perhaps your marriage, divorce, a birth, death, family get-together, something on the job. (Remember, stress is what you think it is.) Leave some space on the page between each entry. Now try to remember what you did or how you reacted in each situation. Did you withdraw, get depressed, enlist help from friends? Maybe after you review your thoughts for all your entries, you'll discover a pattern of coping, perhaps one you'll want to modify or change. If you happen to be able to match up the appearance or growth of your fibroids to any of these events, that's another good clue that making changes in behavior can help make changes in your health.

ALL IN THE FAMILY

As we move through life, accumulating an increasing circle of friends, relatives, acquaintances, and colleagues, we inevitably pick up people who were good for us once but who are no longer contributing to our mental health, creativity, or happiness. Make one list of people who make you feel good, support your health decisions, and are able to listen to what's on your mind; make a second list of people who drain you, disparage you, hurt you. Don't edit for politically incorrect selections like your mother, mate, or boss. Julia Cameron, in *The Artist's Way*, suggests naming these two groups "Warm Fluffy Towels" and "Wet Blankets." Think about spending more time with the warm fluffy towels, and next to each entry, write down a date that you'll call, write, e-mail, or show up for tea.

FOOD AND MOOD

I wonder if the stress of our lifestyles in this country contributes to our national tendency toward being overweight. If you've realized anything about me by now, you know that food is one of my favorite coping strategies. What about you? And are these choices good or bad for your fibroids? Try this: Write the days of the week, one on top of each of seven pages. Before you go to sleep each day, write down what irritated or stressed you out, and what you ate or drank as a result. My friend Andrea eats carrots. This doesn't qualify as a problem (in case you wondered). Don't judge yourself, just list it. At the end of the week, go back and see if you can make any correlations—does stress trigger overeating, one too many glasses of wine, a trip to Mickey D's? Once again, if you see a pattern, you can experiment by making small changes. Like keeping a bag of carrot sticks handy.

WORDPLAY

I swear to you, this actually happened: I had a job interview that consisted in its entirety of the following question: If you were a car, what kind of car would you be? (The answer was a Harley; I didn't get the job.) But, hey, it was fun, so try this: On the left side of a page, list a bunch of categories like music, plants, jewelry, fish, shoes, anything else that comes to mind. You know what to do: On the right side of the page, write down what your fibroid would be if it were a song, a piece of footwear, and so on. Describe it in as much detail as you like. When you're done, look down the right-hand list. If the images are threatening (like sharks and stilettos), maybe you'll decide you want to reimagine your fibroids as something more benign. Or use the images you've come up with to consider your treatment strategy.

Picture This

Picasso said, "Painting is just another way of keeping a diary." Another way to start putting your fibroids in perspective is to picture them—in color, with crayons and a big pad of paper. Sometimes pictures tap into elements of our subconscious that we can't articulate with words, even writing in a journal.

Dr. Bernie Siegel asks his patients to draw a picture of themselves and their disease. He suggests not thinking about it too hard, using plain white paper and a complete spectrum of colored crayons, including black, white, and brown. And no, you don't have to be Georgia O'Keeffe to do this.

So draw a picture of you and your fibroids. Then step back and look at your drawing objectively. What does it say about the person who made it? What would you counsel this woman to do if you thought she needed a new point of view?

Sometimes it can help to put the drawing aside for a few days, or even longer. I was in a career-counseling class a couple of years ago, where the instructor asked us to draw our current job situation. I drew a picture of a sailboat on a rolling sea, with a red flag flying in the breeze—inside a glass ball, like a souvenir snow-shaker. I'd forgotten about it, but looking back, I realize I was expressing a growing feeling of being trapped in my old job, without any real outlet for creativity or freedom of thought. It would take me another year before I made the connection consciously—and quit the job.

I haven't drawn the picture of my fibroids yet, but I have an idea that they'd be big, ugly, and overpowering—as opposed to fist-sized lumps of muscle that aren't nearly as smart, creative, or adorable as I am. At least I hope not.

It's Up to You

Our brains can do so many things. The most obvious—and to me, the most powerful—is the capacity it gives us to make informed choices, choices that feel good not only intellectually but also emotionally. The power of our brains allows us to read, absorb, and process information; the power of our minds allows us to know when a decision feels right.

I remember a call I got from one of the women I'd interviewed for this book. When we'd met, several months before, she was trying to choose between myomectomy and hysterectomy to deal with the uncontrollable bleeding and pressure from her fibroids. Although her doctor had recommended hysterectomy, from the beginning, she still didn't feel right about it. When she called me, she was scheduled for a supracervical hysterectomy, but had just heard about uterine artery embolization. None of the many doctors she'd consulted over the past couple of years had even mentioned this option to her, and she wanted to know more about it before going ahead with her hysterectomy.

I was struck that she hadn't liked the idea of hysterectomy when we'd met, and several months later, she still didn't like it but felt it was her only choice. Her brain had scheduled the surgery, but her mind was telling her she still had to wait.

This felt familiar, because I'd gone through the same process. I was a week away from having a myomectomy. I had an appointment to donate my own blood before the surgery, I was organizing things at work to cover my absence, and arranging to have friends and family stay over for the first few days after surgery. But something just didn't feel right. Actually, it felt horrible. My doctor had warned me that my fibroids might be too large, or the surgery too bloody, and she might wind up having to do a hysterectomy.

Having lost an ovary at the ripe old age of 17, I wasn't prepared—or willing—to lose any more body parts. At that point, in my thirties, I had just decided I might want children, and it seemed like a pretty rotten joke to think I would lose my uterus at precisely that moment. I started crying at the drop of a hat. I was crying even when no hats were dropping. On a weekend away with friends I stood up—too suddenly, perhaps—and for the first time in my life, fainted dead away. Gee, could it have been—stress?

Sobbing in my therapist's office, he looked at me and said, cancel the surgery. I can't, I said, everything's all set. No, he said, it's not set until they're wheeling you into the operating room. But my doctor will be angry, I said. My therapist just looked at me, with that look parents sometimes give their children which says, first, you know better, and second, give me a break.

I canceled the surgery. That was five years ago. And then I started thinking about writing this book. That was my mind's response to what to do about my fibroids. Your mind will have its own response, and whatever you decide, it will be the right thing for you.

◯ *Resources* ◯

IN PUTTING TOGETHER a list of places where you can look for more information, I found myself with both a problem and an opportunity. The opportunity is to guide you to resources that I believe are especially helpful. The problem is that, with a few notable exceptions, most of these resources don't deal with fibroids in a comprehensive way. This is underlined by the fact that I drew on almost 600 separate sources to create this book, weeding out inconsistencies, contrasting study results, putting pieces together.

So I've tried to do something a little bit different when it comes to recommending further reading. Instead of providing you with a laundry list of resources, this is a highly selective list of organizations, books, and Web sites for most of the topics covered in the book. I have no relationship to any of the resources listed here and nothing to gain by recommending one over another.

Is every possible source listed here, for topics as diverse as acupuncture, cancer, and embolization? No. Instead, I've tried to list resources that have proven most helpful to me in terms of finding information specifically about fibroids. I've also tried to stay away from sites selling pharmaceuticals, herbs, or medical devices, although some of these do offer objective information. You'll also see some general sources that I've found particularly helpful for information on nutrition, home products, and other areas.

Several health care facilities and doctors are listed, including some of the doctors who were kind enough to be interviewed for this book. For the most part, I identified these doctors in the first place because I appreciated the way they presented information in their books and/or Web sites. Their listing here is not an endorsement of their respective skills as medical practitioners, as I have no direct experience with them in that capacity.

The Web resources listed should allow you ample opportunity to find additional links. The newsletters and magazines recommended also often offer sources for further reading.

Some caveats: organizations move, phone numbers change. Web sites migrate; please be patient if by the time you read this, any addresses or phone numbers are out of date. As you'd expect, these recommendations are meant to be helpful in your continuing search for information about fibroid treatment, but I am not responsible for the content of any of the resources mentioned here.

Most of all, I encourage you to keep talking: to your friends, to women in chat groups or newsgroups on the Internet, in letters to your state and federal representatives, to your doctors and other health care practitioners. Our best resource is still each other.

A Word about Web Sites

For simplicity, all Web site addresses have been abbreviated. Each address shown should begin with http://. For example, the *New York Times* Web site, listed here as www.nytimes.com, needs to be input to your computer as http://www.nytimes.com.

If there are any slashes in the Web site address, you may have to log on to the home page first, then enter the additional information. For instance, to get to the *Times* section on women (listed below as www.nytimes.com/women), go to http://www.nytimes.com; when you get the main screen, type /women after the address to reach the correct section.

For Web sites where I have not listed information beyond the basic address, you should be able to use the site's navigator to search for information on fibroids. In general, type "fibroids" into the search window, then follow the links.

General Sources for Staying Up to Date on Fibroid Therapies and Research

Center for Uterine Fibroids at Brigham and Women's Hospital in Boston, www.fibroids.net. One of the top U.S. centers for fibroid research.
Fibroid Growth Study, www.niehs.nih.gov/fibroids. While results won't be reported until the entire study is complete, you can click on "News" for other updates on fibroids.
The HERS Foundation, 610-667-7757, www.hersfoundation.com. Information about fibroids and medical care; physician referral service.
Hope for Fibroids, www.hopeforfibroids.org. A not-for-profit organization dedicated to increasing knowledge and awareness about fibroids. Numerous links.
National Uterine Fibroids Foundation, www.nuff.org. A not-for-profit organization dedicated to increasing knowledge and awareness about fibroids. Numerous links.
Uterine Fibroid Research and Education Act. Find out the status by searching *The Congressional Record*, at http://thomas.loc.gov, or the Web sites of the sponsoring legislators, Representative Stephanie Tubbs Jones, www .house.gov/tubbsjones, and Senator Barbara Mikulski, http://mikulski .senate.gov. Contact your state's national legislators via www.house.gov and www.senate.gov.

General Sources for Staying Up to Date on Women's Health

American Board of Obstetrics and Gynecology, www.abog.org/women/ women.html. Find out if your doctor is certified; find an ob/gyn.
HealthWeb, www.healthweb.org. A comprehensive list of noncommercial Web sites on health, sponsored by the National Library of Medicine. Click on "Women's Health."
National Black Women's Health Imperative, 202-548-4000, www.black-womenshealth.org.

National Women's Health Information Center, 800-994-WOMAN, www
.4woman.gov. Click on "news" for daily information on women's health.
The New York Times, www.nytimes.com/women.
ObGyn Net, www.obgyn.net. A comprehensive source of women's health
information.
The Office of Minority Health Resource Center, U.S. Department of Health
and Human Services, 800-444-6472, www.omhrc.gov.

General Medical Research and News

Search for information on fibroids (and many, many other conditions), on:
Medscape, www.medscape.com. Search for recent articles and studies.
The U.S. National Library of Medicine, www.nlm.nih.gov. The world's larg-
est medical library. Includes MedLine, which can access over 9 million
citations of medical and scientific articles.
WebMD, www.webmd.com.

Woman-Centered Medicine

*Our Health, Our Lives: A Revolutionary Approach to Total Health Care
for Women,* Eileen Hoffman, M.D., Pocket Books, 1995.
Woman: An Intimate Geography, Natalie Angier, Houghton Mifflin, 1999.
Women's Bodies, Women's Wisdom, Christiane Northrup, M.D., Bantam
Books, 1994.

Symptoms

HEAVY BLEEDING

Dr. Susan Lark's Heavy Menstrual Flow & Anemia Self Help Book, Susan
M. Lark, M.D., Celestial Arts, 1995.

VON WILLEBRAND'S DISEASE

The National Hemophilia Foundation, 800-42-HANDI, www.hemophilia.
org.

CANCER

Abramson Cancer Institute of the University of Pennsylvania, www
.oncolink.org. Search for information on uterine and other cancers.

Association of Cancer Online Resources, Inc., www.acor.org. A gateway
to over 60 online cancer support groups.
National Cancer Institute, 800-4-CANCER, cancernet.nci.nih.gov.
**The University of Texas M.D. Anderson Cancer Center, Gynecologic
Oncology Center,** www.mdanderson.org/care_centers/gyn.

Medical Therapies

PRESCRIPTION DRUG THERAPY

Rxlist.com, www.rxlist.com. Lists prescribing information for many brand-
name pharmaceuticals. You can find similar information at www.drugs
.com.

UTERINE ARTERY EMBOLIZATION

The Fibroid Corner, www.fibroidcorner.com. The Web site for Dr. Robert
Worthington-Kirsch.
Georgetown University Medical Center, 202-784-3420, www.dml.george
town.edu.
Society of Interventional Radiologists, www.sirweb.org. Information on
UAE and doctor finder.
UAE Fibroid Registry, www.fibroidregistry.org. Find out the latest results
of this comprehensive study on UAE.

MYOMECTOMY

All About Myomectomy, www.myomectomy.net.
The Fibroid Book, Francis L. Hutchins Jr., M.D., The Fibroid Center, 1997.
The Hysterectomy Hoax, Stanley West, M.D., Doubleday, 1994.
Uterine Fibroids: What Every Woman Needs to Know, Nelson H. Stringer,
M.D., Physicians & Scientists Publishing Co., Inc., 1996
WomenCare, 617-441-5550, www.womencare.org. Click on "Services" for
information by Dr. Mitch Levine.

HYSTERECTOMY

The Essential Guide to Hysterectomy, Lauren F. Streicher, M.D., M. Evans
and Company, Inc., 2004
Hysterectomy, Before and After, Winnifred B. Cutler, Ph.D., Harper Paper-
backs, 1990.

Helpful Information Before Surgery

AMA Physician Select, www.ama-assn.org. Information on over 900,000 medical doctors.

HealthGrades.com. Rates hospitals, physicians, and health plans.

Prepare for Surgery, Heal Faster, Peggy Huddleston, Angel River Press, 2002.

Solutions: The Woman's Crisis Handbook, Lauren Hartman, Houghton Mifflin, 1997. Practical advice, including how to handle problems at work due to medical crises.

State health agencies often have information on legal complaints registered against doctors; you can find your state health agency through the FDA at www.fda.gov/oca/sthealth.htm: click on link to state health agencies.

Alternative Medicine

Division for Research and Education in Complementary and Integrative Medical Therapies at Harvard's Osher Institute, www.osher.hms.harvard.edu/news/toc.asp

Dr. Andrew Weil's Self-Healing newsletter, www.drweilselfhealing.com, or 800-523-3296 for subscription information,

Encyclopedia of Healing Therapies, Anne Woodham and Dr. David Peters, Dorling Kindersley, 1997.

Healing Fibroids, Allan Warshowsky, M.D. and Elena Oumano, Simon & Schuster Inc., 2002

Health World Online, www.healthy.net. A good source for articles on alternative therapies for fibroids, including homeopathy, aromatherapy, and herbal medicine.

Natural Healing in Gynaecology: A Manual for Women, Rina Nissim, Pandora, 1996.

Herbs

The American Botanical Council, 512-926-4900, www.herbalgram.org.

The Complete Woman's Herbal: A Manual of Healing Herbs and Nutrition for Personal Well-being and Family Care, Anne McIntyre, Henry Holt & Co., 1995.

PDR for Herbal Medicines™, Joerg Gruenwald Ph.D., editor, Economics Company, 1998.

Tyler's Herbs of Choice, James E. Robbers and Varro E. Tyler, Haworth Press, 1998.

The Woman's Book of Healing Herbs, Sari Harrar and Sara Altshul O'Donnell, Rodale Press, Inc., 1999.

AROMATHERAPY

The Encyclopedia of Essential Oils: The Complete Guide to the Use of Aromatics in Aromatherapy, Herbalism, Health & Well-Being, Julia Lawless, Barnes & Noble Books, 1995.

HYPNOSIS

The American Board of Hypnotherapy, 808-596-7765, www.hypnosis .com.

HOMEOPATHY

The Consumer's Guide to Homeopathy, Dana Ullman, M.P.H., Tarcher/ Putnam, 1996.
Everybody's Guide to Homeopathic Medicine, Stephen Cummings, M.D., and Dana Ullman, Tarcher/Putnam, 1991.
National Center for Homeopathy, 703-548-7790, www.homeopathic.org.

NATUROPATHY

American Association of Naturopathic Physicians, 866-538-2267, or 202-895-1392, www.naturopathic.org.

ACUPUNCTURE

Acupuncture.com, www.acupuncture.com.
American Association of Oriental Medicine, 866-455-7999, or 916-443-4770, www.aaom.org.
Qi: The Journal of Traditional Eastern Health & Fitness, www.qi-journal .com

CHAKRAS

Anatomy of the Spirit: The Seven Stages of Power and Healing, Caroline Myss, Ph.D., Three Rivers Press, 1996.
Hands-On Healing, Jack Angelo, Healing Arts Press, 1997.

AYURVEDA

A Woman's Best Medicine: Health, Happiness and Long Life through Maharishi Ayur-Veda, Nancy Lonsdorf, M.D., Veronica Butler, M.D., and Melanie Brown, Ph.D., Tarcher/Putnam, 1995.

Estrogen

HORMONE REPLACEMENT THERAPY

Dr. Susan Love's Hormone Book: Making Informed Choices About Menopause, Susan M. Love, M.D., with Karen Lindsey, Times Books, 1997.

DES

DES Action USA, 800-DES-9288 or 510-465-4011, www.desaction.org.

ENVIRONMENTAL ESTROGENS

Environmental Defense Fund. Check out names of chemicals you may be working with to see if they're considered endocrine or reproductive threats, at www.scorecard.org.

National Institute of Environmental Health Science, www.niehs.nih.gov. Click on "Environmental Health Perspectives."

Our Stolen Future, Theo Colborn, Dianne Dumanoski, and John Peterson, Myers, Dutton, 1996.

Silent Spring, Rachel Carson, Houghton Mifflin, 1994. The original warning about chemicals in our environment (first released in 1962).

World Wildlife Fund, www.worldwildlife.org. Click on "Global Challenges" for more information about xenoestrogens.

ESTROGENIC CHEMICALS IN FOOD

Food and Drug Administration, Center for Food Safety and Applied Nutrition, 1–888-SAFEFOOD (1-888-723-3366), www.cfsan.fda.gov.

PESTICIDES

Environmental Protection Agency, www.epa.gov. Click on "pesticides."

National Pesticide Information Center, 800-858-7378, http://npic.orst.edu.

HOME PRODUCTS

Natural Cleaning for Your Home: 95 Pure and Simple Recipes, Casey Kellar, Lark Books, 1998. Information on natural cleaning and stain fighting.

The Safe Shopper's Bible, David Steinman and Samuel S. Epstein, M.D., Macmillan, 1995. Information on the safety of household cleaners.

U.S. Consumer Products Safety Commission, 800-638-2772, or 301-504-7923, www.cpsc.gov

Nutrition

Eat, Drink, and Be Healthy: The Harvard Medical School Guide to Healthy Eating, Walter C. Willett, M.D., Free Press, 2001.
Fibroid Tumors & Endometriosis Self Help Book, Susan M. Lark, M.D., Celestial Arts, 1995.
The National Agricultural Library, www.nal.usda.gov/fnic/IBIDS. Information on nutritional supplements.
Sustainable Table, www.sustainabletable.org.
Healthier U.S., www.healthierus.gov/nutrition.html. Government guidelines on health and nutrition. A comprehensive list of nutrition resources and links is at www.cfsan.fda.gov/~dms/nutrlist.html.

Pregnancy

Georgia Reproductive Specialists, 404-843-2229, www.ivf.com. Look for the article by Mark Perloe, M.D., and Linda Gail, "Miracle Babies and Other Happy Endings for Couples with Fertility Problems."
Having Your Baby: A Guide for African-American Women, Dr. Hilda Hutcherson with Margaret Williams, One World/Ballantine Books, 1997.
Intensive Caring: New Hope for High-Risk Pregnancy, Dianne Hales and Timothy R. B. Johnson, M.D., Crown Publishers, Inc., 1990.
What to Expect When You're Expecting, Arlene Eisenberg, Heidi E. Murkoff, Sandee E. Hathaway, B.S.N., Workman Publishing, 1991.
Your Pregnancy: Questions and Answers, Glade B. Curtis, M.D., and Judith Schuler, M.S., Fisher Books, 1995.

INFERTILITY AND MISCARRIAGE

A Woman Doctor's Guide to Miscarriage, Dr. Lynn Friedman with Irene Daria, Hyperion, 1996.
The Ferre Institute, Inc., 607-724-4308, www.ferre.org. A not-for-profit educational organization for infertility and reproductive health
Fertility Friend, www.fertilityfriend.com. A resource for women trying to conceive.
INCIID, InterNational Council on Infertility Information Dissemination, www.inciid.org.
RESOLVE, The National Infertility Association, 301-652-9375, www.resolve .org.
SHARE, Pregnancy and Infant Loss Support, 800-821-6819 or 636-947-6164, www.nationalshareoffice.com.

Mind-Body Medicine, Stress Reduction

Healing Mind, Healthy Woman: Using the Mind-Body Connection to Manage Stress and Take Control of Your Life, Alice D. Domar, Ph.D., and Henry Dreher, A Delta Book/Dell Publishing, 1996.

HealthyPlace.com, http://healthyplace.com, a comprehensive consumer mental health resource.

Love, Medicine & Miracles, Bernie Siegel, M.D., HarperPerennial, 1986.

Resources to Help You Make Creative Life Choices

The Artist's Way: A Spiritual Path to Higher Creativity, Julia Cameron, Tarcher/Perigee Books, 1992.

Creative Visualization, Shakti Gawain, A Bantam New Age Book, 1978, 1982.

Finding the Quiet Mind, Robert Ellwood, The Theosophical Publishing House, 1987.

The Universal Traveler, Don Koberg and Jim Bagnell, William Kaufman, Inc., 1981.

Notes

Opening Quotes

Vollenhoven B, et al., "Representational Difference Analysis: A New and Valuable Tool for Studying the Aetiology of Fibroids," University of Newcastle, Australia, Department of Obstetrics and Gynaecology, Monash University, Monash Medical Centre, Clayton, VIC, 3168, Australia.

"Diseases of Reproduction in Women," National Institutes of Health, www .nih.gov.

Introduction

Researchers believe: The Center for Uterine Fibroids, www.fibroids.net.

The 2000 U.S. Census, www.census.gov.

Stringer NH, *Uterine Fibroids: What Every Woman Needs to Know*, Physicians & Scientists Publishing Co., 1996: 1.

The annual cost: Agency for Healthcare Research and Quality, "34. Management of Uterine Fibroids Volume 1. Evidence Report, Chapter 4," AHRQ Evidence Reports, Numbers 1–60, www.ncbi.nlm.nih.gov.

Fibroids are among the top priorities: "Status of Research on Uterine Fibroids at the National Institutes of Health," September 2003, www4.od.nih .gov/orwh/fibroids2003.pdf.

The Uterine Fibroid Research and Education Act has been proposed in

Congress by Representative Stephanie Tubbs Jones and Senator Barbara Mikulski.

Chapter 1: Fibroids Defined

The most common pelvic tumor: "Disorders of the Uterus: Leiomyomata Uteri," *Journal of Obstetrics & Gynecology,* August 1998.

The most common neoplasms: "Uterine Leiomyomata," ACOG Educational Bulletin 1994; (192).

More than a quarter of a million: This figure comes from adding the 200,000–230,000 hysterectomies attributed to fibroids every year, plus the estimated annual number of myomectomies (20–40,000), uterine artery embolizations (c. 10,000), myolysis, and other procedures.

WHO GETS THEM?

Fibroids create problems for up to half of the women: "How Do I Know I Have Fibroids?," Center for Uterine Fibroids, www.fibroids.net.

Russian study: Vikhlyaeva EM, Khodzhaeva ZS, Fantschenko ND, "Familial Predisposition to Uterine Leiomyomas," *International Journal of Gynaecology and Obstectrics* 1995; 51(2): 127–31.

African-American women are three to five times more likely: "Fast facts About Uterine Fibroids," National Institute of Child Health and Human Development, last modified May 5, 2004, www.nichd.nih.gov/publications/pubs/fibroids/sub1.htm; Baird DD, et al., "High cumulative incidence of uterine leiomyoma in black and white women: Ultrasound evidence," *American Journal of Obstetrics & Gynecology,* Volume 188, Issue 1, January 2003.

145 genes: "Scientists One Step Closer to Cause of Uterine Fibroids," National Institute of Child Health and Human Development, July 22, 2002, www.nih.gov/news/pr/ju12002/nichd-22.htm.

45 percent of the fibroids: Center for Uterine Fibroids, www.fibroids.net; McBride G, "Researchers Take Aim at Uterine Fibroids," *Washington Post,* April 6, 1999; Z09.

WHAT CAUSES FIBROIDS?

Fibroids originate from a single cell: "Disorders of the Uterus: Leiomyomata Uteri," *Journal of Obstetrics & Gynecology* August 1998.

The Human Epigenome Project (HEP), http://www.epigenome.org.

FH: Reuters Health, "Researchers discover gene related to fibroids," February 25, 2003, appearing on www.fibroids.net; original source, *Nature Genetics* 2002; 10.1038/ng849.

Sharon Begley: Begley S, "How a Second, Secret Genetic Code Turns Genes On and Off," *Wall Street Journal*, July 23, 2004.

Scientists at the National Institute of Child Health and Human Development: Office of Research on Women's Health, NIH, DHHS, "Status of Research on Uterine Fibroids," September 2003.

The Human Genome Project: The Wellcome Trust/SG, "Fun facts about the human genome," The Human Genome, February 2, 2001, http://www.wellcome .ac.uk.

WHAT MAKES FIBROIDS GROW?

Normal amounts of estrogen: Parker WH, et al., *A Gynecologist's Second Opinion*, Plume Books, 1996: 19–20.

Use estrogen at a faster rate: Lumsden MA, et al., "The Binding of Steroids to Myometrium and Leiomyomata (Fibroids) in Women Treated with the Gonadotropin-Releasing Hormone Agonist Zoladex (ICI 118630)," *Journal of Endocrinology* 1989; 121(2): 389–96.

According to the Center for Uterine Fibroids: "Theories of Fibroid Formation," Center for Uterine Fibroids, www.fibroids.net.

Discussion about basic fibroblast growth factor; blood vessel changes: Based on information from Stewart EA, et al., "Leiomyoma-Related Bleeding: A Classic Hypothesis Updated for the Molecular Era," *Human Reproduction Update* 1996; 2(4): 295–306.

Progesterone has been targeted: Harrison-Woolrych M, et al., "Fibroid Growth in Response to High-Dose Progestogen," *Fertility and Sterility* 1995; 64(1): 191–92.

Amount of progesterone relative to the estrogen: "Fibroids: Assessing the Options," *Women's Health Advocate* 1996; 3(5): 4–6.

What fibroids are missing: "Fibroid Tumors Lack Critical Structural Protein," National Institute of Child Health and Human Development, June 2, 2004; "What is Collagen?" BioSpecifics Technologies Corporation, www.biospecifics.com.

WHO ARE YOU CALLING A DEGENERATE?

Discussion about degeneration: Based on information from Siccardi DC, "Leiomyomas," Obstetrics & Gynecology, Medstudents, www.med students.com.

Definition of necrosis: Parr JA, et al., *Parr's Concise Medical Encyclopedia*, Applied Science Publishers, 1971: 244.

WHERE DO YOUR FIBROIDS LIVE? MEET YOUR UTERUS

Natalie Angier: Angier N, *Woman: An Intimate Geography*, Houghton Mifflin Company, 1999: 110–11.

"Prostaglandin," *The Columbia Encyclopedia*, Sixth Edition. 2001–05, as found on www.bartleby.com.

Goldfarb H, et al., *The No-Hysterectomy Option*, John Wiley & Sons, 1997: 33.

A unique, natural antibiotic: "Naturally-Occurring Antibiotic Found in Female Urinary/Reproductive Tract," *The Doctor's Guide*, April 15, 1998, www.docguide.com.

Anandamide: Dubuc B, "How Drugs Affect Neutransmitters," *The Brain From Top to Bottom*, www.thebrain.mcgill.ca.

PICTURE THIS

In a sweet . . . description: Parker WH, et al., *A Gynecologist's Second Opinion*, Plume Books, 1996: 3.

Size and weight of uterus: Based partly on information from "Basic Anatomy and Physiology of the Uterus," Center for Uterine Fibroids, www.fibroids.net.

FIBROIDS AND UTERINE REAL ESTATE

Six or seven fibroids: "What are Fibroids?," Center for Uterine Fibroids, www.fibroids.net.

In clusters or singly: "Uterine Fibroids," National Institutes of Health, NIH Pub. No. 0051.

Parasitic leiomyomata: "Uterine Leiomyomata," *ACOG Educational Bulletin* 1994; (192).

Chapter 2: Why You Feel the Way You Do

Between 20 and 50 percent: "How Do I Know I Have Fibroids?," Center for Uterine Fibroids, www.fibroids.net.

UTERINE BLEEDING

About 30 percent: Siccardi DC, "Leiomyomas," Obstetrics & Gynecology, Medstudents, http://atcancer.com.

Fibroid-related bleeding: Stewart EA, et al., "Leiomyoma-Related Bleeding: A Classic Hypothesis Updated for the Molecular Era," *Human Reproduction Update* 1996; 2(4): 295–306.

Heavy bleeding affects the whole body: Wegienka G, et al., "Self-reported heavy bleeding associated with uterine leiomyomata," *Obstetrics & Gynecology* 101:431–437, 2003.

Heavy bleeding also has an economic cost: Côté I, et al., "Work Loss Associated With Increased Menstrual Loss in the United States," *Obstetrics & Gynecology* 100:683–687, 2002.

THE MONTHLY MACHINERY

How do fibroids cause excess bleeding?: West S, *The Hysterectomy Hoax,* Doubleday, 1994: 79; Siccardi DC, "Leiomyomas;" Stewart EA, et al., "Leiomyoma-Related Bleeding."

Some people think . . . the math doesn't add up; how heavy is heavy?: "Uterine Leiomyomata," ACOG *Educational Bulletin* 1994: (192).

Bleeding may have a number of causes: Lark S, *Heavy Menstrual Flow and Anemia Self Help Book,* Celestial Arts, 1995: 10–15; Griffith HW, *Complete Guide to Symptoms, Illness and Surgery,* Berkley Publishing Group, 1995: 424.

ANEMIA

The Centers for Disease Control: "Recommendations to Prevent and Control Iron Deficiency in the United States," Centers for Disease Control, MMWR 47(RR-3); 1–36, 4/3/98.

CRAMPS

One in ten women: Hale E, "Taming Menstrual Cramps," FDA *Consumer Magazine* 1991; 25(5).

Pain may weaken the immune system: "Pain and Women's Health," *National Women's Health Report* 1999: 21(3): 1.

Uterine contractions: Lauersen N, et al., *Listen to Your Body,* Berkley Books, 1982: 45.

PRESSURE ON YOUR BLADDER OR BOWEL

Kidney infection and damage: Siccardi DC, "Leiomyomas." Kidney failure: Courban D, et al., "Acute Renal Failure in the First Trimester Resulting from Uterine Leiomyomas," *American Journal of Obstetrics & Gynecology* 1997; 177(2): 472–73.

FATIGUE

70 percent of women: Chopelas A, "Fibroid Study and Research Program: Causes, Symptoms, Relief and Possible Solutions," 1997.

POLYPS

Information from this section is based in part on "What are Endometrial Polyps?" Center for Uterine Fibroids, www.fibroids.net.

ENDOMETRIOSIS

Weinstein K, *Living with Endometriosis,* Addison-Wesley Publishing Company, 1987: ix.

Over 5 million women: The Endometriosis Association, www.endometriosis assn.org.

18 percent of hysterectomies: *Treatment of Common Non-Cancerous Uterine Conditions: Issues for Research,* Agency for Health Care Policy and Research, 1995, Pub. No. 95–0067.

ADENOMYOSIS

Information in this section is based in part on "What is Adenomyosis?" Center for Uterine Fibroids, www.fibroids.net.

VON WILLEBRAND'S DISEASE

Kadir RA, et al., "Frequency of Inherited Bleeding Disorders in Women," *The Lancet,* 1998; 351(9101): 485–89.

"Hereditary Bleeding Disorder—von Willebrand Disease—Seems to be Widely Undiagnosed and Untreated," Harris Interactive, November 24, 2003, www.harrisinteractive.com.

Chapter 3: My Fibroids, Myself

Northrup C, *Women's Bodies, Women's Wisdom,* Bantam Books, 1994: 650.
Viorst J, *Necessary Losses,* Simon & Schuster, 1986: 265.

THE POWER OF THE UTERUS

Walker BG, *The Woman's Encyclopedia of Myths and Secrets,* Castle Books, 1996. Includes dozens of myths centered around the uterus, fertility symbols, and female sexuality.

WHO'S IN CHARGE HERE?

Feelings of shame: Levinson RL, "Standing Alone at Sinai: Shame and the Unmarried Jewish Woman," appears in Orenstein D, ed., *Lifecycles,* Jewish Lights Publishing, 1994: 111.

You Are Who You Say You Are

Quote by Coco Chanel: *The Quotable Woman,* Running Press, 1991: 39. Quote by Cicely Tyson: *The Quotable Woman,* Running Press, 1991: 93.

Chapter 4: Testing . . . Testing . . .

Sometimes, Less Is More

If you'd like a guideline: Lark S, *Fibroid Tumors & Endometriosis Self Help Book,* Celestial Arts, 1995: 35–59.

The Basics

A 12-week-sized uterus: "Uterine Leiomyomata," *ACOG Educational Bulletin* 1994; (192). Average size of the uterus: Dayman C, ed., *The Human Body,* Dorling Kindersley, 1995: 202.

Sonograms

The Consumer-Patient Radiation Health and Safety Act: SDMS Position Statement, available at www.obgyn.net/us/feature/sdms_act.htm.

American College of Preventive Medicine: Ferrini R, "Screening Asymptomatic Women for Ovarian Cancer: American College of Preventive Medicine Practice Policy Statement," reaffirmed 1/31/2005 through 1/31/2010, www.acpm.org/ovary.htm.

"Saline Sonogram (SSH)," Strong Fertility and Reproductive Science Center/ University of Rochester Medical Center, www.stronghealth.com.

3D and 4D ultrasound: Woo J, "A Short History of the Development of Ultrasound in Obstetrics and Gynecology," www.ob-ultrasound.net.

Magnetic Resonance Imaging

"Safety Guidelines for Conducting Magnetic Resonance Imaging (MRI) Experiments Involving Human Subjects Version 2," Center for Functional Magnetic Resonance Imaging, University of California, San Diego, July 2004.

Open MRIs: "MRI Technology—What You Should Know," NorthEast Medical Rounds, NorthEast Medical Center, www.northeastmedical.org.

Hysterosalpingography

The Atlanta Reproductive Health Center recommends: "A Couple's Guide to Hysterosalpingogram [HSG]," Atlanta Reproductive Health Center, www.ivf.com.

Dr. H. Winter Griffith . . . recommends: Griffith HW. *The Complete Guide to Medical Tests,* Fisher Books, 1988.

Some may give you a local anesthetic: Perloe VI, Gail L, *Miracle Babies and Other Happy Endings for Couples with Fertility Problems,* Atlanta Reproductive Health Center.

Iodine or seafood allergies: "Patient Fact Sheet: Hysterosalpingogram," American Society for Reproductive Medicine, rev. 5/2003.

HYSTEROSCOPY

Petrozza JC, et al., "Hysteroscopy," emedicine.com, updated May 24, 2005.

According to Dr. Fritz Wieser: Wieser F, et al., "Atraumatic Cervical Passage at Outpatient Hysteroscopy," *Fertility and Sterility* 1998; 69(3): 549–51.

LAPAROSCOPY

Your risk: Griffith HW, *The Complete Guide to Symptoms, Illness and Surgery,* Berkley Publishing Group, 1995: 838.

Discussion of CO_2: Goldberg JM, Falcone T, "Gasless Gynecologic Laparoscopy: A Work in Progress," *The Female Patient,* February 1998.

Gasless Laparoscopy: Perez N, et al., "Ureteral Complications after Gasless Laparoscopic Hysterectomy. *Surgical Laparoscopy, Endoscopy & Percutaneous Techniques.* 9(4):300, August 1999; Pryor JP, "Diagnostic Gasless Laparoscopy (DGL) in Penetrating Abdominal," Penn Surgery, University of Pennsylvania, www.uphs.upenn.edu.

RULING OUT CANCER

Fibroids "are not associated with cancer": "Fast Facts about Uterine Fibroids," The National Institutes of Health, updated May 05 2004, www.nichd.nih.gov.

The answer to this question: "Disorders of the Uterus: Leiomyomata Uteri," *Journal of Obstetrics & Gynecology,* August 1998.

A study at the Johns Hopkins University School of Public Health: Norton A, "Cancer fear High Among Women Having Hysterectomy," Reuters Health, June 22, 2005.

Other studies: Center for Uterine Fibroids, www.fibroids.net.

According to the American Cancer Society: "Facts and Figures 1999," American Cancer Society, www.cancer.org/statistics. The incidence of uterine cancer is listed as 22 per 100,000 women; the cervical cancer incidence is listed as 7.4 per 100,000 women. Rates of these cancers for African-American women are twice as high.

Three types of cancer: *What You Need to Know About Cancer of the Uterus,* National Cancer Institute, 1997: 4. NIH Pub. No. 98–1562; "Cancer of the

Uterus," The National Women's Health Information Center, December 2001, www.4woman.org.

CA-125

CA 125: Reuters Health, "CA 125 useful in predicting advanced-stage uterine cancer," May 29, 2003,http://www.oncolink.upenn.edu; "What is CA125," Ask the Experts, http://www.oncolink.upenn.edu.

DOPPLER SCAN

It can tell how fast: Botsis D, Kassanos D, Antoniou G, Karakitsos P, Vitoratos N, "Endometrial Thickness and Doppler Velocimetry in Women with Peri- and Postmenopausal Bleeding, Before Endometrial Sampling," *European Menopause Journal* 1996; 3(2): 42–46; Ferrini R, "Screening Asymptomatic Women for Ovarian Cancer:American College of Preventive Medicine Practice Policy Statement," reaffirmed 1/31/2005 through 1/31/2010, www .acpm.org/ovary.htm.

BIOPSY

Endometrial biopsy: "Looking Inside the Uterus," *Harvard Women's Health Watch,* January 1997; 4(5): 4–5.

D&C

Complications: "Looking Inside the Uterus," *Harvard Women's Health Watch,* January 1997; 4(5): 4–5.

WAVE OF THE FUTURE

"Jefferson Researchers Develop Genetic Test to Identify Uterine Tumors as Malignant or Benign," Thomas Jefferson University, www.jefferson.edu.

TAKING "BLOODS"

Shaheen WH, et al.,"Preoperative Testing," updated November 18, 2004, eMedicine.com.

Chapter 5: Best of the West

FINDING DR. RIGHT

Dr. Judith Reichman: As heard on the *Oprah Winfrey Show,* July 15, 1998.

Male gynecologists: Carlson KJ, et al., "Indications for Hysterectomy," *New England Journal of Medicine 1993; 328(12): 856–60.*

Younger doctors: *Common Uterine Conditions: Options for Treatment,* Agency for Health Care Policy and Research, 1997. AHCPR Pub. No. 98–0003.

Basic questions adapted in part from "A Focus on Fibroids," Alternatives to Hysterectomy, ObGyn.net, www.obgyn.net.

Doctors working in managed care organizations: Grumbach K, et al., "Primary Care Physicians' Experience of Financial Incentives in Managed-Care Systems," *New England Journal of Medicine* 1998; 339(21): 1516–21.

NSAIDs

NSAIDs lower estrogen: Cramer DW, et al., "Basal Hormone Levels in Women Who Use Acetaminophen for Menstrual Pain," *Fertility and Sterility* 1998; 70: 371–73.

STAMP OUT CRAMPS

The advice about hot tea flavors is based on information in McIntyre A, *The Complete Woman's Herbal,* Henry Holt, 1994: 276.

The advice about having an orgasm comes from Graeber L, "Can't They Do Something about Cramps?" *Redbook,* September 1994; 183(5): 74, 76.

THE PILL

A study of over 800 women: Chiaffarino F, et al., "Use of oral contraceptives and uterine fibroids: Results from a case-control study," *British Journal of Obstetrics & Gynaecology,* Vol 106(8) (pp 857–860), 1999.

ORTHO Contraceptives, www.rxmed.com.

Harvard Nurses' Health Study: Marshall LM, et al., "A Prospective Study of Reproductive Factors and Oral Contraceptive Use in Relation to the Risk of Uterine Leiomyomata," *Fertility and Sterility* 1998; 70(3): 432–39; Stewart EA, "Patient information: Fibroids," UptoDate, November 10, 2004, http://patients.uptodate.com.

GnRH AGONISTS

The technical term: Conn PM, et al., "Gonadotropin-Releasing Hormone and Its Analogs," *Annual Review of Medicine* 1994; 45: 391–405.

Ask . . . about minimum doses: Yang Y, et al., "Treatment of Uterine Leiomyoma by Two Different Doses of Mifepristone," *Chung Hua Fu Chan Ko Tsa Chih* 1996; 31(10): 624–26.

What Happens To My Body Without Estrogen?

The side effects of drug-induced estrogen loss were compiled from a number of sources, including: Chrisp P, et al., "Goserelin: A Review of Its Pharmacodynamic and Pharmacokinetic Properties, and Clinical Use in Sex Hormone-Related Conditions," *Drugs* 1991; 41(2): 254–88; Ginsburg J, et al., "Clinical Experience with Tibolone (Livial) Over 8 Years" *Maturitas* 1995; 21(1): 71–76; Auber G, et al., "Use of GnRH Depot Analogue in the Treatment of Uterine Fibroids," *Acta Europaea Fertilitas* 1990 Jul–Aug; 21(4): 185–89; Christiansen JK, "The Facts about Fibroids: Presentation and Latest Management Options," *Postgraduate Medicine* 1993; 94(3): 129–34, 137; Alfini P, et al., "[Treatment of Uterine Fibroma with Goserelin]" *Annali di Ostetricia, Ginecologia, Medicine Pertnatale* 1991; 112(6): 359–67; Chipato T, et al., "Pelvic Pain Complicating LHRH Analogue Treatment of Fibroids," *Australia and New Zealand Journal of Obstetrics and Gynaecology* 1991 Nov; 31(4): 383–84.

Bone mineral loss continued for as long as a year: Nencioni T, et al., Polvani F, "Gonadotropin Releasing Hormone Agonist Therapy and Its Effect on Bone Mass" *Gynecological Endocrinology* 1991; 5(1): 49–56; Adashi EY, "Long-Term Gonadotropin-Releasing Hormone Agonist Therapy: The Evolving Issue of Steroidal "Add-Back" Paradigms," *Keio Journal of Medicine* 1995; 44(4): 124–32.

The Progesterone Parallel

RU486 reduced fibroids by almost 50 percent: Kettel LM, et al., "Clinical Efficacy of the Antiprogesterone RU486 in the Treatment of Endometriosis and Uterine Fibroids" *Human Reproduction* 1994; 9 Suppl 1: 116–20.

RU486 was significantly more effective: Reinsch RC, et al., "The Effects of RU 486 and Leuprolide Acetate on Uterine Artery Blood Flow in the Fibroid Uterus: A Prospective, Randomized Study," *American Journal of Obstetrics & Gynecology* 1994; 170(6): 1623–28.

The FDA approved mifepristone: "Mifeprex (mifepristone) Information," FDA, www.fda.gov/cder/drug/infopage/mifepristone/default.htm; Earll CG, "Frequently Asked Questions: Mifepristone/Mifeprex (RU-486)," Focus on the Family, January 11, 2005 (Updated: August 9, 2005), www.family.org.

In February 2003: "Drug May Shrink Uterine Fibroids, Improve Quality of Life," University of Rochester Medical Center, March 1, 2004, www.urmc.rochester.edu.

Asoprisnil: Carr BR (Ed.), "Progesterone Receptor Antagonists and Selective Progesterone Receptor Modulators (SPRMs)," *Seminars in Reproductive Medicine,* Volume 23, Number 1, 2005; Eisinger SH, et al., "Low-dose

mifepristone for uterine leiomyomata," *Obstetrics & Gynecology,* 2003
Feb; 101(2):243–50.

BUT HEY, IT'S TEMPORARY

Most studies report: Williams JA, et al., "Effect of Nafarelin on Uterine
Fibroids Measured by Ultrasound and Magnetic Resonance Imaging "
European Journal of Obstetrics, Gynecology, and Reproductive Biology
1990; 34(1–2): 111–17; Cagnacci A, et al., "Role of Goserelin-depot in the
Clinical Management of Uterine Fibroids," *Clinical and Experimental
Obstetrics & Gynecology* 1994; 21(4): 263–65; Golan A, "GnRH Analogues
in the Treatment of Uterine Fibroids," *Human Reproduction* 1996; 11
Suppl 3: 33–41.

40 percent of the women remained symptom-free: van Leusden HA, "Symptom-Free Interval after Triptorelin Treatment of Uterine Fibroids: Long-
Term Results," *Gynecological Endocrinology* 1992; 6(3): 189–98.

This biochemical castration: Conn PM, et al., "Gonadotropin-Releasing Hormone and Its Analogs," *Annual Review of Medicine* 1994; 45: 391–405.

UTERINE ARTERY EMBOLIZATION

As of year-end 2004: Broder MS, et al., "Comparison of Long-Term Outcomes of Myomectomy and Uterine Artery Embolization," *Obstetrics &
Gynecology* 2002: 100:864–868.

How successful is UAE: Goodwin SC, et al., Reporting Standards for Uterine
Artery Embolization for the Treatment of Uterine Leiomyomata, *Journal
of Vascular and Interventional Radiology* 14:S467-S476 (2003); Broder MS,
et al., "Comparison of Long-Term Outcomes of Myomectomy and Uterine Artery Embolization," *Obstetrics & Gynecology* 2002; Ravina JH, et
al., [Uterine fibroids embolizations: results about 454 cases"] (translated
from the French), *Gynecol Obstet Fertil* 2003 July–Aug; 31(7–8):597–605;
Gordon CH, et al., "Uterine Artery Embolization: A Minimally Invasive
Technique for the Treatment of Uterine Fibroids," *Journal of Women's
Health and Gender-Based Medicine,* May 2000; 9(4): 357–62.

Caveat emptor: Helliker K, et al., "Hysterectomy Alternative Goes Unmen-
tioned to Many Women," *The Wall Street Journal,* August 24, 2004.

Can you get pregnant? "News From ACOG, Opinion on Uterine Artery
Embolization for Treatment of Fibroids," The American College of
Obstetricians and Gynecologists (ACOG), January 30, 2004, www.medem
.com; Pron G, et al., "Pregnancy after uterine artery embolization for
leiomyomata: the Ontario multicenter trial," *Obstetrics & Gynecology*
2005 Jan;105(1):67–76; Ravina JH, et al., ["Uterine fibroids embolizations:
results about 454 cases"] (article translated from the French), *Gynecol
Obstet Fertil* 2003 July–Aug; 31(7–8):597–605.

Why you might not be a candidate: Andrews RT, "Patient Care and Uterine Artery Embolization for Leiomyomata," *Journal of Vascular and Interventional Radiology* 15:115–120 (2004); Goodwin SC, et al., "Reporting Standards for Uterine Artery Embolization for the Treatment of Uterine Leiomyomata," *Journal of Vascular and Interventional Radiology* 14: S467-S476 (2003); Worthington-Kirsch R, et al., "The Fibroid Registry for Outcomes Data (FIBROID) for Uterine Embolization: Short-Term Outcomes," *Obstetrics & Gynecology* 2005 Jul; 106(1):52–9.

The Ontario study: Pron G, et al., "The Ontario Uterine Fibroid Embolization Trial. Part 2. Uterine fibroid reduction and symptom relief after uterine artery embolization for fibroids," *Fertility & Sterility* 2003 Jan; 79(1):120–7; Pron G, et al., "Tolerance, hospital stay, and recovery after uterine artery embolization for fibroids: the Ontario Uterine Fibroid Embolization Trial," *Journal of Vascular and Interventional Radiology* 2003 Oct; 14(10):1243–50; Pron G, et al., "Hysterectomy for complications after uterine artery embolization for leiomyoma: results of a Canadian multicenter clinical trial," *Journal of the American Association of Gynecolic Laparoscopy* 2003 Feb; 10(1):99–106.

The FIBROID Registry: "About FIBROID," The Cardiovascular and Interventional Radiology Research and Education Foundation, www.fibroidregistry .org/about.htm; Worthington-Kirsch R, et al., "The Fibroid Registry for Outcomes Data (FIBROID) for Uterine Embolization: Short-Term Outcomes," *Obstetrics & Gynecology*, 2005 Jul; 106(1):52–9.

Complications and Side Effects: Andrews RT, et al., Patient Care and Uterine Artery Embolization for Leiomyomata, *Journal of Vascular and Interventional Radiology* 15:115–120 (2004); Siskin GP, et al., "Outpatient Uterine Artery Embolization for Symptomatic Uterine Fibroids: Experience in 49 Patients," *Journal of Vascular and Interventional Radiology* March 2000; 11(3): p.305–311; Toaff ME "Uterine Artery Embolization (UAE) for Uterine Fibroids," last updated 1/1/05, www.althysterectomy.org; Bates B, "Outpatient Treatment of Fibroids: Skepticism Mounts Over Embolization Procedure," *Ob.Gyn. News*, March 1, 2001; Goodwin SC, et al., "Reporting Standards for Uterine Artery Embolization for the Treatment of Uterine Leiomyomata," *Journal of Vascular and Interventional Radiology*; Aungst M, et al., "Necrotic Leiomyoma and Gram-Negative Sepsis Eight Weeks After Uterine Artery Embolization," *Obstetrics & Gynecology*, November 2004; Vol. 104, No. 5, Part 2: pp. 1161–1164; Dietz DM, et al., "Necrosis After Uterine Artery Embolization," *Obstetrics & Gynecology*, November 2004; Vol. 104, No. 5, Part 2: pp. 1159–1161.

Can Your Fibroids Come Back? Broder MS, et al., "Comparison of Long-Term Outcomes of Myomectomy and Uterine Artery Embolization," *Obstetrics & Gynecology*, 2002: 100:864–868, www.acog.org.

Focused Ultrasound Surgery

Up to ten thousand times more powerful: "Conditions," *The Times* (London), November 5, 2003.

2 percent of cases: Altman K, "Treating Troubling Fibroids Without Surgery," *New York Times*, November 23, 2004.

Elizabeth Stewart, et al., "MRI-guided focused U/S: novel therapy for leiomyomata." *Contemporary Ob/Gyn* 2003; 48:22–30; "First Non-Invasive Uterine Fibroids Therapy Shows Promise," July 15, 2003, www.brighamand womens.org.

Early results: Hindley J, et al., "MRI guidance of focused ultrasound therapy of uterine fibroids: early results." *AJR Am J Roentgenol.* 2004 Dec; 183(6):1713–9; "FDA Approves New Device to Treat Uterine Fibroids," FDA Talk Paper, October 22, 2004.

Myolysis and Cryomyolysis

Doctors at Yale: Zreik TG, et al., "Cryomyolysis, A New Procedure for the Conservative Treatment of Uterine Fibroids," *Journal of the American Association of Gynecologic Laparoscopists* 1998; 5(1): 33–38.

An Italian study: Ciavattini A, et al., "Laparoscopic Cryomyolysis: an alternative to myomectomy in women with symptomatic fibroids," *Surg Endosc,* 2004 Dec; 18(12):1785–8.

What about Endometrial Ablation?

Lost in the hoopla: "FDA Approves New Device to Treat Excessive Menstrual Bleeding," *HHS News,* December 12, 1997.

With a myomectomy: Loffer FS, "Improving results of hysteroscopic submucosal myomectomy for menorrhagia by concomitant endometrial ablation," *J Minim Invasive Gynecol,* 2005 May–June; 12(3):254–60.

Myomectomy

One myomectomy is performed in the United States for every five hysterectomies: The Center for Uterine Fibroids estimates that there are 18,000 myomectomies per year; Berger GS, "Outpatient Abdominal Myomectomy: Analysis of 150 Consecutive Cases," advance copy, estimates the annual number of myomectomies as 44,000.

Take heart: Hutchins FL Jr, "Abdominal Myomectomy as a Treatment for Symptomatic Uterine Fibroids," *Obstetrics & Gynecology Clinics of North America* 1995; 22(4): 781–89.

Why Won't a Doctor Recommend a Myomectomy?

Many of the arguments against myomectomy appeared in the following articles: "Hysterectomy vs. Myomectomy: Frequently Asked Questions," an interview with Chris Grover, MD, Assistant Clinical Professor of Obstetrics & Gynecology at University of California, San Francisco, and University of California, Davis, Salu Communications, Inc.; Mayfield E, "Choosing a treatment for uterine fibroids," *FDA Consumer Magazine*, 1993; 27(9). Also see *Uterine Fibroids: What Every Woman Needs to Know*, Stringer NH, Physicians & Scientists Publishing Co., 1996: 88–91.

A review of over 40 studies: Agency for Healthcare Research and Quality, "34. Management of Uterine Fibroids Volume 1. Evidence Report, Chapter 4," AHRQ Evidence Reports, Numbers 1–60, www.ncbi.nlm.nih.gov.

Your fibroids grow back; a 2002 article: Broder MS et al., "Comparison of Long-Term Outcomes of Myomectomy and Uterine Artery Embolization," *Obstetrics & Gynecology* 2002: 100:864–868.

A doctor skilled in myomectomy: Hutchins FL Jr, "Abdominal Myomectomy as a Treatment for Symptomatic Uterine Fibroids," *Obstetrics & Gynecology Clinics of North America* 1995; 22(4): 781–89.

A five-year study: Iverson RE Jr, et al., "Relative Morbidity of Abdominal Hysterectomy and Myomectomy for Management of Uterine Leiomyomas," *Obstetrics & Gynecology* 1996; 88(3): 415–19.

Vaginal Myomectomy

Resection won't work: "Hysteroscopes and Gynecologic Laparoscopes, Submission Guidance for a 510(k)," March 7, 1996. Prepared by Obstetrics-Gynecology Devices Branch, Office of Device Evaluation, Center for Devices and Radiological Health. U.S. Food and Drug Administration, www.fda.gov.

Fluid overload: Brooks PG, "Resectoscopic Myoma Vaporizer," *Journal of Reproductive Medicine* 1995; 40 (11): 791–95.

Only about 10 percent: "VersaPoint System for Fibroid Removal Cleared by FDA," Doctors Guide Web site, posted November 4, 1996, www.pslgroup.com.

Laparoscopic Myomectomy

Most women getting laparoscopy: Mais V, et al., "Laparoscopic versus Abdominal Myomectomy: A Prospective, Randomized Trial to Evaluate Benefits in Early Outcome," *American Journal of Obstetrics & Gynecology* 1996; 174(2): 654–58.

The description of the laparoscopic procedure is based on information found in Hill DA, "Laparoscopy," published on www.obgyn.net; and Griffith HW, *The Complete Guide to Medical Tests,* Fisher Books, 1988.

A 2005 article: Hurst BS, "Laparoscopic myomectomy for symptomatic uterine myomas," *Fertility and Sterility* 2005 Jan; 83(1):1–23.

Dr. Camran Nezhat: Nezhat C, "The 'Cons' of Laparoscopic Myomectomy in Women Who May Reproduce in the Future," *International Journal of Fertility and Menopausal Studies* 1996; 41(3): 280–83.

Side effects: Härkki-Sirén P, et al., "Finnish National Register of Laparoscopic Hysterectomies: A Review and Complications of 1,165 operations," *American Journal of Obstetrics & Gynecology* 1997; 176(1 Pt 1): 118–22; Härkki-Sirén P, Sjöberg J, et al., "Urinary Tract Injuries after Hysterectomy" *Obstetrics & Gynecology* 1998; 92(1): 113–18.

A smaller uterus helps: Galen DI, et al., "Outpatient Laparoscopic Hysterectomy: A Review of 50 Patients," *Journal of the American Association of Gynecologic Laparoscopists* May 1994, Vol 1, No. 3.

ABDOMINAL MYOMECTOMY

Many doctors prefer: Goldfarb HA, Greif J, *The No-Hysterectomy Option: Your Body–Your Choice,* John Wiley & Sons, 1997: 139–40.

Hutcherson H, Williams M, *Having Your Baby: A Guide for African-American Women,* One World/Ballantine Books, 1997: 10.

UAE and abdominal myomectomy: Broder MS, et al., "Comparison of Long-Term Outcomes of Myomectomy and Uterine Artery Embolization," *Obstetrics & Gynecology,* 2002: 100:864–868; Razavi MK, et al., "Abdominal myomectomy versus uterine artery embolization in the treatment of symptomatic uterine leiomyomas," *AJR Am J Roentgenol* 2003 Jun; 180(6):1571–5; Wysoki MG, "Uterine fibroid embolization reduces pain, may enhance women's sex lives," March 15, 2002, Yale-New Haven Hospital, www.ynhh.org.

HYSTERECTOMY

From a medical point of view: Davies A, et al., "Indications and Alternatives to Hysterectomy," *Baillieres Clinical Obstetrics and Gynaecology* 1997; 11(1): 61–75.

Hysterectomy statistics: Keshavarz H, et al., "Hysterectomy Surveillance—United States, 1994–1999," CDC, July 12, 2002; Bren L, "Alternative to Hysterectomy: New Technologies, More Options," *FDA Consumer,* November–December 2001, www.fda.gov.

Estimated hospital costs: "AHRQ Women's Health Highlights,Hysterectomy and Other Treatments for Uterine Conditions, Women's Health Highlights: Recent Findings," www.ahrq.gov.

A panel of physicians: McKeown LA, "More Hysterectomies, More Inappropriate Reasons," WebMD Medical News, January 31, 2000.

Ovaries, UCLA study: Associated Press, "Ovary Removal for Hysterectomy Unnecessary?" August 1, 2005.

A Maryland study: Kjerulff KH, et al., "Hysterectomy and Race," *Obstetrics & Gynecology* 1993, Nov; 82(5): 757–64.

In Denmark: Settnes A, et al., "Hysterectomy in a Danish Cohort. Prevalence, Incidence and Socio-Demographic Characteristics," *Acta Obstetricia et Gynecologica Scandinavica* 1996; 75(3): 274–80.

A public education campaign: Lilford R, editorial, "Hysterectomy: Will It Pay the Bills in 2007?" *BMJ* 1997; 314: 160.

As much as 30 percent: UPI, "Knowing options lowers hysterectomy rate," May 27, 2005, www.sciencedaily.com.

OH, OH, OVARIES

Dr. Susan Love: Love S., "New Looks at Old Questions," *The New York Times*, June 6, 2004.

According to the CDC: Keshavarz H, et al., "Hysterectomy Surveillance— United States, 1994–1999," CDC, July 12, 2002.

Love SM, Lindsey K, *Dr. Susan Love's Hormone Book*, Times Books 1997: 7,78–79,85.

Northrup C, *Women's Bodies, Women's Wisdom*, Bantam Books, 1994: 197–98.

West S, *The Hysterectomy Hoax*, Main Street Doubleday Books, 1994: 173–74.

RISKS

A whole new set of problems: Davies A, et al., "Indications and Alternatives to Hysterectomy," *Baillieres Clinical Obstetrics and Gynaecology* 1997; 11(1): 61–75; Carlson KJ, et al., "The Maine Women's Health Study: I. Outcomes of Hysterectomy," *Obstetrics & Gynecology* 1994; 83(4): 556–72.

Dr. Nelson Stringer: Stringer NH, *Uterine Fibroids: What Every Woman Meeds to Know*, Physicians & Scientists Publishing Co., 1996: 76.

25 percent of all women get seriously depressed: "The Hysterectomy-Depression Connection," Sapient Health Network, www.webmd.com.

Angier N, *Woman*, Houghton Mifflin, 1999: 90.

SUPRACERVICAL HYSTERECTOMY

Munro MG, "Supracervical Hysterectomy: . . . a Time for Reappraisal," *Obstetrics & Gynecology* 1997; 89(1): 133–39.

A comparison: Learman LA, et al., "A randomized comparison of total or supracervical hysterectomy: surgical complications and clinical outcomes," *Obstet Gynecol.* 2003 Sep; 102(3):453–62.

VAGINAL HYSTERECTOMY

A typical cut-off: Polet R, et al., "Laparoscopically Assisted Vaginal Hysterectomy (LAVH)—An Alternative to Total Abdominal Hysterectomy," *South African Medical Journal* 1996; 86(9 Suppl): 1190–94; Magos A, et al., "Vaginal Hysterectomy for the Large Uterus," *British Journal of Obstetrics and Gynaecology* 1996; 103(3): 246–51.

Goldfarb HA, Greif J, *The No-Hysterectomy Option*, John Wiley & Sons, 1997: 139–40.

Chapter 6: But Wait, There's More

Dr. David Eisenberg: Eisenberg D, et al., "Trends in Alternative Medicine in the United States 1990–1997," *JAMA* Nov. 11, 1998, www.ama-assn.org; Centers for Complementary and Alternative Medicine Research, NIH Guide, release date September 24, 1998, RFA OD 98008.

Nissim R, *Natural Healing in Gynecology*, Pandora, 1996: 2.

Harkey MR, et al., "Variability in commercial ginseng products: an analysis of 25 preparations," *Am J Clin Nutr*, 2001, vol. 73, pp. 1101–1106.

The New England Journal of Medicine: Angell M, Kassirer JP, "Alternative Medicine—The Risks of Untested and Unregulated Remedies," *New England Journal of Medicine* 1998; 339(12): 839–41.

WESTERN HERBALISM

Regulation: Dietary Supplement Health and Education Act of 1994, www.fda.gov.

According to Patricia Eagon, an herb researcher: Fackelmann K, "Researchers Study Herbal Remedies for Hot Flashes," *Science News* 1998; 153(25): 392.

300 plants: Xavier Center for Bioenvironmental Research at Tulane University, http://e.hormone. tulane.edu.

Controversial remedies for women with fibroids: The information was compiled from the following references: Love SM, et al., *Dr. Susan Love's Hormone Book*, Times Books, 1997; Harrar S, et al., *The Woman's Book of Healing Herbs*, Rodale Press, 1999; Woodham A, et al., *Encyclopedia of Healing Therapies*, Dorling Kindersley, 1997; McIntyre A, *The Complete Woman's Herbal*, Henry Holt, 1995; Goldstein SR, *The Estrogen Alternative*, G.P. Putnam's Sons, 1998; Fackelmann K, "Researchers study herbal remedies for hot flashes," *Science News* 1998; 153(25): 392, "Herbs With Estrogen Action May Raise Cancer Risk," Healthcare News, April 23, 2002, www.fhshealth.org.

I Yam What I Yam

The FDA is not happy: Cruse AE, "WARNING LETTER," Public Health Service, Food and Drug Administration, January 25, 2005.

Cooper A, et al., Studies: "Systemic Absorption of Progesterone from Progest Cream in Postmenopausal Women," *The Lancet* 1998; 351: 1255–56; Hermann AC, et al., "Over-the-counter progesterone cream produces significant drug exposure compared to a food and drug administration-approved oral progesterone product," *J Clin Pharmacol.* 2005 Jun; 45(6):614–9.

Traditional Chinese Medicine (TCM)

Each of these organs: Lee Y, "Acupuncture: It's More Than Just Needles," The National Council on Women's HealthGrowth that's . . . stifled: Martin RW, "Tumors, Cysts, Fibroids, Cancer: Is Your Wood Overgrown?" A series of four articles appearing on America Online/Alt.Med.

Yin and yang: Stone A, "Chinese Medicine's Treatments for Women," www.herbldoc.com.

Acupuncture

Acupunture can slow the growth: Mehl-Madrona L, "Treatment of Fibroids with Complementary Medicine," www.healing-arts.org/mehl-madrona; Mehl-Madrona L., "Complementary medicine treatment of uterine fibroids: a pilot study," *Altern Ther Health Med.* 2002 Mar–Apr; 8(2):34–6,38–40, 42, 44–6.

The World Health Organization: Loeliger W, "Complementary Medicine: Acupuncture Part II," GBMC Alternative and Complementary Health Center; "Review and Analysis of Reports on Controlled Clinical Trials," World Health Organization, 1996, www.who.int.

Chinese Herbalism

Study results: Mehl-Madrona L, "Treatment of Uterine Fibroids with Complementary Medicine," www.healing-arts.org/mehl-madrona; Null G, *The Woman's Encyclopedia of Natural Healing,* Seven Stories Press, 1996: 106; *American Journal of Chinese Medicine,* 1992; (20)3–4: 313–17; Akase T, et al., "A comparative study of the usefulness of toki-shakuyaku-san and an oral iron preparation in the treatment of hypochromic anemia in cases of uterine myoma," *Yakugaku Zasshi.* 2003 Sep; 123(9):817–24.

"Complementary and Alternative Healing University," alternativehealing
.org; Gao Y, et al., [Clinical study on effect of Tripterygium wilfordii Hook.
f. on uterine leiomyoma][Article in Chinese], *Zhonghua Fu Chan Ke Za
Zhi*. 2000 Jul; 35(7):430–2; Pyatt DW, "Hematotoxicity of the Chinese
Herbal Medicine Tripterygium wilfordii Hook f in CD34-Positive Human
Bone Marrow Cells," *Molecular Pharmacology*, 57:512–518 (2000). Vol. 57,
Issue 3, 512–518, March 2000.

A survey of women: Chopelas A, "Fibroid Study and Research Program:
Causes, Symptoms, Relief and Possible Solutions," 1997, originally published on Intradesign.com.

BODYWORK

Common scents: Keville K, Green M, "Reproductive System," Aromatherapy,
HealthWorld Online, www.healthy.net.

Massage: "Touch Therapy," *Food and Fitness Advisor*, The Center for Women's
Healthcare, Weill Medical College of Cornell Univeristy, 1999; 2(5): 6.

Reflexology: Dougans I, *The Complete Illustrated Guide to Reflexology*,
Element Books, 1996: 161,168.

Sitz baths: Nissim R, *Natural Healing in Gynecology*, Pandora, 1996: 155,190.

Castor oil packs: Martin RW, "Tumors, Cysts, Fibroids, Cancer Is Your Wood
Overgrown?" A series of four articles on AOL Alt.Med.

HOMEOPATHY

15 different types of personalities: Woodham A, Peters D, *Encyclopedia of
Healing Therapies*, Dorling Kindersley, 1997: 129.

Ullman D, *The Consumer's Guide to Homeopathy*, Tarcher/Putnam, 1996.

Reichenberg-Ullman J, "Healing Uterine Fibroids," Healthy World Online
Net, www.healthy.net.

Null, Gary, *The Woman's Encyclopedia of Natural Healing*, Seven Stories Press,
1996: 96. Cummings S, Ullman D, *Everybody's Guide to Homeopathic
Medicine*, Tardier/Putnam, 1997: 175.

NATUROPATHY

The primary resource for this section is Woodham A, Peters D, *Encyclopedia
of Healing Therapies*, Dorling Kindersley, 1997: 118–19.

AYURVEDA

The primary resource for this section is Lonsdorf N, Butler V, Brown M, *A
Woman's Best Medicine: Health, Happiness, and Long Life through Maharishi Ayur-veda*, Tarcher/Putnam, 1995.

TAPPING INTO YOUR CHAKRAS

The primary resource for this section is Angelo J, *Hands-On Healing*, Healing Arts Press, 1994.

BRINGING BALANCE TO YOUR FIBROID-FIGHTING PROGRAM

Hutchins FL Jr, *The Fibroid Book*, The Fibroid Center, 1997: 80.

Chapter 7: A Question of Estrogen

Latin translation: Traupman JC, *The New College Latin and English Dictionary*, Bantam Books 1966: 204.

Our bodies make three major forms of estrogen; 200 different kinds of estrogen: Peyser M, "The Estrogen Dilemma," *Newsweek* 1999 Spring/Summer (Special Issue): 35–37.

Estrogen doesn't work in a vacuum: Flake GP, et al., "Etiology and Pathogenesis of Uterine Leiomyomas: A Review," *Environmental Health Perspectives*, Volume 111, Number 8, June 2003.

OUR BODIES, OUR ESTROGEN

10 percent of premenopause levels: Peyser M, "The Estrogen Dilemma," *Newsweek* 1999 Spring/Summer (Special Issue): 35–37.

Puberty in reverse . . . reactivating fibroids: Love SM, Lindsey K, *Dr. Susan Love's Hormone Book*, Times Books, 1997: 3, 146.

SORTING OUT THE HRT OPTIONS

Women's Health Initiative: "Study Updates, WHI Hormone Program Update," 2004, Women's Health Initiative, www.whi.org; "Update on the Health Effects of Postmenopausal Hormones," *NHSN NEWS, The Nurses' Health Study Annual Newsletter*, Volume 11, 2004.

Tibolone: de Aloysio D, et al., "Bleeding Patterns in Recent Postmenopausal Outpatients with Uterine Myomas: Comparison between Two Regimens of HRT," *Maturitas* 1998; 29(3): 261–64; Ang WC, et al., "Effect of hormone replacement therapies and selective estrogen receptor modulators in postmenopausal women with uterine leiomyomas: a literature review," *Climacteric.* 2001 Dec; 4(4):284–92.

Hunter DS, et al., "Influence of Exogenous Estrogen Receptor Ligands on Uterine Leiomyoma: Evidence from an in Vitro/in Vivo Animal Model for Uterine Fibroids," *Environmental Health Perspectives Supplements*, Volume 108, Number S5, October 2000.

One researcher noted: Flake GP, et al., "Etiology and Pathogenesis of Uterine Leiomyomas: A Review," *Environmental Health Perspectives*, Volume 111, Number 8, June 2003.

"Estrace," 2/15/05, Drug Information Online, drugs.com.

"Premarin," 1/23/04, Drug Information Online, drugs.com.

Minimal dose of progestin: Palomba S, et al., "Effect of different doses of progestin on uterine leiomyomas in postmenopausal women," *Eur J Obstet Gynecol Reprod Biol.* 2002 May 10; 102(2):199–201.

Transdermal HRT : Palomba S. et al, "Transdermal hormone replacement therapy in postmenopausal women with uterine leiomyomas," *Obstet Gynecol.* 2001 Dec; 98(6):1053–8.

A three-year study: Yang CH, et al., "Effect of hormone replacement therapy on uterine fibroids in postmenopausal women—a 3-year study," *Maturitas.* 2002 Sep 30; 43(1):35–9.

SERMs

Raloxifene: Jirecek S, et al., "Raloxifene prevents the growth of uterine leiomyomas in premenopausal women," *Fertil Steril.* 2004 Jun; 81(6):1719–20; Palomba S, et al., "Effects of raloxifene treatment on uterine leiomyomas in postmenopausal women," *Fertil Steril.* 2001 Jul; 76(1):38–43.

Henig RM, "Behind the Buzz on Designer Estrogens, Questions Linger," *New York Times*, June 21, 1998: WH4.

A cautionary tale: Epstein S, Cody P, "New Drug Poses Risk of Ovarian Cancer," DES Action *Voice* 1998, No. 76: 1; Goldstein SR, Ashner L, *The Estrogen Alternative*, G.P. Putnam's Sons, 1998: acknowledgments,59; "Evista Warnings," Rx List, Page last Updated 12/08/2004, www.rxlist.com.

Love SM, et al., *Dr. Susan Love's Hormone Book*, Times Books, 1997: 270–71.

Plant Estrogens: Do Carrots Have Cravings?

Phytoestrogens are much weaker: Baird DD, Epidemiology Branch, Environmental Diseases and Medicine Program, Division of Intramural Research, National Institute of Environmental Health Sciences, http://dir.niehs .nih.gov.

Three popular phytoestrogens: Fackelmann K, "Researchers Study Herbal Remedies for Hot Flashes," *Science News* 1998; 153(25): 392.

the ABCs of DDT, PCBs, and APEs

Carson R, *Silent Spring*, Houghton Mifflin, 1994 (first published in 1962).

How chemical estrogens can affect our bodies: Raloff I, "Does Yo-Yo Dieting

Pose Cancer Threat?" Science News Online, March 15, 1997; Fact Sheet #10, "Q & As from the Cornell University Program on Breast Cancer and Environmental Risk Factors in New York State," March 1998; "Endocrine Disrupting Chemicals and Women's Health Outcomes," *NIH Guide* 24(38), National Institute of Environmental Health Sciences, Office of Research on Women's Health, 1995; Golan R, *Optimal Wellness*, Ballantine Books, 1995: 366.

Moore T, *Care of the Soul*, HarperCollins, 1992: 171.

Since 1993: Boyd V, et al., "Women's Health Research at NIEHS," *Environmental Health Perspectives*, 1993; 101(2).

Tulane/Xavier Center for Bioenvironmental Research: www.e.hormone.tulane.edu.

Testimony before the Senate Committee: Recent Testimony of Interest to the National Cancer Institute, "Cancer, Genetics, and the Environment," Department of Health and Human Services, Statement of Francis Collins, Director, National Center for Human Gene Research, Richard Klausner, Director, National Cancer Institute, Kenneth Olden, Director, National Institute of Environmental Health Sciences, before the Senate Committee on Labor and Human Resources, March 6, 1996.

Laboratory studies: Newbold RR, et al., "Advances in Uterine Leiomyoma Research: Conference Overview, Summary, and Future Research Recommendations," *Environmental Health Perspectives Supplements* Volume 108, Number S5, October 2000.

Al Gore: From the Foreword of Colborn T, *Our Stolen Future*, Dutton, 1996.

Dr. Andrew Weil recommends: "Hormone Mimics," *Dr. Andrew Weil's Self-Healing*, February 1999: 1,6,7.

LEARNING OUR LESSONS: DES

New research: 1999 National DES Research Conference, DES Action, www.desaction.org; Newbold RR, et al., "Increased Tumors But Uncompromised Fertility in the Female Descendants of Mice Exposed Developmentally to Diethylstilbestrol," *Carcinogenesis* 19: 1655–63; Newbold RR, et al., "Advances in Uterine Leiomyoma Research: Conference Overview, Summary, and Future Research Recommendations," *Environmental Health Perspectives Supplements*, Volume 108, Number S5, October 2000.

TEACH YOUR CHILDREN WELL

In 1995: "Endocrine Disrupting Chemicals and Women's Health Outcomes," *NIH Guide* 24(38), National Institute of Environmental Health Sciences, Office of Research on Women's Health, 1995.

Chapter 8: Nothing to Eat but Food

DAIRY PRODUCTS

Both . . . advise women: Northrup C, *Women's Bodies, Women's Wisdom,* Bantam Books 1994: 599; Lark S, *Fibroid Tumors & Endometriosis Self Help Book,* Celestial Arts 1995: 84.

Milk products are considered very "yin": Golan R, *Optimal Wellness,* Ballantine Books, 1995: 366.

Ann Chopelas says: Chopelas A, "Fibroid Study and Research Program: Causes, Symptoms, Relief and Possible Solutions," 1997, originally published on Intradesign.com.

About one-third of our cows: "The Issue: rBGH," The Sustainable Table, www.sustainabletable.org; McKenzie J, "Is Cow's Milk Additive Safe? Consumer Group Launches Action Against FDA," December 15, 1998, ABCNEWS.com.

According to the FDA: Report on the Food and Drug Administration's Review of the Safety of Recombinant Bovine Somatotropin, www.fda.gov.

Canada: "Safe Milk? Ask the FDA," DES Action *Voice,* Spring 1999, No. 80: 4. Quotes a study from the *Breast Cancer Action Newsletter* that links high levels of IGF-1 to a seven-fold increase in breast cancer among women under 50.

MEAT AND POULTRY

The FDA: *Monitoring for Residues in Food Animals,* CI'M Memo-19, FDA Center for Veterinary Medicine, Communications and Education Branch, DHHS Pub. No. (FDA)94–6001).

A study in Italy: "Uterine Fibroids May Be Associated with a Diet High in Red Meat and Low in Green Vegetables and Fruits," *Highlights in Obstetrics & Gynecology,* ACOG news release, August 31, 1999.

THE FACTS ON FAT

Two basic kinds of fat: "Essential Fatty Acids: Getting Back in Balance," *Women's Health Advocate,* May 1998, 5(3): 4–5.

Free radicals: LaMont S, "Fiber, Fat and Breast Cancer Prevention," AOL alt .med; "Fishing for Omega-3s," *Food and Fitness Advisor,* April 1999: 1.

Dr. Andrew Weil: "Good Fats, Bad Fats," *Dr. Andrew Weil's Self-Healing,* December 1998: 1,6,7.

SUGAR AND SPICE AND EVERYTHING NICE

Too much sugar: Chopelas A, "Fibroid Study and Research Program: Causes, Symptoms, Relief and Possible Solutions," 1997, originally published on Intradesign.com.

The average American: Lark S, *Fibroid Tumors & Endometriosis Self Help Book,* Celestial Arts, 1995: 88.

Complex carbohydrates: "The 'Sugar Busters' Diet," *Dr. Andrew Weil's Self-Healing,* October 1998: 7.

COFFEE, BOOZE, AND RED DYE #3

Indirect ways that caffeine may have an impact: Lark S, *Fibroid Tumors & Endometriosis Self Help Book,* Celestial Arts, 1995: 88–89; Baker K, "Anemia, What Every Woman Should Know," AOL.alt.med.

Beer: Wise LA, et al., "Risk of uterine leiomyomata in relation to tobacco, alcohol and caffeine consumption in the Black Women's Health Study," *Human Reproduction,* 2004 Aug; 19(8):1746–54.

Aspartame: Chopelas A, "Fibroid Study and Research Program: Causes, Symptoms, Relief and Possible Solutions," 1997, originally published on Intradesign.com.

SOY AHOY

Lark S, *Fibroid Tumors & Endometriosis Self Help Book,* Celestial Arts, 1995: 78,88.

Brody J, *The New York Times Book of Health,* The New York Times Book Company, 1997: 127, 135.

An added boost: "Soy Intake May Reduce Risk of Uterine Cancer—New Cancer Research Study," August 29, 1997, Doctors Guide Web site, www.docguide.com; "Northern California Cancer Center Publishes Study in JNCI Finding Phytoestrogen-rich Diet Associated with Lower Risk of Endometrial Cancer," *Journal of the National Cancer Institute,* August 5, 2003.

MMM, PASS THE FIBER

Increasing dietary fiber: LaMont S, "Fiber, Fat and Breast Cancer Prevention," AOL alt.med.

Dietary fiber is the express bus: McDougall JA, "Hormone Dependent Diseases," www.drmcdougall.com.

EAT YOUR VEGGIES

Think in color: Pettus E, "Can Breast Cancer Be Prevented?" Country Living's *Healthy Living,* January 1999: 62

V IS FOR VITAMINS

The chart was compiled for your reference from Lark S, *Fibroid Tumors & Endometriosis Self Help Book,* Celestial Arts, 1995; Weil A, *Natural Health, Natural Medicine,* Houghton Mifflin Company, 1995; Golan R, *Optimal Wellness,* Ballantine Books, 1995; Warshowsky A, et al., *Healing Fibroids,* Simon & Schuster New York 2002; Wilson ML, et al., "Herbal and dietary therapies for primary and secondary dysmenorrhoea," *Cochrane Database Syst Rev.* 2001; (3):CD002124, among other sources.

LEAN AND MEAN: FIBROIDS AND BODY WEIGHT

What it boils down to: Flake GP, et al., "Etiology and Pathogenesis of Uterine Leiomyomas: A Review," *Environmental Health Perspectives,* Volume 111, Number 8, June 2003.

Marshall LM, et al., "Risk of Uterine leiomyomata among Premenopausal Women in Relation to Body Size and Cigarette Smoking," *Epidemiology,* 1998; 9(5): 511–17.

Sato F, et al., "Body Fat Distribution and Uterine Leiomyomas," *Epidemiology,* 1998; 8(3): 176–80.

Shikora SA, et al., "Relationship Between Obesity and Uterine Leiomyomata," *Nutrition,* 1991; 7(4): 251–55.

Some women do report: Chopelas A, "Fibroid Study and Research Program: Causes, Symptoms, Relief and Possible Solutions" 1997, originally published on Intradesign.com.

In a 1998 paper: Beatty D, et al., "Position of the American Dietetic Association and the Canadian Dietetic Association: Women's Health and Nutrition," The American Dietetic Association.

SHAKE IT UP, BABY: FIBROIDS AND EXERCISE

Athletic women: "Uterine Fibroids," National Institutes of Health, NIH pub 0051.

Gentle exercise: Lark S, *Fibroid Tumors & Endometriosis Self Help Book,* Celestial Arts, 1995: 64.

TAKE A CHILL PILL, LIL: FIBROIDS AND STRESS

Chopelas A, "Fibroid Study and Research Program: Causes, Symptoms, Relief and Possible Solutions," 1997, originally published on Intradesign.com.

Stress does three other things: Lark S, *Fibroid Tumor & Endometriosis Self Help Book,* Celestial Arts, 1995: 153.

The impact of violence: "The NHS II Stress Study," *NHSN NEWS, The Nurses' Health Study Annual Newsletter,* Volume 10, 2003.

GET YOUR ZZZS, LOUISE: FIBROIDS AND SLEEP

Discussion of melatonin, including information from Dr. Russel Reiter: "Nighttime Light and Cancer," *Women's Health Advocate*, 1999, 5(12): 1–2.

LET THE SUN SHINE IN: FIBROIDS AND THE GREAT OUTDOORS

A Cherokee belief: Cantrell R, "The Fundamentals of Health," AOL Alt .Med.

Chapter 9: Sex and the Single Fibroid

Kolata G, "Women and Sex: on This Topic, Science Blushes," *New York Times*, June 21, 1998: 3.

LADIES, START YOUR ENGINES

Paralyzed women: Angier N, *Woman*, Houghton Mifflin, 1999: 84.
You know the feeling: Cardoso SH,"How the Brain Organizes Sexual Behavior," *Brain & Mind*, September/November 1997, www.epub.org.br.
Inverted penis: McGregor DK, *From Midwives to Medicine*, Rutgers University Press, 1998: 34–35.
G-spot: Perry JD, "Effects of Clitoral and G-Spot Stimulation on Pelvic Muscles," InContiNet, www.incontinet.com.

THE ROLE OF THE CERVIX

Frankenhauser uterovaginal plexus: Hasson HM, "Cervical Removal at Hysterectomy for Benign Disease—Risks and Benefits," *Journal of Reproductive Medicine*, 1993 Oct; 38(10): 781–90.
Beta-endorphins: Cutler WB, *Hysterectomy, Before and After,* HarperPerennial, 1988: 103.
A thin mucus: Goldfarb HA, Greif J, *The No-Hysterectomy Option*, John Wiley & Sons, 1997: 32.
The vagus nerve: Cardoso SH, "How the Brain Organizes Sexual Behavior," *Brain & Mind*, September/November 1997, www. epub.org.br.

SEX AFTER UAE

Sex after UAE: A.C. Lai, et al., "Sexual Dysfunction after Uterine Artery Embolization," *Journal of Vascular and Interventional Radiology*, June 2000; 11(6): p.755–8; Walker AG, "Embolization gaining ground as uterine fibroid treatment," *The Medical Post,* April 10, 2001, Volume 37 Issue 14; Goodwin SC, et al., "Reporting Standards for Uterine Artery Embolization for the Treatment of Uterine Leiomyomata," *Journal of Vascular and Interventional Radiology,* 14:S467-S476 (2003).

Georgetown University: "Uterine Fibroid Embolization doesn't hurt, may help women's sex lives," Society of Interventional Radiology, February 19, 2001, www.sirweb.org.

Self-esteem: Medical outcomes study, provided by Dr. James Spies, Georgetown University Medical Center; submitted for publication.

Sex after Myomectomy

Bialystock, Poland: Szamatowicz J, Laudanski T, Bulkszas B, Akerlund M, "Fibromyomas and Uterine Contractions," *Acta Obstetricia et Gynecologica Scandinavica* 1997; 76(10): 973–76.

Sex After Hysterectomy

Dr. M. E. Davis: Howe L, "The Uterus, Still a Mystery" originally appeared on Wellness Web, March 19, 1998, www.wellweb.com.

Sexuality after a hysterectomy: Dargent D, *Contraception, Fertilité, Sexualité,* 1996; 24(5): 347–49; Goldstein I, "Sexual Dysfunction after Hysterectomy," Boston University School of Medicine, Last Edited 5/13/2003, www. bumc.bu.edu; Meston C, "The Effects of Hysterectomy on the Subjective and Physiological Sexual Function of Women with Benign Uterine Fibroids," *Archives of Sexual Behavior,* Vol. 33, No. 1, February 2004, pp. 31–42. Plenum Publishing Corporation, as found on www.athena institute.com.

Your male partner: Castleman M, "Can Hysterectomy Affect a Man?" originally appeared on Sex Matters, July 8, 1999, www.onhealth.com.

50 to 60 percent: Raboch J, et al., "[Sex Life Following Hysterectomy]," *Geburtshilfe und Frauenheilkunde* 1985; 45(1): 48–50; Helstrom L, et al., "Sexuality After Hysterectomy: A Factor Analysis of Women's Sexual Lives Before and After Subtotal Hysterectomy," *Obstetrics & Gynecology* 1993; 81(3): 357–62; Sakai K, et al., *Nippon Sanka Fujinka Gakkai Zasshi* 1983; 35(6): 757–63.

33 percent to 46 percent: Zussman L, et al., "Sexual Response after Hysterectomy-Oophorectomy: Recent Studies and Reconsideration of Psychogenesis," *American Journal of Obstetrics & Gynecology,* 1981; 140(7): 725–29.

Gates Foundation: "Hysterectomy," Physical Conditions That Affect Sexual Function, Sexual Anatomy and Physiology, Sexuality and Sexual Health, 2003, www.engenderhealth.org.

Even kissing: Choi YS, et al., "[A Study on the Relationship between Pre- and

Post-Hysterectomy Sexual Behavior Differences and the Sexual Satisfaction of Women Who Have Had a Hysterectomy]," *Taehan Kanho. Korean Nurse* 1989 28(1): 67–76.

Dr. Judith Reichman, as heard on the *Oprah Winfrey Show*, July 15, 1998.

Does the type of hysterectomy you have make a difference?: Ellstrom MA, et al., "A randomized trial comparing changes in psychological well-being and sexuality after laparoscopic and abdominal hysterectomy," *Acta Obstet Gynecol Scand.* 2003 Sep; 82(9):871–5; Zobbe V, et al., "Sexuality after total vs. subtotal hysterectomy," *Acta Obstet Gynecol Scand.* 2004 Feb; 83(2):191–6; Kim DH, et al., "Alteration of sexual function after classic intrafascial supracervical hysterectomy and total hysterectomy," *J Am Assoc Gynecol Laparosc.* 2003 Feb; 10(1):60–4; Roovers J, *British Medical Journal*, Oct. 4. 2003; vol 327: pp 774–779.

Dr. Anne Walling: Walling AD, "Does Hysterectomy Have an Impact on Sexuality?" *American Family Physician*, June 1, 2004.

A French survey: Ayoubi JM, et al., "Respective consequences of abdominal, vaginal, and laparoscopic hysterectomies on women's sexuality," *Eur J Obstet Gynecol Reprod Biol.* 2003 Dec 10; 111(2):179–82.

The Role of the Ovaries

A third of the time: Angier N, *Woman*, Houghton Mifflin, 1999: 120.

A study of almost 700 women: Nathorst-Boos J, von Schoultz B, "Psychological Reactions and Sexual Life after Hysterectomy with and without Oophorectomy," *Gynecologic and Obstetric Investigation* 1992; 34(2): 97–101.

That Big Sex Organ Called . . . Your Brain

A self-fulfilling prophecy: Lalinec-Michaud M, et al., "Anxiety, Fears and Depression Related to Hysterectomy," *Canadian Journal of Psychiatry* 1985; 30(1): 44–47.

Nurses are the most valuable source: Krueger JC, et al., "Relationship Between Nurse Counseling and Sexual Adjustment after Hysterectomy," *Nursing Research*, 1979; 28(3): 145–50.

Chapter 10: And Baby Makes Three

"Diseases of Reproduction in Women," NIH, www.nih.gov.

Dr. Marjorie Greenfield: "Ask Dr. Greenfield," June 12, 2001, www.drspock.com.

ACOG: "Uterine Fibroids," Medical Library, American College of Obstetricians and Gynecologists, February 2005, www.medem.com.

A fun fact: Flake GP, et al., "Etiology and Pathogenesis of Uterine Leiomyomas: A Review," *Environmental Health Perspectives*, Volume 111, Number 8, June 2003.

How Can Fibroids Complicate Pregnancy?

The information in this section was compiled from the following references: Hales D, et al., *Intensive Caring: New Hope for High Risk Pregnancy*, Crown Publishers, 1990: 10, 146; Siccardi DC, "Leiomyomas," Obstetrics and Gynecology, www.medstudents.com; Hutcherson H, et al., *Having Your Baby: A Guide for African-American Women*, One World/Ballantine Books, 1997: 209; "Uterine Leiomyomata," *ACOG Educational Bulletin* 1994; (192).

Can Fibroids Cause Infertility?

20 percent of couples: Hales D, et al., *Intensive Caring: New Hope for High-Risk Pregnancy*, Crown Publishers, 1990: 10, 32.

60 pregnant women: Hasan F, et al., "Uterine Leiomyomata in Pregnancy," *International Journal of Gynaecology and Obstetrics* 1991; 34(1): 45–48.

Parker WH, Parker RL, *A Gynecologist's Second Opinion*, Plume Books, 1996: 29.

Women aged 35–39: Hamilton BE, et al., "Births: Preliminary data for 2003," National vital statistics reports; vol. 53 no. 9, National Center for Health Statistics.

Four major ways in which fibroids might interfere: sources include Lark S, *Fibroid Tumors & Endometriosis Self Help Book*, Celestial Arts, 1995: 13; Hutcherson H, et al., *Having Your Baby: A Guide for African-American Women*, One World/Ballantine Books, 1997: 208,209.

Other problems that can affect fertility: Maderas L, *Womancare*, Avon Books, 1984: 435. Lauersen N, Whitney S, *It's Your Body: A Woman's Guide to Gynecology*, Berkley Books, 1983: 345.

Fibroids And IVF

Having fibroids reduces your chance of success: Small-Pal, EJ, et al., "Uterine Leiomyomas and Infertility," *Female Patient*, December 2002; Rackow BW, et al., "Fibroids and in-vitro fertilization: which comes first?" *Curr Opin Obstet Gynecol.* 2005 Jun; 17(3):225–31.

A Brazilian study: Oliveira FG, et al., "Impact of subserosal and intramural uterine fibroids that do not distort the endometrial cavity on the outcome of in vitro fertilization-intracytoplasmic sperm injection," *Fertil Steril.* 2004 Mar; 81(3):582–7.

An Australian study: Healy DL, "Impact of Uterine Fibroids on ART

Outcome," *Environmental Health Perspectives* Volume 108, Supplement 5, October 2000.

WHAT ABOUT MISCARRIAGE?

University of North Carolina at Chapel Hill: "Small uterine fibroids are associated with an increased risk of miscarriage," *Women's Health News*, Apr. 13, 2004, www.News-Medical.Net.

15 to 30 percent: Hales D, et al., *Intensive Caring: New Hope for High-Risk Pregnancy*, Crown Publishers, 1990: 228.

If a fibroid causes miscarriage: Friedman L, et al., *A Woman Doctor's Guide to Miscarriage*, Hyperion, 1996: 4.

OH, YOU'VE GOT THAT GLOW: FIBROIDS AND PREGNANCY

10 percent of the time: Katz VL, et al., "Complications of Uterine Leiomyomas in Pregnancy," *Obstetrics & Gynecology*, 1989; 73(4): 593–96; Bilich K, "Fibroids During Pregnancy," Discovery Health, Reporting by Richard H. Schwarz, MD, Content courtesy of *American Baby*, May 2, 2005, http://health.discovery.com.

The CDC: "Safe Motherhood: Preventing Pregnancy-Related Illness and Death," National Center for Chronic Disease Prevention and Health Promotion, page last reviewed July 20, 2005, www.cdc.gov.

Is your pregnancy high risk: Hales D, et al., *Intensive Caring: New Hope for High-Risk Pregnancy*, Crown Publishers, 1990: 2, 194, 208–9, 211, 289–90.

The American Nurses Association: Slupik RI, ed., *American Medical Association Complete Guide to Women's Health*, Random House, 1996: 424.

Carneous degeneration: Hasan F, et al., "Uterine Leiomyomata in Pregnancy," *International Journal of Gynaecology and Obstetrics* 1991; 34 (1): 45–48.

Hutcherson H, et al., *Having Your Baby: A Guide for African-American Women*, One World/Ballantine Books, 1997: 209, 210, 211, 270–71.

Hospitalization for pain relief: Dildy GA 3rd, et al., "Indomethacin for the Treatment of Symptomatic Leiomyoma Uteri during Pregnancy," *American Journal of Perinatology* 1992; 9(3): 185–89.

Fibroids can increase three to five times: Siccardi DC, "Leiomyomas," *Obstetrics & Gynecology*, Medstudents, www.medstudents.com.

The most severe possibility: Goodman RM, *Planning for a Healthy Baby: A Guide to Genetic and Environmental Risks*, Oxford University Press, 1986: 58, 230–31.

Placenta previa: Chan PD, et al., *Current Clinical Strategies: Gynecology and Obstetrics*, Current Clinical Strategies Publishing, 1997: 107, 108, 122.

Premature rupture: Eisenberg A, et al., *What to Expect When You're Expecting*, Workman Publishing, 1991: 359–60, 365.

FIBROIDS AND DELIVERY

Preterm labor: Hales D, et al., *Intensive Caring: New Hope for High Risk Pregnancy*, Crown Publishers, 1990: 209, 211.

About 12 percent: "Preterm Labor," March of Dimes Pregnancy & Newborn Health Education Center, June 2005, http://search.marchofdimes.com.

Tocolytic: Hutcherson H, et al., *Having Your Baby: A Guide for African-American Women*. One World/Ballantine Books, 1997: 271.

If you've had a myomectomy: Sudik R, et al., "Fertility and Pregnancy Outcome after Myomectomy in Sterility Patients," *European Journal of Obstetrics, Gynecology, and Reproductive Biology*, 1996; 65(2): 209–14.

AFTER MYOMECTOMY

Estimates of delivery rates: Small-Pal, EJ, et al., "Uterine Leiomyomas and Infertility," *Female Patient*, December 2002; Campo S et al., "Reproductive outcome before and after laparoscopic or abdominal myomectomy for subserous or intramural myomas," *Eur J Obstet Gynecol Reprod Biol.* 2003 Oct 10; 110(2):215–9.

Vaginal delivery: Kumakiri J, et al., "Pregnancy and delivery after laparoscopic myomectomy," *J Minim Invasive Gynecol.* 2005 May–Jun; 12(3):241–6.

A second opinion: Babaknia A, et al., "Pregnancy Success Following Abdominal Myomectomy for Infertility," *Fertility and Sterility*, 1978; 30(6): 644–47.

BUT DON'T FIBROIDS COME BACK AFTER MYOMECTOMY?

Microscopic fibroids . . . continue to grow: Uterine Myomas (Fibroids), originally published on the Medfem Clinic website, www.medfem.co.za/Fibroids.html.

An Italian study: Candiani GB, et al., "Risk of Recurrence After Myomectomy," *British Journal of Obstetrics and Gynaecology*, 1991; 98(4): 385–89.

AFTER GNRH

Small studies: Vollenhoven BJ, et al., "An Open Study of Luteinizing Hormone Releasing Hormone Agonists in Infertile Women with Uterine Fibroids," *Gynecological Endocrinology*, 1993; 7(1): 57–61; Kuhlmann M, et al., "Uterine Leiomyomata and Sterility: Therapy with Gonadotropin-

Releasing Hormone Agonists and Leiomyomectomy," *Gynecological Endocrinology*, 1997; 11(3): 169–74.

Asherman's Syndrome

Friedman L, et al., *A Woman Doctor's Guide to Miscarriage*, Hyperion, 1996: 63–64.

After UAE, Myolysis, and Cryomyolysis

Uterine Rupture: Vilos GA, et al., "Pregnancy Outcome after Laparoscopic Electromyolysis," *Journal of the American Association of Gynecologic Laparoscopists*, 1998: 5(3): 289–92.

Chapter 11: Reach Out and . . .

Tannen D, *You Just Don't Understand*, Ballantine Books, 1990: 25.
Dr. Cynthia Morton notes: Kiewra K, "Gene Dreams," *BWH* 1997.

Lucy, You Have Some 'Splainin' to Do

Write It Out: Cameron J, *The Artist's Way*, Tarcher/Perigee Books, 1992: 37–38.
Rabbi Harold Kushner: from a speech given at *Spirituality and Healing in Medicine*, a conference presented by the Harvard Medical School Department of Continuing Education and the Mind/Body Medical Institute CareGroup, Beth Israel Deaconess Medical Center, December 12–14, 1998, Boston, Mass.
Caring conversation can change . . . your brain: Kotulak R, *Inside the Brain*, Andrew and McMeel, 1996: 22–23.

Paging Dr. Freud . . .

Take this little quiz: Ridgeway V, et al., "Psychological Preparation for Surgery: A Comparison of Methods," *British Journal of Clinical Psychology* 1982; 21(Pt 4): 271–80.

That Old-Time Religion

Dean Ornish, M.D., quoted in Country Living's *Healthy Living*, February 1999: 59.

Chapter 12: Know Thyself

Dr. David G. Myers: from a speech given at *Spirituality and Healing in Medicine*, a conference presented by the Harvard Medical School Department of Continuing Education and the Mind/Body Medical Institute CareGroup, Beth Israel Deaconess Medical Center, December 12–14, 1998, Boston, Mass.

Domar AD, et al., *Healing Mind, Healthy Woman*, A Delta Book, 1996: 4.

Siegel B, *Love, Medicine and Miracles*, HarperPerennial, 1986: 97.

East and West, We've All Got Stress

Two-thirds of all visits to the doctor: "You Say Ta-may-toe . . . ," *Esquire*, December 1998: 152.

It's not that we want to get sick: Blakeslee S, "Placebos Prove So Powerful Even Experts Are Surprised," *New York Times*, October 13, 1998.

Our bodies release hormones under stress: Horn C, et al., "7 Surefire Strategies for Stress," *Natural Health*, 4/99: 121.

Women dealing with infertility: Domar AD, et al., *Healing Mind, Healthy Woman*, A Delta Book, 1996: 233.

The Pleasure Principle: Moore T, *Care of the Soul*, HarperPerennial, 1992: 164.

If you're already predisposed: Lee K, "Women Who Were Determined to Heal," *Essence*, July 1997, 28(3): 22–29.

Can stress make fibroids grow?: "Stress and Cancer: Mind, Body, and Immunity," *Women's Health Advocate*, 11/98, 5(8): 4.

Trouble In Mind

West African saying: Applewhite A, Evans WR III, Frothingham A, eds., *And I Quote*, St. Martin's Press, 1992: 70.

Chopra D, *The 7 Spiritual Laws of Success*, Amber-Allen Publishing and New World Library, 1994: 74–5.

Say Amen, Sister: Faith in a Higher Power

A 1998 survey: "Survey of the American Public, HMO Professionals and Family Physicians to Determine General Attitudes Toward Spirituality as a Component of the Healing Process," 1998 Yankelovich Partners survey.

58 percent of us: Matthews DA, author of *The Faith Factor*, "Is Religion Good for Your Health?" a paper presented at *Spirituality and Healing in Medicine*, a conference presented by the Harvard Medical School Department of Continuing Education and the Mind/Body Medical Institute

CareGroup, Beth Israel Deaconess Medical Center, December 12–14, 1998, Boston, Mass.

A 2004 survey: Walker D, "Prayer and Spirituality in Health: Ancient Practices, Modern Science," *CAM at the NIH*, Volume XII, Number 1: Winter 2005

Larson, DB, "Spirituality and Medical Outcomes," discussion of a paper presented at *Spirituality and Healing in Medicine*, a conference presented by the Harvard Medical School Department of Continuing Education and the Mind/Body Medical Institute CareGroup, Beth Israel Deaconess Medical Center, December 12–14, 1998, Boston, Mass.

At Duke University: Koenig HG, et al., "Use of Hospital Services, Religious Attendance, and Religous Affiliation," *Southern Medical Journal*, 1998; 91(10): 925–32.

A study of Muslim patients: Benedict O, "Medicine's Neglected Spirit," *Science and Spirit*, 9(3): 3.

Even remote prayer: Van Bieme D, "A Test of the Healing Power of Prayer," *Time*, October 12, 1998; 152(15): 72.

Prayer team: Harris WS, et al., "A randomized, controlled trial of the effects of remote, intercessory prayer on outcomes in patients admitted to the coronary care unit," *Arch Intern Med.* 1999 Oct 25; 159(19):2273–8.

Mary Baker Eddy quote appears in Applewhite A, et al., eds., *And I Quote*, St. Martin's Press, 1992: 191.

People with a strong faith in God: "The Power of Prayer," *Natural Health*, April 1999: 34.

Satchel Paige quote appears in Applewhite A, et al., eds., *And I Quote*, St. Martin's Press, 1992: 112.

BELIEVE YOU ME: POSITIVE EXPECTATIONS

Six impossible things: Carroll L, *The Annotated Alice*, Bramhall House Edition: 251.

A physical effect: "The Placebo Effect," Mind-Body-Health.net, 2003; "Mind-Body Medicine: An Overview," National Center for Complementary and Alternative Medicine. updated August 2005.

A study of women: Elcombe S, et al., "The Psychological Effects of Laparoscopy on Women with Chronic Pelvic Pain," *Psychological Medicine*, 1997; 27(5): 1041–50.

Patients with AIDS: Mehl-Madrona LE, et al., "Faith in Treatment Influences Efficacy among AIDS Patients," Presented at the annual meeting (1997) of the National Institute for the Clinical Application of Behavioral Medicine.

Dr. Dan Molerman: Blakeslee S, "Enthusiasm of Doctor Can Give Pill Extra Kick," *New York Times*, October 13, 1998.

DECISIONS, DECISIONS

Koberg D, et al., *The Universal Traveler*, William Kaufman, 1981: 17, 41.
Chopra D, *The 7 Spiritual Laws of Success*, Amber-Allen Publishing and New World Library, 1994: 42,57–59.

THE POWER OF POSITIVE THINKING

Is the glass half empty: "Mind-Body Medicine: An Overview," National Center for Complementary and Alternative Medicine, updated August 2005.

THE RELAXATION RESPONSE

Herrigel E, *Zen in the Art of Archery*, Vintage Books, 1989: ix.
The relaxation response: Domar AD, et al., *Healing Mind, Healthy Woman*, A Delta Book, 1996; Benson H, "Spirituality and Healing in Medicine . . . The Genesis of the Course," a paper presented at *Spirituality and Healing in Medicine,* a conference presented by the Harvard Medical School Department of Continuing Education and the Mind/Body Medical Institute CareGroup, Beth Israel Deaconess Medical Center, December 12–14, 1998, Boston, Mass.
Ellwood R, *Finding the Quiet Mind,* Theosophical Publishing House, 1983: 7, 103.
University of Wisconsin: "Meditation Helps With Anxiety and General Health," Feb. 7, 2003, HealthyPlace.com.

YOU'RE GETTING SLEEEEEPY, VERRRY . . .

Before anesthesia was invented: Herrara S, "No-Hoax Hypnotherapy," Country Living's *Healthy Living,* February 1999: 88.
One practioner suggests: Bronson C, "Reproductive Issues in Women," www.provide.net.
Koberg D, et al., *The Universal Traveler,* William Kaufman, 1981: 116.
Tannen D, *You Just don't Understand,* Ballantine Books, 1990: 128.

CREATIVE VISUALIZATION

Gawain S, *Creative Visualization,* Bantam Books, 1978: 2.
Chopelas A, "Fibroid Study and Research Program: Causes, Symptoms, Relief and Possible Solutions," 1997, originally published on Intradesign.com.

Journaling

We might place: Moore T, *Care of the Soul*, HarperPerennial, 1992: 164.

Writing for twenty minutes: Goode E, "Your Mind May Ease What's Ailing You," *New York Times*, April 18, 1996: 6; "Written word helps wounds heal," BBC NEWS, 9/6/2003, http://news.bbc.co.uk.

Journals to evaluate reactions to stress and food were used in Dr. Lewis Mehl-Madrona's integrated treatment program for women with fibroids: Mehl-Madrona L, "Treatment of Uterine Fibroids with Complementary Medicine," www.healing-arts.org/mehl-madrona.

Julia Cameron: Cameron J, *The Artist's Way*, Tarcher/Perigee Books, 1992: 199.

Picture This

Picasso said: Cameron J, *The Artist's Way*, Tarcher/Perigee Books, 1992: 17.

Bernie Siegel asks: Siegel BS, *Love, Medicine and Miracles*, HarperPerennial, 1986: 114.

∽ *Acknowledgments* ⌒

I OFTEN LOOK at the acknowledgment pages in books out of idle curiosity; maybe I know somebody. But this time, on these pages, you will know somebody—at least one. Bear with me and you'll see what I mean.

I wouldn't have started this project at all if it weren't for my agent, Andrea Pedolsky, who listened to me talk about getting five different opinions from five different doctors on how to treat my fibroids, and saw a book that could help other women going through similar experiences. She and her partner, Nicholas Smith, took a risk and saw me through the long process of developing the proposal and manuscript with enormous generosity, dedication, and friendship. Andrea is a wonderfully talented editor and agent; I feel lucky to also count her as a friend.

Matthew Lore, at Marlowe & Company, has been an enthusiastic and generous supporter of this book from the beginning; for this second edition, I especially appreciate his commitment to keeping the content up to date. I'd like to thank Sue McCloskey, my editor for the second edition, and three women who helped make the first edition better than I could have made it alone: Cassandra Conyers, Donna Galassi, and especially Dianna Delling.

And because there's so much more to life than fibroids, I offer my thanks and gratitude to John Ciongoli, for his deep reserves of caring and support, and to the friends who are a constant ballast in my life, among them, Rochelle Cohen, Don Cohen, Carey Earle, Cathleen Rittereiser, Howard Matz, Stephen Altman, Tonya Hinch (and all the ladies in the theater club), Susan Carr, Amber Wood, Mary Athanis, Katherine Kurs, John Hudson, Lia Bass, Anne Kohn, Sandi Borger, Elizabeth Rubin, Mark Kaufman, Sharon Linnea, David Leipziger, Bobbi Berenbaum, Fern Flamberg, Danny Flamberg, Lis and Tom Hogan, Matt and Marla Herman; the kids in my life, Zachary, Allie, Josh, Lilly, and Marlene; and my parents, who never miss an opportunity to make sure the bookstores they visit have at least one copy of each of my books on the shelves.

Dr. Nelly Szlachter has helped me through years of fibroid management—and is still the only doctor I know of who shows up for surgery wearing a leather skirt and pearls. Dr. Milton Wainberg has helped me understand and manage my feelings about fibroids—and so many other things—for more years than I can count.

And although they are long gone from this life, I continue to draw inspiration, hope, and courage from the strength, wisdom, and joie de vivre of two people I still love dearly: my grandmother Erna Siegel and my friend, teacher, and rebbe, Marshall T. Meyer.

I would like to thank the doctors and other health care professionals who generously spent time with me to provide their insights about fibroids, research, and current treatments. These are, in alphabetical order, Dr. Linda Abend; Dr. Gary S. Berger; Ann Chopelas, Ph.D.; Nora Coffey, Director, HERS Foundation; Dr. Patricia Conrad; Dr. Joseph Feste; Dr. Carlos G. Forcade; Dr. Scott C. Goodwin; Dr. Malcolm Griffiths; Dr. Leon Hoffman; Dr. Dan Javit; Dr. Mitch Levine; Dr. Lewis Mehl-Madrona; Dr. David L. Olive; Dr. Mark Perloe, Dr. J. Victor Reyniak; Dr. James B. Spies; the late Dr. Nelson Stringer; Dr. Hans van der Slikke; Dr. Frank Vogel; Dr. Brian Walsh; Dr. Allan Warshowsky; Dr. Stanley West; Dr. Robert Worthington-Kirsch; and Dr. Ricardo A. Yazigi.

I'd especially like to thank Dr. Eileen Hoffman for her enthusiasm and encouragement for this project and for writing the foreword; Dr. Cynthia Morton, Director of Cytogenetics at Brigham and Women's Hospital, Boston, Massachusetts, for her unfailing help and generousity; James deFrancisco, who took on the challenges of researching this second edition with exceptional diligence and vigor; and Fran Janik, who took the best picture of me, *ever.*

And the women. Originally, I'd thought this book would simply tell the tales of women living with—or without—their fibroids. Obviously, it's become more comprehensive since that first idea. But the book still contains the stories of dozens of women, all of whom spoke to me extensively and intimately about their lives, medical decisions, and emotions, in hopes of helping others. (Since almost all of them had concerns about their privacy, I've respected it here, and many names have been changed—but the stories all are true.) I thank all of them for giving of themselves and making this book come to life.

And finally, I'd like to thank you, for reading, for understanding, perhaps for sharing your new knowledge about fibroids with someone else, and becoming one of the growing network of women to advocate for more, and better, solutions to women's unique health issues.

With best wishes for health, happiness, and peace of mind,
Johanna Skilling

Index